MR Imaging of the Athlete

Guest Editor

GEORGE KOULOURIS, MBBS,
GrCertSpMed, MMed, FRANZCR

MAGNETIC RESONANCE IMAGING CLINICS OF NORTH AMERICA

www.mri.theclinics.com

November 2009 • Volume 17 • Number 4

SAUNDERS an imprint of ELSEVIER, Inc.

W.B. SAUNDERS COMPANY
A Division of Elsevier Inc.

1600 John F. Kennedy Boulevard • Suite 1800 • Philadelphia, Pennsylvania 19103-2899

http://www.theclinics.com

MRI CLINICS OF NORTH AMERICA Volume 17, Number 4
November 2009 ISSN 1064-9689, ISBN 13: 978-1-4377-1239-1, ISBN 10: 1-4377-1239-8

Editor: Joanne Husovski
Developmental Editor: Theresa Collier

Magnetic Resonance Imaging Clinics of North America (ISSN 1064-9689) is published quarterly by Elsevier Inc., 360 Park Avenue South, New York, NY 10010-1710. Months of issue are February, May, August, and November. Application to mail at periodicals postage rates is pending at New York, NY and at additional mailing offices. Subscription prices are $309.00 per year (domestic individuals), $455.00 per year (domestic institutions), $150.00 per year (domestic students/residents), $345.00 per year (Canadian individuals), $571.00 per year (Canadian institutions), $448.00 per year (international individuals), $571.00 per year (international institutions), and $217.00 per year (international and Canadian students/residents). International air speed delivery is included in all *Clinics* subscription prices. All prices are subject to change without notice. **POSTMASTER:** Send address changes to *Magnetic Resonance Imaging Clinics*, Elsevier Health Sciences Division, Subscription Customer Service, 3251 Riverport Lane, Maryland Heights, MO 63043. Customer Service (orders, claims, online, change of address): Elsevier Health Sciences Division, Subscription Customer Service, 3251 Riverport Lane, Maryland Heights, MO 63043. Tel:1-800-654-2452 (U.S. and Canada); 314-447-8871 (outside U.S. and Canada). Fax: 314-447-8029. E-mail: journalscustomerservice-usa@elsevier.com (for print support); journalsonlinesupport-usa@elsevier.com (for online support).

Reprints. For copies of 100 or more of articles in this publication, please contact the Commercial Reprints Department, Elsevier Inc., 360 Park Avenue South, New York, NY 10010-1710. Tel.: 212-633-3812; Fax: 212-462-1935; E-mail: reprints@elsevier.com.

Magnetic Resonance Imaging Clinics of North America is covered in the *RSNA Index of Imaging Literature*, *MEDLINE/PubMed (Index Medicus)*, and *EMBASE/Excerpta Medica*.

Contributors

GUEST EDITOR

**GEORGE KOULOURIS, MBBS,
GrCertSpMed, MMed, FRANZCR**
Director, Melbourne Radiology Clinic,
East Melbourne, Australia

AUTHORS

STEVEN ALATAKIS, MBBS, FRANZCR
Radiologist, Department of Diagnostic
Imaging, Southern Health, Monash Medical
Centre, Clayton South, Victoria, Australia

DIANE BERGIN, MD
Consultant Radiologist, Department of
Radiology, Galway University Hospital,
Galway, Ireland

GREGORY A. COWDEROY, MBBS, FRANZCR
Consultant Radiologist, Radiology
Department, Queensland Diagnostic
Imaging, Brisbane Private Hospital,
Brisbane, Australia

**STEPHEN J. EUSTACE, MD, MSc,
MB, FFRRCSI**
Director, Institute of Radiological Sciences;
and Newman Professor of Radiology,
University College Dublin; Professor of
Radiology, Department of Radiology,
Mater Misericordiae University Hospital;
Department of Radiology, Cappagh
National Orthopaedic Hospital; Department
of Radiology, Santry Sports Surgery
Clinic, Santry Demense, Dublin, Ireland

GREGORY C. FANELLI, MD
Department of Orthopedic Surgery, Geisinger
Medical Center, Danville, Pennsylvania

BRUNO M. GIUFFRE, MBBS, FRANZCR
Consultant Radiologist; and Clinical
Associate Professor, Department
of Radiology, Royal North Shore Hospital,
University of Sydney, Sydney, Australia

CATHERINE L. HAYTER, MBBS
Radiology Registrar, Department of
Radiology, Royal North Shore Hospital,
University of Sydney, Sydney, Australia

**PHILIP A. HODNETT, MD, FFRRCSI,
MRCPI, MMedSci**
Fellow in Musculoskeletal Radiology, Division
of Radiology, Mater Misericordiae University
Hospital, Dublin, Ireland

BRIAN A. HOGAN, MB, FFRRCSI
Fellow, Department of Radiology, Santry Sports
Surgery Clinic, Santry Demense, Dublin, Ireland

EOIN C. KAVANAGH, MD, MB, FFRRCSI
Consultant Musculoskeletal Radiologist,
Department of Radiology, Mater Misericordiae
University Hospital, Dublin, Ireland

**GEORGE KOULOURIS, MBBS,
GrCertSpMed, MMed, FRANZCR**
Director, Melbourne Radiology Clinic, East
Melbourne, Australia

JAMES LINKLATER, MBBS, FRANZCR
Castlereagh Sports Imaging, North Sydney
Orthopaedic and Sports Medicine Centre,
Crows Nest, NSW, Australia

DAVID A. LISLE, MBBS, FRANZCR
Consultant Radiologist, Queensland
Diagnostic Imaging; The Royal Children's
Hospital; Associate Professor of Medical
Imaging, Division of Medical Imaging,
University of Queensland Medical School,
Brisbane, Australia

PETER J. MACMAHON, MD, MRCPI
Specialist Registrar in Radiology,
Department of Radiology, Mater
Misericordiae University Hospital,
Dublin, Ireland

W. JAMES MALONE, DO
Director Musculoskeletal Imaging,
Department of Radiology, Geisinger
Medical Center, Danville, Pennsylvania

NINA MARSHALL, MBBS, FRANZCR
Lecturer in Radiology, Royal College of
Surgeons in Ireland, Beaumont Hospital,
Dublin, Ireland

MICHAEL R. MOYNAGH, MD
Specialist Registrar in Radiology,
Department of Radiology, Mater
Misericordiae University Hospital,
Dublin, Ireland

PARM NAIDOO, MBBS, FRANZCR
Radiologist, Department of Diagnostic
Imaging, Southern Health, Monash Medical
Centre, Clayton South, Victoria, Australia

PAUL T. O'CONNELL, MBBS, FRANZCR
Consultant Radiologist, Queensland
Diagnostic Imaging, St Andrews Hospital,
Brisbane, Australia

SYLVIA A. O'KEEFFE, MB, FFRRCSI
Fellow, Department of Radiology, Mater
Misericordiae University Hospital,
Dublin, Ireland

MARTIN J. SHELLY, MD, MRCPI
Specialist Registrar in Radiology,
Department of Radiology, Mater
Misericordiae Hospital, Dublin, Ireland

GARY J. SHEPHERD, MBBS, FRANZCR
Musculoskeletal Imaging Fellow, Qscan
Radiology Clinics, Brisbane, Australia

FRANCO VERDE, MD
Resident, Department of Radiology,
Geisinger Medical Center, Danville,
Pennsylvania

DAVID WEISS, MD
Department of Radiology, Geisinger Medical
Center, Danville, Pennsylvania

Contents

Overuse and impingement syndromes in the shoulders of athletes are predominantly caused by instability of the glenohumeral joint. Glenohumeral joint instability is usually acquired from repetitive overuse of the rotator cuff and shoulder girdle muscles, or injury of the static and dynamic stabilizers of the glenohumeral joint. Congenital hypermobility of the joint may also contribute to these syndromes in some individuals. The throwing action may lead to a cascade of injuries to the static and dynamic stabilizers of the posterosuperior glenohumeral joint, caused by the repetitive, high-energy nature of the action rather than a specific injury. Injury to the anterosuperior stabilizers of the glenohumeral joint may also lead to anterosuperior impingement syndrome. The role of MR in overuse and impingement syndromes of the shoulder is to accurately diagnose the underlying structural changes and serves to assist the clinician in instituting the appropriate conservative or surgical treatment for individual athletes.

Athletes who partake in overhead or throwing activities frequently suffer from shoulder pain. Glenohumeral instability plays an important role in sports-related shoulder pain. Shoulder instability can be traumatic, atraumatic, or microtraumatic in origin. In athletes, atraumatic and microtraumatic instabilities can lead to secondary impingement and chronic damage to intra-articular structures. MR arthrography is the modality of choice for assessing glenohumeral instability and diagnosing labroligamentous injuries. This article reviews imaging of instability-related injuries in athletes, with special emphasis on MR imaging.

MR imaging is a useful modality for evaluating athletes presenting with elbow pain. Osteochondral injuries and ligamentous injuries are well seen on MR imaging. Ligamentous injuries may be associated with clinical instability syndromes, the secondary signs of which may be evident on MR images. Enthesopathies and distal biceps tendon injuries are common clinical problems that may be seen in both professional and recreational athletes. Nerve compression syndromes may be investigated using MR imaging; however, the usual aim of imaging is to exclude an underlying space-occupying lesion. This article reviews the basic anatomy of the elbow joint and discusses the common osteochondral injuries, ligamentous injuries, instability syndromes, and tendinous pathologies at the elbow joint. The role of imaging in compressive neuropathies is briefly discussed.

Traumatic and overuse injuries of the hand and wrist are common in athletes. Increasingly, MR imaging is being used to complement clinical and radiographic assessment in the diagnosis and management of these injuries. MR imaging is able to image accurately the bones, tendons, ligaments, nerves, and other small structures of the hand and wrist. This article provides an overview of traumatic and overuse injuries of the hand and wrist in athletes and a review of the MR imaging appearances.

Groin pain is a commonly encountered problem in musculoskeletal radiology. The diagnosis can be difficult to establish, based on the complex interconnected anatomy at the pubic symphysis and surrounding structures. The differential diagnosis is therefore broad, and diagnostic imaging is crucial in reaching the correct diagnosis, thus allowing appropriate therapy to be instituted. This article reviews the relevant anatomy and differential diagnoses encountered in overuse injuries of the groin. The common mechanisms of injury, presenting symptoms, and imaging findings for each diagnosis are addressed.

The aim of this article is to emphasize the importance of MR imaging in the evaluation of chronic hip pain and overuse injuries. Image interpretation of the hip can be difficult because of the complex anatomy and the varied pathology that athletes can present with, such as labral and cartilaginous injuries, surrounding soft tissue derangement involving muscles or tendons, and osseous abnormalities. The differential diagnosis in adults is diverse and includes such common entities as stress fracture, avulsive injuries, snapping-hip syndrome, iliopsoas bursitis, femoroacetabular impingement syndrome, tendinosis, and tears of the gluteal musculature.

Traumatic lesions of the hip in athletes may be clinically challenging because of the overlap in clinical presentation due to differing pathologies and the presence of multiple injuries. Imaging of the hip in the athlete has undergone a recent resurgence of interest and understanding related to the increasing accessibility and use of hip arthroscopy, which expands the treatment options available for intra-articular pathology. MR imaging and MR arthrography have a unique role in diagnosis of these pathologies, guiding the surgeon, arthroscopist, and referring clinician in their management of bony and soft tissue injury.

The primary stabilizers of the knee can be functionally compartmentalized into the cruciate ligaments, the medial and posteromedial stabilizers, and the lateral and posterolateral stabilizers. This complex anatomy provides global knee stability. This article familiarizes the reader with the normal MR imaging appearance of these structures, and the changes following injury. The posteromedial and posterolateral corners are emphasized because recent research has improved the understanding of their importance, and their repair and reconstruction are becoming more common. Accurate identification of injury is important to ensuring optimal patient outcome.

Overuse injuries are a common cause of morbidity in athletes. They occur after repetitive microtrauma, abnormal joint alignment, and poor training technique without appropriate time to heal. Overuse injuries are frequent in the knee joint because of the numerous attachment sites for lower limb musculature and tendons surrounding the joint. MR imaging is regarded as the noninvasive technique of choice for detection of internal derangements of the knee. This article describes the characteristic findings on MR of the common overuse injuries in the knee, including patellar tendinopathy, iliotibial band syndrome, cartilage disorders, medial plica syndrome, and bursitis.

This article addresses the role of MR imaging in the evaluation of meniscal injuries, with emphasis placed on the common meniscal injuries, including horizontal, longitudinal, radial, and flap tears. An understanding of typical meniscal postoperative findings, together with those factors responsible for the misinterpretation of meniscal abnormalities, is essential for the accurate assessment of MR imaging in the athlete. This article also reviews the common articular cartilage injuries identified in the knee. MR imaging is the imaging modality of choice for the assessment of the menisci and articular cartilage, with the ready availability of MR imaging allowing for the rapid assessment of the injured athlete.

Although most muscle injuries in the athlete are diagnosed clinically, MR imaging is an excellent noninvasive diagnostic adjunct to clinical examination, which allows the site and severity of muscle injury to be assessed accurately, influencing therapy and overall outcome. There has been a rapid expansion in the clinical use of MR imaging during the past decade. MR imaging conveys unparalleled anatomic resolution and high sensitivity in the detection of acute and chronic muscle abnormalities. This article discusses the spectrum of muscle injuries, emphasizing the important role of MR imaging in their diagnosis and management.

Impingement is defined as a painful limitation of motion. Impingement lesions as identified on MR imaging of the ankle may relate to a range of soft tissue or bony

Contents

pathologies that can be interpreted as predisposing to painful limitation of motion, accepting that the diagnosis of impingement remains clinical and not radiological. Typically, impingement lesions are classified according to their location and whether the underlying pathology is osseous or soft tissue in nature. Most commonly, impingement lesions relate to posttraumatic synovitis and intra-articular fibrous bands–scar tissue, capsular scarring, or bony prominences, the latter either developmental or acquired. Well-recognized sites of impingement around the ankle include the anterolateral, centroanterior, anteromedial, posteromedial, and posterior sites. This article reviews the anatomy in these regions and focuses on common causes of impingement around the ankle; their pathogenesis, clinical features, and management; the approach to imaging of these lesions with MR imaging and their imaging features; and the relevant imaging differential diagnoses.

Magnetic Resonance Imaging Clinics of North America

RELATED INTEREST

Clinics in Sports Medicine October 2008 (Vol. 27, No. 4)
Shoulder Problems in Athletes
Benjamin Shaffer, MD, *Guest Editor*

THE CLINICS ARE NOW AVAILABLE ONLINE!

Access your subscription at:
www.theclinics.com

Preface

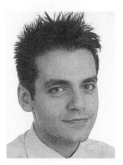

George Koulouris, MBBS,
GrCertSpMed, MMed, FRANZCR
Guest Editor

Musculoskeletal MRI continues to be an ever-expanding field of rapid development and progress, particularly with the increased introduction of 3-Tesla scanners into imaging centers. Elite athletes benefit the most from the recent advancements in our field because of the ready and often immediate access they have to MRI, with most musculoskeletal radiologists enthusiastic to provide their imaging expertise and service. The recreational athlete and the mature athlete have also benefited from the improved resolution of MRI. Mature athletes are particularly susceptible to injury, given their age and their need to be active for the purposes of disease prevention. It is therefore essential that this issue of *Magnetic Resonance Imaging Clinics of North America* caters to all these athletes. In this issue, emerging themes such as groin pain and muscle injuries are visited, and there is a comprehensive review of each joint. It is hoped that this issue will serve as a quick reference guide to help answer many routine musculoskeletal imaging dilemmas and also to stimulate further debate and research into areas where controversy exists. I am exceedingly proud of the work that the authors have presented in this issue, and I would like to take this opportunity to thank them for their tremendous effort to make this edition a success. I trust that this will be as informative reading for the reader as it has been for myself.

George Koulouris, MBBS
GrCertSpMed, MMed, FRANZCR
Melbourne Radiology Clinic
3-6/100 Victoria Parade
East Melbourne, VIC 3002, Australia

E-mail address:
GeorgeKoulouris@melbourneradiology.com.au

Magn Reson Imaging Clin N Am 17 (2009) xiii
doi:10.1016/j.mric.2009.06.011

Overuse and Impingement Syndromes of the Shoulder in the Athlete

Gregory A. Cowderoy, MBBS, FRANZCR[a],*,
David A. Lisle, MBBS, FRANZCR[b,c,d], Paul T. O'Connell, MBBS, FRANZCR[e]

KEYWORDS

- Impingement • Instability • Tendinosis • Labrum
- Bursitis • Imaging

Instability of the glenohumeral joint and fixed anatomic and pathologic variations of the coracoacromial arch lead to the most common overuse syndrome of the shoulder, subacromial impingement. Subacromial impingement is a cause of bursitis and tendinosis of the supraspinatus tendon and, if left untreated, may progress to tearing of the tendon.

Internal impingement of the glenohumeral joint refers to a complex combination of abnormalities, predominantly seen in throwing and overhead activities. Impingement at the posterosuperior corner of the glenohumeral joint in the fully cocked throwing position is the most common type of internal impingement. Anterosuperior impingement is also seen with excessive adduction and internal rotation of the humerus.

Little Leaguer's shoulder occurs in adolescent pitchers. It is caused by a stress injury of the proximal humeral growth plate. This injury is relatively specific to baseball and is not seen commonly in the author's practice, with cricket being the dominant national ball game in Australia. Osteolysis of the lateral end of the clavicle is also discussed.

ANATOMY AND BIOMECHANICS

The glenohumeral joint has a large range of movement compared with all other joints. This range of movement is achieved at the expense of osseous stability, with the humeral head approximating a golf ball balanced on a tee, the glenoid. The lack of bony stability is compensated for by a complex system of fixed and dynamic soft tissue stabilizers, including the glenoid labrum, the capsule and its ligaments, the rotator cuff, and the long head of biceps.

The glenoid labrum forms a fibrocartilaginous rim that deepens the glenoid fossa, providing improved static stability, further supported by static stabilizers, the superior, middle, and inferior glenohumeral ligaments. These ligaments reinforce the anterior and inferior capsule of the joint, resisting anterior and inferior dislocation. The rotator cuff muscles and tendons further envelope the glenohumeral joint, contracting and relaxing in a coordinated manner to keep the humeral head centered on the glenoid. These are the main dynamic stabilizers of the joint.

[a] Radiology Department, Queensland Diagnostic Imaging, Brisbane Private Hospital, 259 Wickham Terrace, Brisbane Q 4000, Queensland, Australia
[b] Queensland Diagnostic Imaging, Brisbane Q 4000, Australia
[c] The Royal Children's Hospital, Brisbane, Australia
[d] Division of Medical Imaging, University of Queensland Medical School, Herston, Brisbane Q 4029, Australia
[e] Queensland Diagnostic Imaging, St Andrews Hospital, Brisbane, Australia
* Corresponding author.
E-mail address: gcowderoy@gmail.com (G.A. Cowderoy).

Magn Reson Imaging Clin N Am 17 (2009) 577–593
doi:10.1016/j.mric.2009.06.003

The long head of biceps tendon provides additional dynamic stabilization of the anterosuperior corner of the joint. The tendon arises from the supraglenoid tubercle, reinforcing the superior glenoid labrum and forming the biceps labral anchor. The tendon passes anterolaterally over the humeral head as an intra-articular structure. It passes through the anterior capsule of the glenohumeral joint at the biceps (rotator) interval between the subscapularis and supraspinatus tendons, taking with it a synovial sleeve from the glenohumeral joint into the bicipital groove. The tendon changes from a horizontal orientation within the joint to a vertical orientation in the bicipital groove. This change in direction is facilitated by

a ligamentous pulley within the biceps interval formed by the coracohumeral and superior glenohumeral ligaments (**Fig. 1**). This biceps pulley also provides fixed stabilization of the long head of biceps tendon and is crucial to stabilizing the anterosuperior glenohumeral joint. The joint achieves further stability through maintaining negative intra-articular pressure. The humeral head is held firmly in the shallow glenoid fossa by this vacuum effect. Disruption of the static stabilizers of the joint may compromise this effect, resulting in further destabilization.

The coracoacromial arch, formed by the coracoid process, acromion, and the coracoacromial ligament, provides fixed protection and support

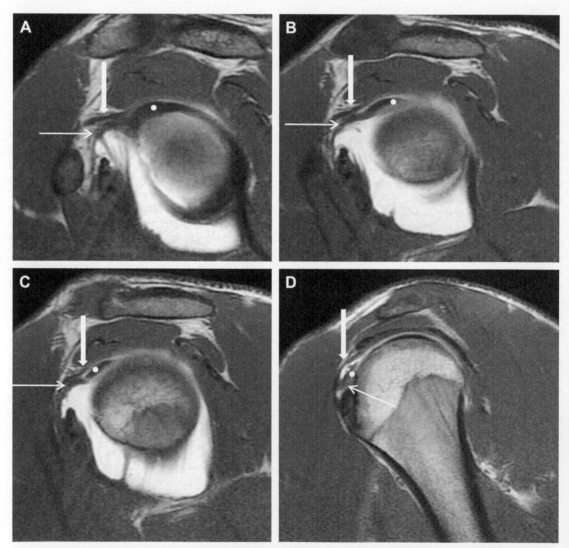

Fig. 1. (*A–D*) The normal biceps pulley consisting of the coracohumeral ligament (*thick arrow*), superior glenohumeral ligament (*thin arrow*) and long head of biceps tendon (*white dot*). The superior glenohumeral ligament wraps under the biceps tendon as it passes from the biceps labral anchor (*A*) anterolaterally toward the bicipital groove (*D*). The coracohumeral ligament forms the roof of the biceps pulley.

to the anterosuperior aspect of the glenohumeral joint. The coracoacromial ligament arises from the anteroinferior margin of the acromion. It passes anteromedially to insert on the lateral border of the coracoid process. It forms a fibro-osseous tunnel through which the supraspinatus, long head of biceps, and the subscapularis tendons pass.

IMPINGEMENT

The classification of shoulder impingement syndromes has evolved since Neer's[1] 1972 publication. Shoulder impingement was first described in the literature much earlier by Meyer[2] in 1931. A contemporary classification of shoulder impingement syndromes is shown in **Box 1**.

Shoulder impingement syndromes can occur external to or within the glenohumeral joint. The supraspinatus tendon, long head of biceps tendon, biceps interval, and the subacromial bursa are compressed between the humeral head and the coracoacromial arch in the most common form of external impingement, subacromial impingement. The subscapularis tendon and the subcoracoid bursa may be compressed between the coracoid process and the humeral head with subcoracoid impingement.

The articular surface of the posterior supraspinatus tendon and the anterior infraspinatus tendon impinge against the posterosuperior glenoid labrum in abduction and external rotation in the commonest form of internal impingement. This is a normal finding in most people (**Fig. 2**). It is only with instability of the humeral head in the ABER (abduction and external rotation) position that pathologic impingement and tissue damage occurs. This is most commonly seen in high-level throwing athletes.

Anterosuperior internal impingement occurs with adduction and internal rotation of the humerus. The anterior supraspinatus tendon, the subscapularis tendon, the long head of biceps tendon, the coracohumeral ligament, and the superior glenohumeral ligament impinge on the anterosuperior glenoid labrum in this less common form of internal impingement.

External Impingement Syndromes

Subacromial impingement

Subacromial impingement syndrome is a clinical diagnosis. The clinical presentation of subacromial impingement usually consists of a painful arc with abduction and flexion of the shoulder. Imaging findings supporting this diagnosis may be found on radiographs, ultrasound, CT, and MR imaging. Direct evidence of impingement may be seen on dynamic ultrasound examination. In some cases of subacromial impingement, imaging findings will be negative.

Subacromial impingement is classified as being primary if a structural cause in the coracoacromial arch is present that impedes the movement of the underlying soft tissues with abduction or flexion. Secondary subacromial impingement occurs because of instability of the glenohumeral joint, allowing compression of the supraspinatus tendon and its adjacent soft tissues between the humeral head and the normal coracoacromial arch with abduction or flexion.

Primary subacromial impingement Primary subacromial impingement is caused by pathology or normal variations in the coracoacromial arch and the acromioclavicular joint. These structures impinge directly on the subacromial bursa, supraspinatus tendon, biceps interval, and long head of biceps tendon with abduction and flexion of the shoulder. The acromial shape has been classified by Bigliani and colleagues[3] as follows: type 1 is flat, type 2 is curved, and type 3 is hooked (**Fig. 3**).

Type 3 acromial morphology has been associated with an increased incidence of supraspinatus tendinosis and impingement. Morrison and Bigliani[4] found that 80% of full thickness supraspinatus tendon tears showed a type 3 acromial morphology on outlet views of the shoulder. More recently, doubt has been cast on the relationship of acromial shape to subacromial impingement.[5] A type 2 or 3 acromion alone is unlikely to primarily cause subacromial impingement. It may, however, in the presence of multidirectional or microinstability, contribute to the condition.

The most common cause of primary subacromial impingement is spur formation at the anteroinferior margin of the acromion. This occurs with ossification of the acromial insertion of the

---

Box 1
Classification of impingement syndromes of the shoulder
External impingement
Subacromial
Primary
Secondary
Subcoracoid
Internal impingement
Posterosuperior
Anterosuperior

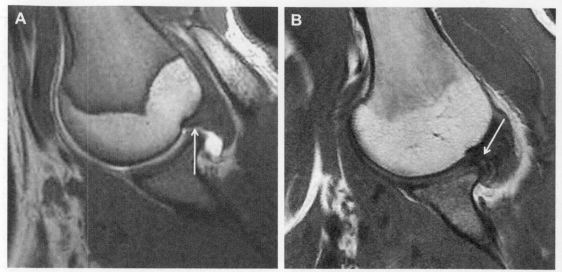

Fig. 2. (*A*) T1 arthrogram. (*B*) Proton density–weighted nonarthrogram of abduction and external rotation view through posterosuperior glenoid. It is normal for the articular surface of the posterosuperior rotator cuff to contact the glenoid labrum in abduction and external rotation (*arrow*).

coracoacromial ligament. Spurs do not usually develop until middle age and are not commonly the cause of impingement in young athletes.

A persistent os acromiale also has been associated with the development of subacromial impingement syndrome.[6,7] It is present in 8% of the population and is bilateral in 33%.[8] The acromion ossifies during adolescence from three centers: the meta-acromion, the mesoacromion, and the preacromion (**Fig. 4**). Failure of fusion may occur between any or all of these ossification centers.

Os acromiale most commonly occurs from failure of fusion between the meta-acromion and the mesoacromion. Caution must be exercised in reporting an os acromiale in the young athlete, because the normal acromial physis can be present up to 25 years of age.[9] Abnormal movement of the os acromiale may cause a stress injury at its junction with the acromion. This condition will have clinical and imaging findings that overlap with those of subacromial impingement (**Fig. 5**).[10] Movement of the os acromiale can cause osteophyte formation on

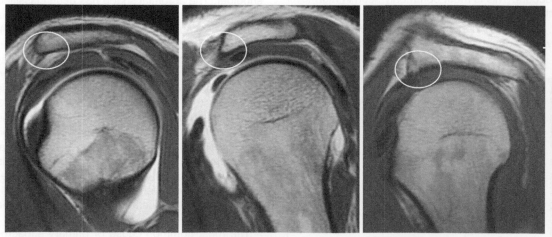

| Type 1 - Flat | Type 2 - Curved | Type 3 - Hooked |

Fig. 3. Sagittal T1 images lateral to acromioclavicular joint show the Bigliani classification of acromial morphology. Type 3 acromial morphology has been associated with a high incidence of supraspinatus pathology.

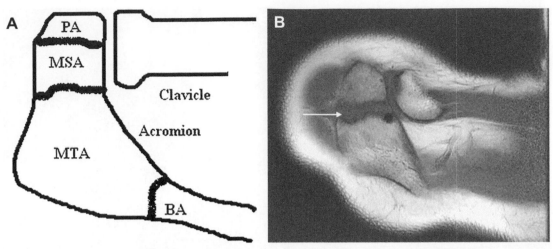

Fig. 4. (A) The acromion ossifies from up to three centers: preacromion (PA), mesoacromion (MSA), and meta-acromion (MTA). The ossification centers unite with each other and the basiacromion (BA) by 25 years of age. (B) Axial T1 image through the right shoulder shows failure of osseous union between the mesoacromion and the meta-acromion (arrow), the most common type of an os acromiale.

the margins of the pseudarthrosis, which impinge on the subacromial space, but usually not until middle age. Depression of the os acromiale during deltoid contraction has been postulated as a further cause of impingement.[9]

Evidence of acromioclavicular joint pathology causing subacromial impingement is controversial.[9–11] Acromioclavicular joint injury and subacromial impingent are common in athletes and may be seen coincidentally. MR can be useful in identifying capsular or bony impingement on the supraspinatus at the acromioclavicular joint when the clinical syndrome is present (Fig. 6).

Subacromial spur formation, acromioclavicular joint degeneration and marginal osteophyte formation, associated with subacromial impingement in the population older than 40 years, usually does not develop in the young adult.

Secondary subacromial impingement Secondary impingement from instability of the humeral head within the glenoid during activity is the most

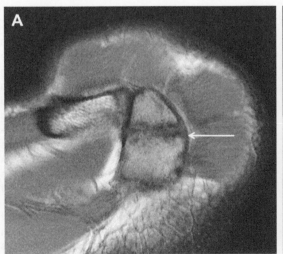

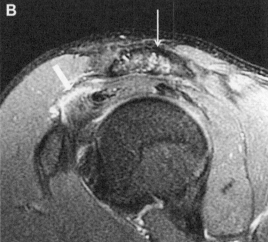

Fig. 5. Stress reaction at the junction of the os acromiale and the acromion caused by motion of the os acromiale secondary to deltoid contraction. This condition manifests as subcortical irregularity on either side of the pseudoarthrosis on the (A) axial proton density–weighted image (arrow) and bone marrow edema on the (B) sagittal T2-weighted imaging with fat saturation (arrow). Note the subacromial bursitis (thick arrow) and underlying supraspinatus tendinosis caused by impingement associated with the mobile os.

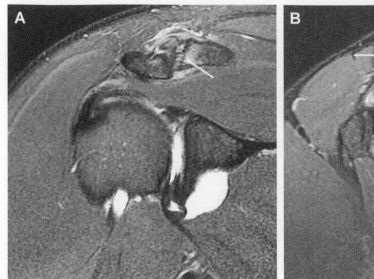
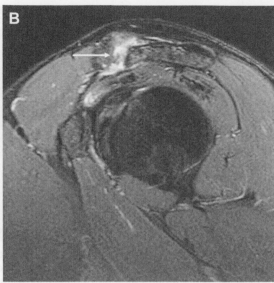

Fig. 6. (A) Coronal T2- and (B) sagittal T2-weighted images show bone marrow edema and capsular thickening of the acromioclavicular joint consistent with arthrosis (arrow), which may contribute to subacromial impingement and supraspinatus tendinosis. The acromioclavicular joint disease can cause a variable degree of shoulder pain that may be difficult to differentiate from pain associated with impingement.

common form of impingement in adolescents and young adults. It is seen in the athlete involved in overhead activities, such as basketball, tennis, and swimming. Decentering of the humeral head during abduction and flexion is more likely if capsular and ligamentous laxity is present. This mechanism may be a normal state in some genetically predisposed individuals or may be the result of recurrent energetic stretching of these structures during sport or activity.

Imbalance in the strength or coordination of the rotator cuff muscles and the long head of biceps muscle commonly contributes to the development of glenohumeral instability and capsular laxity. Compression of the subacromial soft tissues between the humeral head and the coracoacromial arch results in secondary subacromial impingement. This low-grade dynamic instability of the shoulder has been termed *multidirectional instability* or *atraumatic multidirectional bilateral instability* (AMBRI).[12–14] This condition is treated conservatively with physiotherapy to correct the imbalance in rotator cuff function. Surgical decompression of the subacromial space will often exacerbate the problem by further destabilizing the glenohumeral joint.

The term *microinstability* has been recently used to describe subtle instability from injury of the anterosuperior structures of the glenohumeral joint. The structures involved include the biceps labral anchor, superior labrum, coracohumeral and superior glenohumeral ligaments, biceps interval,

and anterosuperior rotator cuff. The resulting anterosuperior instability may then cause subacromial impingement syndrome.

Subacromial impingement causes a cascade of abnormalities, as first popularized by Neer.[15] Subacromial–subdeltoid bursitis is followed by the development of supraspinatus tendinosis, which if left untreated will lead to partial and eventually full thickness tearing of the supraspinatus tendon.

Subacromial bursitis

The subacromial–subdeltoid bursa is a large structure overlying the rotator cuff and facilitates its movement under the coracoacromial arch. The first imaging change of impingement is thickening of and mildly increased signal in the bursa on water-weighted MR sequences (Fig. 7). Bursal thickness of 2 mm or greater has been used to as a cutoff measurement to indicate abnormality,[16] although symptomatic impingement is often seen with bursal thickness less than this. A normal bursa on MR imaging or ultrasound is a barely perceptible line between the rotator cuff and the subdeltoid fat plane.

Bursal thickening often precedes symptoms of subacromial impingement, and is often seen in the asymptomatic contralateral shoulder. This symmetric thickening of the burse should not be misinterpreted as normal. Fluid may be seen within the subacromial–subdeltoid bursa if impingement continues. More than a trace of fluid in the bursa should instigate a careful search

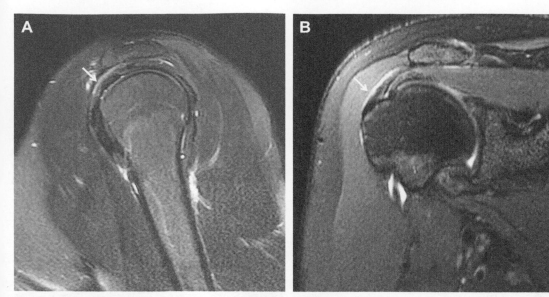

Fig. 7. (A) Early or mild bursitis may have no imaging findings. Subtle thickening and increased signal under the anterior acromion and coracoacromial ligament (*arrow*) on water-weighted sequences is often the first evidence of impingement. (B) With further impingement, the edema and bursal thickening increases over the supraspinatus tendon (*arrow*).

for a full-thickness tear of the rotator cuff (**Fig. 8**). Bursitis from an inflammatory arthropathy may be seen in adolescents or young adults, and usually results in more marked synovial hypertrophy than is seen with mechanical impingement. Intravenous contrast should be used to highlight the synovial proliferation if inflammatory arthritis is suspected.

Tendinosis

Neer[15] described the pathologic continuum of acute supraspinatus tendinosis progressing to chronic tendinosis, partial thickness tearing, and eventual full-thickness tearing of the tendon with chronic subacromial impingement.

In athletes, the early stages of this continuum commonly begin with subacromial bursitis and

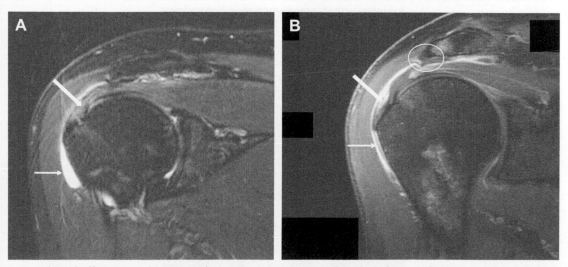

Fig. 8. A bursal effusion may be seen with ongoing impingement alone but always indicates a possible full-thickness supraspinatus tear. (A) Coronal T2-weighted image with fat saturation shows a bursal effusion (*arrow*) and supraspinatus tendinosis (*thick arrow*). (B) Similar imaging sequence in a different patient shows a bursal effusion (*arrow*) and bursal surface partial-thickness tear of supraspinatus tendon (*thick arrow*) secondary to a subacromial spur (*circle*).

progress to supraspinatus tendinosis. The tendon becomes thickened and shows increased signal on T2 and proton density sequences (Fig. 9). The tendon thickening exacerbates the subacromial impingement and accelerates the progress toward a tendon tear unless treatment is instituted (Fig. 10).

Treatment may include oral anti-inflammatory medication or a subacromial injection of corticosteroid; however, this will not provide long-term relief if the underlying instability is not corrected. A structural cause for instability, such as a labral or rotator cuff tear, will require surgery. In the absence of a surgical lesion, physiotherapy is required to correct the strength and balance of the dynamic stabilizers of the shoulder.

MR imaging technique

Adequate assessment of subacromial impingement may be obtained using a nonarthrographic technique. Coronal oblique proton density, T2 with fat saturation sequences, sagittal T1 and T2 with fat saturation sequences, and an axial proton density sequence provide a well-balanced mix of structural information with good tissue and fluid contrast.

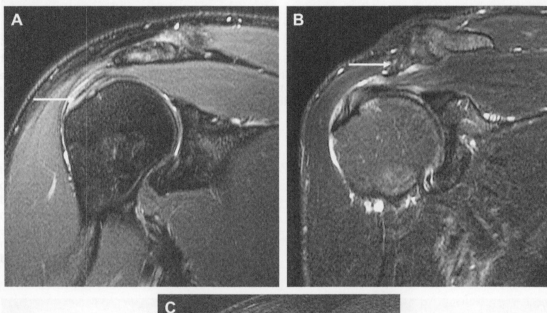

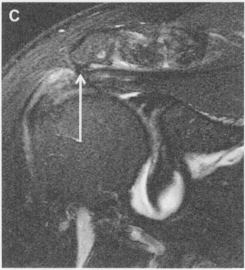

Fig. 9. (A) Supraspinatus tendinosis is best visualized on fat-saturated T2 sequences as increased signal and thickening of the tendon (arrow). (B) Lateral downsloping of the acromion (arrow) is a known cause of impingement, in this case resulting in subacromial bursitis and supraspinatus tendinosis. (C) A thickened subacromial bursa often impinges against a prominent origin of the coracoacromial ligament (arrow).

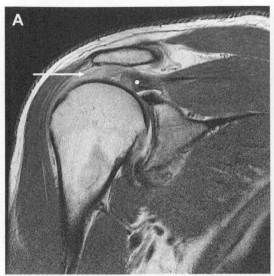 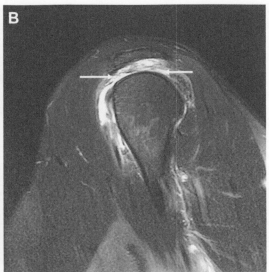

Fig. 10. (A) Coronal proton density–weighted image shows absence of normal tendon signal (*arrow*) consistent with a full-thickness tear of the supraspinatus tendon from chronic subacromial impingement. The tendon edge is retracted medially (*dot*). (B) Sagittal T2-weighted image also shows the defect between the two arrows.

Findings include:

- Spur formation on the undersurface of the acromion; this is most common at the origin of the coracoacromial ligament
- Osteophyte or capsular hypertrophy of the acromioclavicular joint compressing the supraspinatus
- Acromial morphology on the sagittal images
- Fluid, thickening, or abnormal signal in the subacromial–subdeltoid bursa
- Supraspinatus tendinosis; thickening of and increased signal in the supraspinatus tendon on water-weighted sequences
- Bicipital tendinosis and fluid in the biceps tendon sheath
- Bursal surface partial-thickness tears of the supraspinatus tendon
- Full-thickness supraspinatus tendon tears

Subcoracoid impingement

Uncommonly, the subscapularis tendon and its superficial bursa become compressed between the anterior glenohumeral joint and the coracoid process. The normal coracohumeral interval measures approximately 1 cm on axial MR images, with a large range of 4 to 18 mm found in a control group.[17] The measurement is 3 mm less on average in women than in men. A group of patients who had clinically diagnosed subcoracoid impingement showed an average coracohumeral interval of 6.2 mm, with a range of 2 to 9 mm.[17] Features believed to contribute to a reduced coracohumeral interval include a long or prominent coracoid process, the shape of the coracoid, and a prominent lesser tuberosity of the humeral head; however, Giaroli and colleagues[17] showed that the morphology of the coracoid and the lesser tuberosity has no apparent predictive value in diagnosing subcoracoid impingement.

The measurement of the coracohumeral interval changes significantly with the imaging plane and with rotation of the humeral head. It changes with movement of the shoulder and the degree of glenohumeral stability. A full-thickness supraspinatus tear or a biceps pulley injury will cause microinstability and anterosuperior translation of the humeral head, resulting in a reduced coracohumeral interval.[18] Although dynamic ultrasonography may be useful in directly assessing the subscapularis tendon passing under the coracoid, it is subjective and requires considerable operator experience. Subcoracoid impingement typically remains a clinical diagnosis. Imaging findings may corroborate the clinical diagnosis or offer an alternative diagnosis for the symptoms (**Fig. 11**).

Findings include:

- Subcoracoid stenosis; coracohumeral interval 6 mm or less
- Large lesser tuberosity of the humerus
- Large coracoid process
- Subscapular tendinosis
- Partial or full thickness tear of the subscapular tendon
- Subcoracoid bursitis
- Anterior subacromial-subdeltoid bursitis

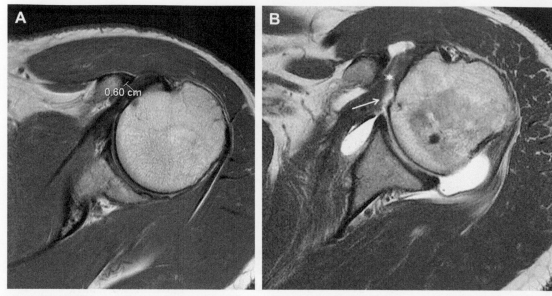

Fig. 11. (*A*) Axial proton density–weighted image shows a stenotic subcoracoid space. Note that measurement of the subcoracoid space varies with different imaging planes and position of the arm. (*B*) Axial T1 arthrogram shows subscapularis tendinosis (*star*) and partial-thickness undersurface tearing of the tendon (*arrow*) caused by chronic subcoracoid impingement.

Internal Impingement

Internal impingement syndromes of the glenohumeral joint refer to impingement of the supporting soft tissues of the glenohumeral joint between the humeral head and the glenoid. Posterosuperior and anterosuperior impingement are the two recognized internal impingement syndromes.

Posterosuperior impingement

The posterosuperior glenoid labrum contacts or is immediately adjacent to the articular surface of the posterior supraspinatus tendon and the anterior infraspinatus tendon when the arm is held in abduction and external rotation. This relationship is normal in common upper limb positions, such as those seen in throwing, swimming, and overhead activities (see **Fig. 2**).

Posterosuperior impingement (PSI) refers to impingement of the supraspinatus and infraspinatus tendons, the adjacent capsule and bursa between the humeral head and the posterosuperior glenoid. PSI is caused by abnormal biomechanics and excess activity and may lead to tendinosis and tearing of the articular surfaces of the tendons and a tear of the glenoid labrum. Multidirectional instability caused by congenital or acquired capsular laxity may predispose individuals to PSI. The throwing athlete is most at risk for developing PSI , because the arm is cocked into maximum abduction and external rotation before the rapid forward release of the upper limb.

Throwing shoulder The term *throwing shoulder* refers to a constellation of conditions, including glenohumeral internal rotation deficit (GIRD),[19] a posterior superior labrum anterior to posterior (SLAP) tear,[20] SICK scapula syndrome,[21] and articular surface partial-thickness tears of the posterior supraspinatus tendon and the anterior infraspinatus tendon. A combination of these conditions leads to pain and loss of performance in the throwing athlete, which may result in and have been previously considered part of the PSI syndrome. In the baseball pitcher, this is referred to as a *dead arm*.[19–21]

Glenohumeral internal rotation deficit Forceful follow-through when throwing causes tensile loading of the posterior shoulder capsule and the posterior band of the inferior glenohumeral ligament. Unrestricted repetition of this action may cause thickening and contracture of these structures, restricting internal rotation and adduction of the glenohumeral joint (**Fig. 12**).

When GIRD has developed, the tight posterior band of the inferior glenohumeral ligament forms a sling under the humeral head as the arm is placed into the ABER position, forcing it to move posterosuperiorly within the glenoid. The posterosuperior shift of the humeral head shifts the articular contact point toward the posterosuperior margin of the glenoid. This movement is believed to cause the subarticular sclerosis and cyst formation in the glenoid at this site in these athletes. It

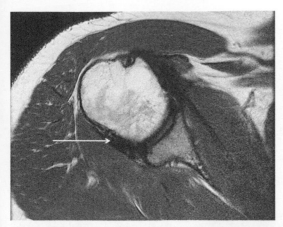

Fig. 12. Repetitive forceful throwing or pitching may injure the posterior limb of the inferior glenohumeral ligament and the posterior joint capsule at the end of the follow-through. This injury can result in thickening and contraction of these structures (*arrow*), as noted on this axial proton density–weighted image, which limits the degree of adduction and internal rotation of the humerus. With abduction and external rotation, the thickened posterior band forms a sling under the humeral head, causing posterosuperior subluxation.

also clears the greater tuberosity of the posterosuperior glenoid, allowing extended external rotation in the cocked throwing position. Pseudolaxity of the anteroinferior capsule caused by the posterosuperior subluxation of the humeral head also allows excessive external rotation. The extended abduction and external rotation may result in increased power in the throwing action, but places additional stress on the biceps labral anchor, the superior labrum, the rotator cuff tendons, and the balance of the rotator cuff muscles.

SICK scapula syndrome The SICK scapula syndrome refers to a condition in throwing athletes resulting from overuse and fatigue of the muscles of the shoulder girdle. The acronym refers to scapular malposition, inferior medial border prominence, coracoid pain and malposition, and dyskinesis of scapular movement.

This condition initially manifests as tilting of the scapula from its normal plane. This syndrome is classified as type 1 with prominence of the inferomedial border of the scapula and type 2 with prominence of the medial border of the scapula, both of which are associated with posterosuperior labral lesions. Type 3 SICK scapula has prominence of the superomedial border and is associated with lesions of the rotator cuff and subacromial impingement.[21] The combination of GIRD and SICK scapula increases the likelihood

of posterosuperior impingement, posterosuperior labral tears, and rotator cuff pathology.

The peel-back lesion Posterosuperior movement of the humeral head during abduction and external rotation occurs with a tight posterior glenohumeral capsule, multidirectional instability, or GIRD and is exacerbated with abnormal tilting of the scapula as occurs with the development of SICK scapular syndrome. The posterosuperior translation of the humeral head during cocking of the throwing arm forces the long head of biceps tendon superiorly and rotates it posteriorly, causing a peel-back action on the biceps labral anchor and the posterosuperior labrum. These abnormal forces lead to a posterior type 2 SLAP tear, also known as a peel-back lesion (**Fig. 13**).[20]

The rotator cuff The repetitive contact of the articular surface of the posterior supraspinatus tendon and the anterior infraspinatus tendon against the posterosuperior glenoid during abduction and external rotation was initially believed to be the cause of the partial-thickness articular surface tears seen in these tendons with posterosuperior impingement.[22] Apposition of the posterosuperior labrum with the articular surface of the supraspinatus and infraspinatus tendons with abduction and external rotation has been repeatedly shown to be normal.[23–25] More recently, it has been postulated that the articular surface tears seen in the posterior supraspinatus and anterior infraspinatus tendons in throwing athletes are caused by excessive external rotation of the tendons, resulting in torsional overload and shear failure of the articular surface fibers (**Fig. 14**).

Overuse injury of the shoulder in the throwing athlete is a multifactorial condition that includes the elements discussed earlier. Impingement of the soft tissues of the posterosuperior corner of the shoulder between the humeral head and the glenoid most likely occurs only after the labrum and the rotator cuff have been damaged, rather than being the primary abnormality. MR plays an important role in recognizing the abnormalities associated with the symptomatic throwing shoulder and alerting the attending physician to the evolving syndrome. Conservative treatment may be instituted if a labral or rotator cuff tear has not occurred, or surgical treatment may be tailored to best address the structural damage and the glenohumeral instability.

MR imaging technique
The findings of posterosuperior impingement are most clearly shown with an MR arthrogram (**Fig. 15**). With improvements in coil technology and increasing experience, MR assessment of

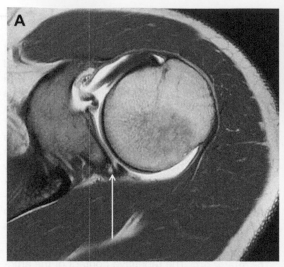

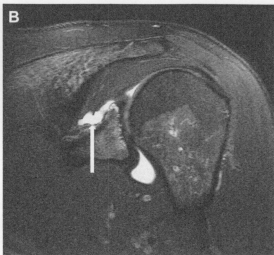

Fig. 13. The Peel back lesion. (A) A posterior SLAP lesion (*arrow*) is demonstrated on this axial T1 arthrogram image. (B) Coronal T2 fat-saturated arthrogram image shows a paralabral cyst (*thick arrow*), which is often seen in association with the tear. This may compress the suprascapular nerve in the spinoglenoid notch, causing denervation of infraspinatus.

internal impingement can be adequate using non-arthrographic techniques.

In the authors' institutions, an MR arthrogram is used when assessing for possible internal impingement with the following protocol: TI axial, ABER, and sagittal sequences, with the sagittal series extending medially through the rotator cuff musculature, and coronal oblique TI and T2 sequences, both with fat saturation.

Findings include:

- Sclerosis and subarticular cyst formation in the posterosuperior glenoid
- Exaggerated subcortical cyst formation in the bare area of the humeral head deep to the infraspinatus tendon
- Partial-thickness articular surface tears in the posterior supraspinatus tendon and the anterior infraspinatus tendon

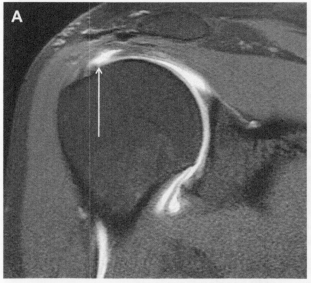

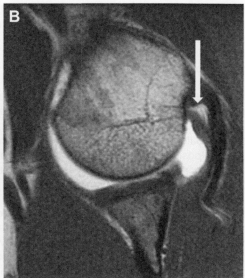

Fig. 14. Rotator cuff tears in posterosuperior impingement. (A) Coronal T1 fat-saturated arthrogram shows a partial-thickness articular surface tear of the posterior supraspinatus and anterior infraspinatus tendons (*arrow*). (B) Occasionally, this tear is best appreciated on the abduction and external rotation view (*thick arrow*). Note the posterior decentering of the humeral head on the abduction and external rotation view that is commonly seen in posterosuperior impingement.

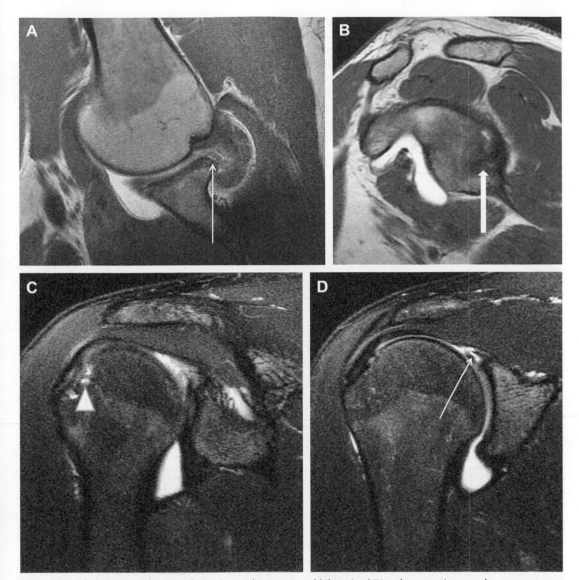

Fig. 15. (A) T1 abduction and external rotation arthrogram and (B) sagittal T1 arthrogram images show a posterosuperior labral tear with articular surface irregularity of the posterior supraspinatus tendon (*arrow*), and sclerosis and cortical irregularity of the posterosuperior glenoid (*thick arrow*). Coronal T2 fat-saturated arthrogram shows (C) exaggerated subcortical cyst formation deep to the infraspinatus tendon (*arrowhead*) and (D) a posterior type 2 SLAP tear (*arrow*). All of these findings are characteristic of posterosuperior impingement.

- Posterosuperior labral tear
- Posterosuperior decentering of the humeral head on the ABER view
- Posterior capsular thickening in the throwing athlete

Anterosuperior impingement

Anterosuperior impingement (ASI) is an uncommon clinical diagnosis in athletes who experience anterior shoulder pain and weakness with horizontal adduction and internal rotation of the shoulder. It was initially postulated that the subscapularis tendon and the biceps pulley were caught between the humeral head and the glenoid, with adduction and internal rotation of the shoulder resulting in injury of these structures and the glenoid labrum.[26] Contact of the anterosuperior labrum and the articular surface of the rotator cuff in adduction and internal rotation has been shown to be physiologic.[27] The intact long head of biceps tendon and its pulley are significant anterosuperior stabilizers of the shoulder.

Habermeyer and colleagues[28] showed that ASI can occur only after biceps pulley injury, with resultant medial subluxation of the long head of biceps tendon. This effect causes microinstability with anterosuperior translation of the humeral head. The increasing medial subluxation/dislocation of the biceps tendon causes tearing of the distal subscapularis tendon, which contributes further to instability and anterosuperior translation of the humeral head. A tear of the distal articular surface of the supraspinatus tendon is often present in patients who have ASI, although it is likely to be associated with the injury that results in the biceps pulley lesion rather than as a result of ASI. ASI cannot occur until the anterosuperior stabilizers have been compromised. However, once ASI occurs, the injuries to the subscapularis tendon, biceps interval, and anterior labrum

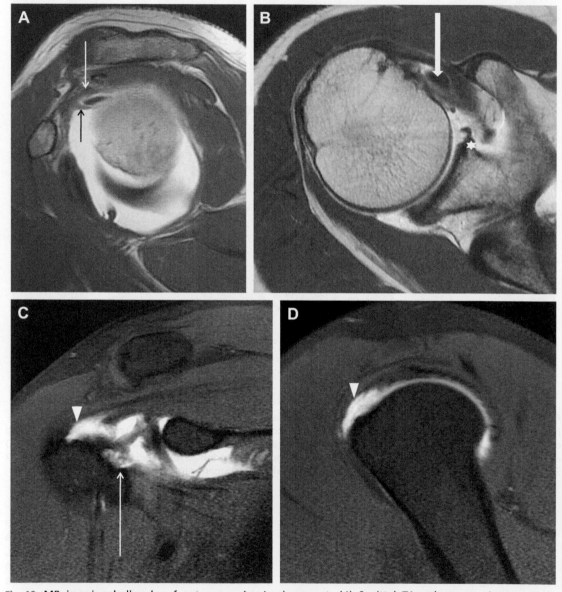

Fig. 16. MR imaging hallmarks of anterosuperior Impingement. (*A*) Sagittal T1 arthrogram. Anterosuperior impingement (ASI) does not occur without injury of the biceps pulley. The biceps pulley consists of the coracohumeral ligament (*white arrow*) and the superior glenohumeral ligament (*black arrow*). (*B*) Axial T1 arthrogram. A torn biceps pulley results in medial subluxation of the long head of biceps tendon into subscapularis tendon (*thick arrow*) and a tear of the anterosuperior labrum (*star*). Coronal (*C*) and sagittal (*D*) T1 fat-saturated arthrographic images show an articular surface partial-thickness tear of the anterior supraspinatus tendon (*arrowhead*) and superior margin of subscapularis insertion (*long arrow*).

typically progress from the underlying impinge-ment (**Fig. 16**). ASI and acromioclavicular joint arthrosis are associated,[26,28] but the mechanism of this association is unclear.

Findings include:

- Injury of the biceps pulley
- Partial-thickness tear of the articular surface of the anterior supraspinatus tendon
- Medial subluxation of the long head of biceps tendon
- Partial-thickness tears of the distal subsca-pularis tendon. These may be articular surface, bursal surface, or intrasubstance from the biceps tendon dissecting directly into the distal tendon. The type of tear is dependent on the specific biceps pulley injury
- Tearing of the anterosuperior labrum
- Acromioclavicular joint arthrosis

Little Leaguer's shoulder

"Little Leaguer's" shoulder is a stress injury of the proximal humeral physis seen in adolescent throwing athletes, most commonly baseball pitchers. The average age of onset is 14 years, which has been attributed to rapid skeletal growth associated with this age.[29] The patient presents with pain and tenderness in the proximal humerus with throwing. This condition responds well to re-fraining from pitching until symptoms have completely resolved. An average of three months rest has been recommended with gradual resump-tion of activity.[30]

MR imaging findings of Little Leaguer's shoulder include (**Fig. 17**):

- Widening of the proximal humeral physis
- Increased signal on the margins of the physis on water-weighted sequences
- Periosteal edema

Osteolysis of the lateral end of the clavicle

Cahill described 46 cases of osteolysis of the lateral end of the clavicle in athletes[31] who presented with pain and tenderness of the acromioclavicular joint. Radiographic changes include osteopenia, loss of cortical definition, and subcortical cyst formation in the lateral end of the clavicle. The cause of this condition is not certain. Increased vascularity at the lateral end of the clavicle, injury to the articular cartilage, reactive synovitis, avascular necrosis, and stress fractures in the distal end of the clavicle have all been proposed as causes of this condition.[32,33]

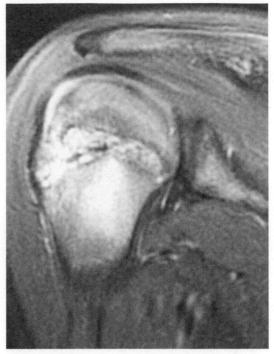

Fig. 17. Coronal T2 fat-saturated image shows widening (*arrow*) and abnormal signal along the proximal humeral physis, features consistent with Little Leaguer's shoulder. (*Courtesy of* Meghan Blake, MD, Radnet Medical Imaging, San Francisco, CA.)

MR findings in osteolysis of the lateral end of the clavicle include (**Fig. 18**):

- Increased fluid signal in the distal clavicle
- Cortical thinning and irregularity at the lateral end of the clavicle
- Small subcortical cysts

SUMMARY

Overuse and impingement syndromes in the shoulders of athletes are predominantly caused by instability of the glenohumeral joint. Glenohum-eral joint instability is usually acquired from repetitive overuse of the rotator cuff and shoulder girdle muscles, or injury of the static and dynamic stabilizers of the glenohumeral joint. Congenital hypermobility of the joint may also contribute to these syndromes in some individuals. The throwing action may lead to a cascade of injuries to the static and dynamic stabilizers of the poster-osuperior glenohumeral joint, caused by the repet-itive, high-energy nature of the action rather than a specific injury.

Injury to the anterosuperior stabilizers of the gle-nohumeral joint may also lead to anterosuperior

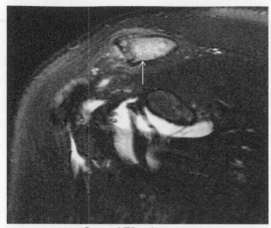

Coronal T2 arthrogram

Fig. 18. Oedema, subcortical cyst fation and cortical irreguormlarity of the lateral end of the clavicle [*arrow*] is not uncommonly seen in the athlete with pain at the AC joint. This may develop following trauma or due to overuse of the shoulder.

impingement syndrome. The role of MR in overuse and impingement syndromes of the shoulder is to accurately diagnose the underlying structural changes and assist clinicians in instituting the appropriate conservative or surgical treatment for individual athletes.

REFERENCES

1. Neer CS II. Anterior acromioplasty for the chronic impingement syndrome in the shoulder. J Bone Joint Surg Am 1972;54:41–50.
2. Meyer AW. The minuter anatomy of attrition lesions. J Bone Joint Surg Am 1931;13:341–60.
3. Bigliani LU, Morrison DS, April EW. The morphology of the acromion and its relationship to rotator cuff tears. Orthop Trans 1986;10:228.
4. Morrison DS, Bigliani LU. The clinical significance of variations in acromial morphology. Orthop Trans 1987;11:234.
5. Chang EY, Moses DA, Babb JS, et al. Shoulder impingement: objective 3D shape analysis of acromial morphologic features. Radiology 2006;239: 497–505.
6. Swain R, Wilson F, Harsha D. The os acromiale: another cause of impingement. Med Sci Sports Exerc 1996;28:1459–62.
7. Bigliani L, Norris R, Fischer J, et al. The relationship between the unfused acromial epiphysis and subacromial lesions. Orthop Trans 1983;7:138.
8. Sammarco VJ. Os acromiale: frequency, anatomy and clinical implications. J Bone Joint Surg Am 2000;82:394–400.
9. Park JG, Lee JK, Phelps CT. Os acromiale associated with rotator cuff impingement: MR imaging of the shoulder. Radiology 1994;193:255–7.
10. Pagnani M, Mathis C, Solman C. Painful os acromiale (or unfused acromial apophysis) in athletes. J Shoulder Elbow Surg 2006;15:432–5.
11. Petersson CJ, Gentz CF. Ruptures of the supraspinatus tendon. The significance of distally pointing acromioclavicular osteophytes. Clin Orthop 1983; 174:143–8.
12. Silliman J, Hawkins R. Current concepts and recent advances in the athletes shoulder. Clin Sports Med 1991;10:693–705.
13. Silliman J, Hawkins R. Classification and physical diagnosis of instability of the shoulder. Clin Orthop Relat Res 1993;291:7–19.
14. Lippitt S, Harryman D. Diagnosis and management of AMBRI syndrome. Tech Orthop 1991;6:61–73.
15. Neer CS II. Impingement lesions. Clin Orthop 1983; 173:70–7.
16. van Holsbeeck M, Strouse PJ. Sonography of the shoulder: evaluation of the subacromial-subdeltoid bursa. AJR Am J Roentgenol 1993;160:561–4.
17. Giaroli EL, Major NM, Lemley DE, et al. Coracohumeral interval imaging in subcoracoid impingement syndrome on MRI. AJR Am J Roentgenol 2006; 186:242–6.
18. MacMahon PJ, Taylor DH, Duke D, et al. Contribution of full-thickness supraspinatus tendon tears to acquired subcoracoid impingement. Clin Radiol 2007;62:556–63.
19. Burkhart SS, Morgan CD, Kibler WB. The disabled throwing shoulder: spectrum of pathology, part I: pathoanatomy and biomechanics. Arthroscopy 2003;19:404–20.
20. Burkhart SS, Morgan CD, Kibler WB. The disabled throwing shoulder: spectrum of pathology, part II: evaluation and treatment of SLAP lesions in throwers. Arthroscopy 2003;19:531–9.
21. Burkhart SS, Morgan CD, Kibler WB. The disabled throwing shoulder: spectrum of pathology, part III: the SICK scapula, scapula dyskinesis, the kinetic chain and rehabilitation. Arthroscopy 2003;19:641–61.
22. Walch G, Boileau P, Noel E, et al. Impingement of the deep surface of the supraspinatus tendon on the posterior-superior glenoid rim: an arthroscopic study. J Shoulder Elbow Surg 1992;1:238–45.
23. Halbrecht JL. Internal impingement of the shoulder: comparison of findings between the throwing and nonthrowing shoulders of college baseball players. Arthroscopy 1999;15:253–8.
24. Barber FA, Morgan CD, Burkhart SS, et al. Labrum/ biceps/cuff dysfunction in the throwing athlete. Arthroscopy 1999;15:852–7.
25. McFarland EG, Hsu CY, O'Neil O. Internal impingement of the shoulder: a clinical and arthroscopic analysis. J Shoulder Elbow Surg 1999;8:458–60.

26. Gerber C, Sebesta A. Impingement of the deep surface of the subscapularis tendon and the reflection pulley on the anterosuperior glenoid rim: a preliminary report. J Shoulder Elbow Surg 2000;9:483–90.

27. Struhl S. Anterior internal impingement: an arthroscopic observation. Arthroscopy 2002;18:2–7.

28. Habermeyer P, Magosch P, Pritsch M, et al. Anterosuperior impingement of the shoulder as a result of pulley lesions: a prospective arthroscopic study. J Shoulder Elbow Surg 2004;13:5–12.

29. Hatem SF, Recht MP, Profitt B. MRI of Little Leaguer's shoulder. Skeletal Radiol 2006;35:103–6.

30. Carson WG Jr, Gasser SI. Little Leaguer's shoulder. A report of 23 cases. Am J Sports Med 1998;26: 575–80.

31. Cahill BR. Osteolysis of the distal part of the clavicle in male athletes. J Bone Joint Surg Am 1982;64: 1053–8.

32. Kassarjian A, Llopis E, Palmer WE. Distal clavicular osteolysis: MR evidence for subchondral fracture. Skeletal Radiol 2007;36:17–22.

33. Patten RM. Atraumatic osteolysis of the distal clavicle: MR findings. J Comput Assist Tomogr 1995; 19:92–5.

Imaging Shoulder Instability in the Athlete

Diane Bergin, MD

KEYWORDS

- Imaging • Shoulder instability • Glenohumeral instability
- Magnetic resonance arthrography • Labral tear

In the last decade, understanding of the biomechanics and physiology of the athletic shoulder and of shoulder-stabilizing forces has significantly improved.[1–3] It is now understood that instability related to sports activities is associated with secondary impingement, muscular dysfunction, and damage to intra-articular structures that can be detrimental to athletes' performance and ultimately to their careers.[2,3]

For athletes whose sport requires repetitive overhead motion, such as baseball, softball, volleyball, and swimming, glenohumeral instability is recognized as an important cause of ongoing shoulder pain and dysfunction.[1,2] The term "shoulder instability" refers to a spectrum of disorders including dislocation, subluxation, and laxity of the shoulder joint.[1–3] Dislocation is defined as complete loss of the humeral articulation with the glenoid fossa as a result of acute trauma. Subluxation is a partial loss of the articulation causing symptoms, and is typically caused by repetitive trauma. As with subluxation, laxity is defined as a partial loss of the glenohumeral articulation; however, patients with shoulder laxity are frequently asymptomatic.

The high degree of mobility of the shoulder joint makes it inherently prone to instability.[3] Functional stability of the glenohumeral joint is achieved through static and dynamic stabilizers.[2] The static stabilizers include negative intra-articular pressure, size, shape, and orientation of the glenoid fossa and the capsulolabral complex. Dynamic stabilizers include the rotator cuff and the long head of the biceps tendon.[2] Repetitive throwing action places high stress loads on the capsulolabral complex and rotator cuff.[2]

Minor repetitive injury to these structures can become symptomatic and produce significant functional impairment. Joint laxity may develop as a consequence of the injury to these tissues, leading to even more damage and further instability. It is now understood that in the throwing athlete, these injuries are not usually the consequence of a single event of dislocation but are the result of multiple episodes of microtrauma, producing a gradual increase of shoulder pain at some point in the throwing position.[3–5]

This article reviews the basic normal anatomy and pathophysiology of shoulder instability in the athlete, and reviews the magnetic resonance (MR) imaging findings in the more common instability patterns seen in these patients.

IMAGING TECHNIQUE

Imaging of glenohumeral instability and the underlying structural abnormalities has significantly evolved.[4–12] Imaging techniques such as conventional radiography, computed tomography (CT), arthrography, and most recently MR imaging are used to evaluate the shoulder.[12–15] Conventional radiography is the initial imaging study for evaluating the patient with persistent shoulder pain and instability. Radiographs can demonstrate joint space narrowing, glenohumeral joint dislocation, high-riding humerus (suggestive of large rotator cuff tears), fractures such as Hill-Sachs and Bankart lesions, osteophytes, erosions, sclerosis, subchondral cysts, abnormal bone density, and joint and soft tissue ossification and calcification.

CT and MR arthrography, with inherent distension of the joint, are used to evaluate the capsular

Department of Radiology, Galway University Hospital, Galway, Ireland
E-mail address: diane.bergin@hse.ie

Magn Reson Imaging Clin N Am 17 (2009) 595–615
doi:10.1016/j.mric.2009.06.002

and labral structures of the shoulder.[13–16] Studies using conventional unenhanced MR imaging in the evaluation of glenohumeral instability have produced mixed results in the detection of labral tears, with sensitivities and specificities ranging from 44% to 100% and 66% to 95%, respectively.[13,15] MR arthrography has reported sensitivities of 86% to 91% and specificities of 86% to 98%, and is the modality of choice when evaluating the labrum and glenohumeral ligaments.[11,12] Labral tears are detected best when a joint effusion is present or with MR arthrography.[13–15] Small osseous fragments and cartilage lesions are better seen with CT.[15] Due to limited soft tissue contrast, CT arthrography is less useful for evaluation of soft tissues such as the labrum or rotator cuff, and is typically reserved for patients who cannot undergo MR imaging due to contraindications such as the presence of a cardiac pacemaker or cochlear implant.

MAGNETIC RESONANCE ARTHROGRAPHIC TECHNIQUE

Direct MR arthrography is performed routinely in the author's practice in athletes with clinical evidence of shoulder instability or with idiopathic shoulder pain. With MR arthrography the intra-articular fluid distends the joint and outlines labral and capsular structures as well as the undersurface of the rotator cuff.[13,15,16] Under fluoroscopic guidance, 12 to 18 mL of a 2.5 mmol/L solution of a gadolinium chelate is injected into the mid to lower one-third of the glenohumeral joint using a classic anterior approach (**Fig. 1**), a 22-gauge spinal needle, and sterile technique. Intra-articular position of the needle tip is confirmed by application of a small amount of iodinated contrast medium. Alternative methods of intra-articular joint injection include the posterior approach or injection at the level of the rotator cuff interval under fluoroscopic guidance.[17–20] Intra-articular injection using ultrasound guidance has also been described.[20,21]

The relative small bore size and circumferential gantry of most standard MR closed systems allows limited alternatives for patient positioning when imaging the shoulder. The shoulder typically is imaged with the patient supine and the arm extended along the side. Hand position may be neutral (thumb pointing upward) or externally rotated during imaging of the shoulder.[18] With a dedicated shoulder coil, transverse, coronal oblique, and sagittal oblique T1-weighted spin-echo (SE) sequences are obtained (**Table 1**). Fat suppression is applied in the coronal oblique and transverse planes, and may also be applied in

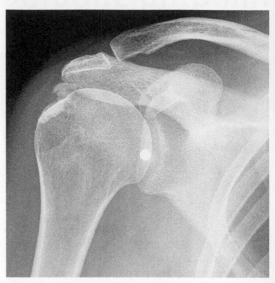

Fig. 1. Anteroposterior radiograph with marker indicating standard site of needle placement for intra-articular injection at the junction of the mid and lower one-third of the humeral head. Calcific supraspinatus tendinosis incidentally noted.

the sagittal oblique plane. Non-fat-suppressed T1-weighted images should be acquired in one plane to evaluate the bone marrow and to detect fatty infiltration of muscle. The examination is supplemented by the acquisition of a coronal oblique T2-weighted (echo time, 150 ms) turbo or fast spin-echo (TSE or FSE) sequence with spectral fat saturation. T2-weighted sequences are used to detect rotator cuff tears that do not involve the articular surface, paralabral cysts, bursitis, cartilage abnormalities, and marrow and muscle edema. Axial acquired images extend from the top of the acromion through the inferior margin of the inferior axillary recess.

For patients with anterior instability or suspected posterosuperior glenoid impingement (PSI), a T1-weighted SE sequence in the abduction and external rotation (ABER) position is obtained.[22,23] This position is acquired in a transverse oblique orientation along the long axis of the humerus with the elbow flexed and the patient's hand behind his head or neck (**Fig. 2**).[22] The ABER position is used primarily during MR arthrography to enhance detection of subtle tears of the anteroinferior labrum, such as Perthes lesions.[23] This position also opens the articular surface of the supraspinatus and infraspinatus tendons.[22] Subtle shoulder subluxation, not demonstrated with the arm at the patient's side, may be evident in this position.

The newly described adduction internal rotation (ADIR) position is more limited in scope but can be used to evaluate anterior labroligamentous

Table 1
Shoulder MR arthrography protocol

Plane	Sequence	TR	TE	ET
3-Plane loci				
1. Axial	T1 fs	600	20	4
2. Cor	T1 obl fs	600	20	4
3. Cor	T2 obl fs	3000	55	8
4. Ax	T2 FSE	3000	55	8
5. Sag obl	T1	600	20	4
6. ABER	T1 fs	600	20	3

Field of view: 12 to 14. Slice thickness = 3 to 4 mm; no skip. NEX = 3. Matrix = 224 × 256 up to 512.
Abbreviations: ABER, abduction and external rotation; Ax, axial; Cor, coronal; fs, fat-suppressed; FSE, fast spin echo; obl, oblique; Sag, sagittal.

periosteal sleeve avulsion (ALPSA) lesions of the anterior inferior labrum.[24] In this position, the hand of the affected arm is placed behind the back. Kinematic imaging is feasible on new more spacious MR units. Internal and external rotation of the shoulder is used to assess posterior and anterior labral tears, respectively, and for assessment of subcoracoid impingement.[25–32] An open magnet allows for dynamic abduction external rotation of the shoulder.[32–34] The diagnostic value of these additional sequences during clinical imaging time has yet to be determined.[31–35]

Complications of direct MR arthrography are rare[36,37] and include infection, bleeding, allergy, and synovitis. If a patient is known to have an allergy to iodinated contrast or anesthetic, he or she may be premedicated with steroid before the procedure. Gadolinium is an uncommon allergen, although mild to severe reactions have been reported. To date, there has been no report of nephrogenic systemic fibrosis (NSF) caused by intra-articular injection of gadolinium as there have been with the intravenous injections of gadolinium.[38] The relatively tiny volume of gadolinium used in MR arthrography would make NSF very unlikely as a potential complication. Bleeding related to MR arthrography is unusual if blood-thinning medications have been appropriately handled with a normal preprocedure International Normalized Ratio (INR). Infection is rare following arthrography performed with the sterile technique. Joint pain may be encountered a few hours after the procedure and may last for up to a week, most likely related to joint distension and synovitis.[37]

Intravenous or indirect MR arthrography has been described for evaluating the shoulder for instability.[39,40] A standard intravenous injection of gadolinium is injected approximately 10 to 20 minutes before the MR examination, followed by imaging with a protocol identical to that of the direct MR arthrogram. This technique does not require fluoroscopy or intra-articular injection, increasing patient acceptance. The gadolinium outlines the labrum and undersurface of the tendons. A major disadvantage of this technique is a lack of joint distension if there is no preexisting effusion. It is also more difficult to be certain about the significance of sites of contrast enhancement because intravenous contrast flows to vascularized tissues, including the subacromial-subdeltoid bursa, labral base, and degenerated or vascularized portions of the tendons of the rotator cuff. Sommer and colleagues[39] and Maurer and colleagues,[40] comparing nonenhanced MR

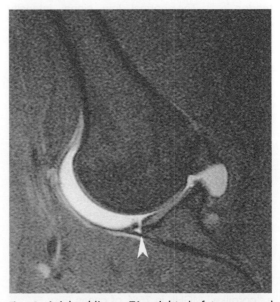

Fig. 2. Axial oblique T1-weighted fat-suppressed image weighted in the abduction external rotation position, demonstrating anteroinferior Bankart type labral tear (*arrowhead*).

imaging with indirect MR arthrography in patients with suspected labral tears, reported significant improvement in sensitivity and specificity for labral pathology with the latter technique.

MR arthrography has been firmly established as the imaging modality of choice for demonstrating structural soft tissue abnormalities associated with glenohumeral instability.

MAGNETIC RESONANCE IMAGING ANATOMY AND NORMAL VARIANTS

The glenohumeral capsular mechanism is fundamental in shoulder stability, and abnormalities of this mechanism play a central role in joint instability.[41,42] The anterior complex includes the supraspinatus muscle and tendon, subscapularis muscle and tendon, the rotator cuff interval, anterior capsule, glenohumeral ligaments, synovial membrane, the anterior labrum, and osseous glenoid.[42] The posterior complex includes the infraspinatus muscle and tendon, teres minor muscle and tendon, posterior capsule, synovial membrane, posterior labrum, and osseous glenoid.[41] The labrum is a fibrous connective tissue that stabilizes the shoulder joint by deepening the shallow glenoid fossa and increases the contact area for the humeral head.[42,43] The intact labrum acts as a pressure seal, allowing negative pressure to occur within the shoulder joint during motion, aiding in the dynamic stabilization of the joint. The labrum anchors the glenohumeral ligaments as well as the long head of the biceps tendon.[42–45] The normal low signal intensity labrum lies on hyaline articular cartilage that is of intermediate signal intensity on T1-weighted and T2-weighted MR images (**Fig. 3**). Glenoid cartilage is of intermediate signal intensity on FSE images. The hyaline cartilage can be thin or absent near the center of the ovoid glenoid fossa in a region referred to as the bare area.[43] The labrum can be triangular or round, as well as anteriorly cleaved, notched, or even absent in asymptomatic individuals.[44,45] Absence of the anterosuperior labrum may be congenital (known as the Buford complex). This condition is seen in 1% to 2% of shoulder arthroscopies and is associated with a "cordlike" middle glenohumeral ligament (MGHL) (**Fig. 4**).[43,44] Another labral variant seen in 11% to 15% of shoulders in the anterosuperior region of the glenoid labrum is the sublabral foramen.[45,46] This foramen or hole is seen at the base of the anterosuperior labrum, and is also associated with a "cordlike" MGHL in 75% of cases (**Fig. 5**).[45,46] Although not common, both the Buford complex and the sublabral foramen can extend into the anteroinferior portion of the labrum.[46] The sublabral

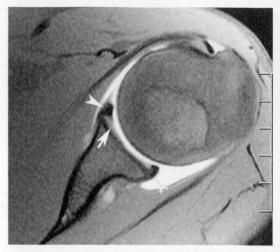

Fig. 3. Normal labrum. Axial T1 fat-suppressed image of MR arthrogram shows low signal labrum (*arrowhead*) and intermediate signal cartilage (*arrow*).

recess is a normal recess that can exist between the superior labrum and the glenoid articular cartilage.[47,48] This anatomic variant is smooth, 1 to 2 mm in width, and does not extend to the top of the labrum (**Fig. 6**). The sublabral recess is not associated with a paralabral cyst, as are some superior labral tears.[47–50]

The glenohumeral ligaments are thin, ligamentous structures that are best assessed with capsular distension created by a large joint effusion or dilute intra-articular contrast in the shoulder joint.[51–54] The superior, middle, and inferior glenohumeral ligaments are infoldings of the capsule. Each ligament contributes to stability of the glenohumeral joint, depending on the position

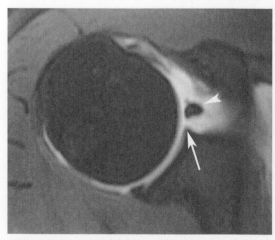

Fig. 4. Buford complex. Absent anteroinferior labrum (*arrow*) and cordlike middle glenohumeral ligament (*arrowhead*).

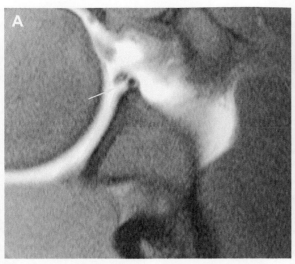
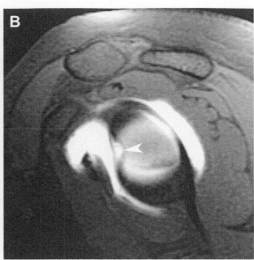

Fig. 5. Axial (*A*) and sagittal (*B*) T1 fat-suppressed image of MR arthrogram shows contrast deep to the anterosuperior labrum consistent with a sublabral foramen (*arrow* and *arrowhead*).

of the arm. The superior glenohumeral ligament (SGHL) extends from the supraglenoid tubercle anteriorly to the insertion of the long head of the biceps tendon, and inserts onto the fovea capitis line superior to the lesser tuberosity of the humerus. The SGHL is seen on axial images adjacent to the origin of the long head of the biceps tendon. The SGHL lies medial and parallel to the coracoid, and is located in the rotator cuff interval, just underneath the extra-articular coracohumeral ligament (**Fig. 7**). The SGHL and coracohumeral ligament together form a sling around the intra-articular portion of the biceps tendon in the rotator interval. The SGHL varies in thickness and is present 90% to 97% of the time in cadavers. The coracohumeral ligament (CHL) is an extracapsular structure located superior to the long head of the biceps tendon (**Fig. 8**). The coracohumeral ligament arises from the coracoid process and divides into a medial and lateral limb. The medial limb attaches to the subscapularis tendon. The lateral limb attaches to the anterior margin of the subscapularis tendon as well as the greater tuberosity of the humeral head.

The MGHL has a variable origin from the glenoid, scapula, anterior labrum, biceps tendon, inferior glenohumeral ligament (IGHL), or superior glenohumeral ligament.[51] The MGHL attaches to the anterior aspect of the proximal humerus just below the attachment of the SGHL, and can be absent in up to 27% of individuals.[51,53,54] Absence of this ligament is not associated with increased incidence of instability, but the subscapular recess may be enlarged, and the IGHL usually originates more superiorly than when the MGHL is present. The MGHL arthroscopically is attached to the anterior surface of the scapula, medial to the

articular margin. The MGHL lies obliquely, posterior to the superior margin of the subscapularis muscle, and blends with the anterior capsule (**Fig. 9**); it is attached distally to the anterior aspect of the proximal humerus, below the attachment of the SGHL.[51] Using MR arthrography, the scapular insertion of the MGHL is typically seen at the level of the anterosuperior labrum.[55]

The IGHL is now considered the most important stabilizer of the glenohumeral joint. The IGHL is a complex that originates at the mid to inferior portion of the anterior glenoid labrum. The IGHL drapes for a variable distance from anterior to

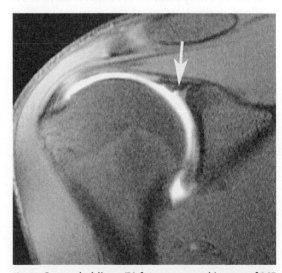

Fig. 6. Coronal oblique T1 fat-suppressed image of MR arthrogram shows contrast deep to the superior labrum (*arrow*) consistent with a smoothly marginated sublabral recess.

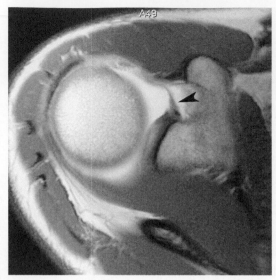

Fig. 7. Axial T1 fat-suppressed image of MR arthrogram shows the superior glenohumeral ligament (*arrowhead*).

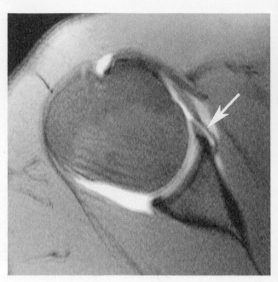

Fig. 9. Axial T1 fat-suppressed image of MR arthrogram shows the middle glenohumeral ligament (*arrow*).

posterior and inserts onto the anatomic neck of the humerus (**Fig. 10**). This ligament is inseparable from the labrum, forming a labroligamentous complex; it is composed of strong, collagenous, thickened anterior and posterior bands, joined by a fibrous thickening of the capsule called the axillary pouch or recess. The IGHL acts as a sling to support the humeral head and prevent abnormal anterior and posterior instability.[56,57] The IGHL reinforces the anterior capsule between the subscapularis muscle and the inferior aspect of the glenoid at or near the origin of the long head of the triceps.

In the throwing position the anterior band of the IGHL is under tension. If the arm is placed in abduction and internal rotation, the posterior band is in more tension than the anterior band. The relative contribution of each individual glenohumeral ligament to joint stability has been the subject of debate. The SGHL and MGHL are absent in a high percentage of individuals, and therefore must not be important structures in maintaining joint stability.[58] Previous studies concluded that the IGHL is the most important structure in the prevention of dislocation with the arm at 90° of ABER.[56,58] The different ligaments contribute to the stability of the glenohumeral joint in a diverse fashion, depending on the position of the arm. The SGHL and the CHL together limit inferior translation of the adducted shoulder and posterior translation of the flexed, adducted, and internally rotated shoulder.[56,58] The MGHL limits anterior translation of the humeral head when the arm is abducted between 60° and 90°. The IGHL complex prevents increased translation of the humeral head on the glenoid. With the arm in abduction, the entire complex moves beneath the humeral head and becomes taut. With internal rotation, the complex moves posteriorly and limits posterior translation. With external rotation, the complex moves anteriorly and limits anterior translation. The long head of the biceps tendon and the coracohumeral and coracoacromial ligaments are also important structures contributing in different ways to the normal biomechanics of the joint. The coracohumeral ligament helps maintain the stability of the long head of the biceps tendon, and the coracoacromial ligament is an important part of the acromial arch.[57]

The anterior fibrous capsule insertion is divided into 3 types, depending on the proximity of the

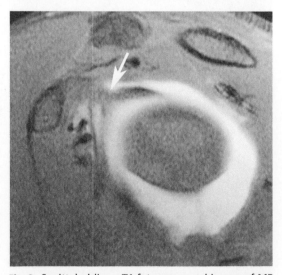

Fig. 8. Sagittal oblique T1 fat-suppressed image of MR arthrogram shows the coracohumeral ligament (*arrow*).

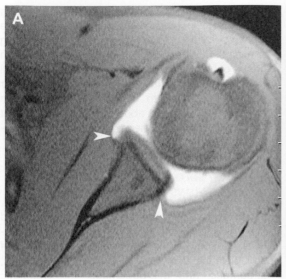
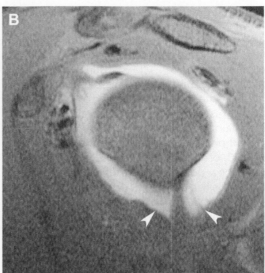

Fig. 10. Axial (A) and sagittal (B) oblique T1 fat-suppressed image of MR arthrogram shows the anterior and posterior bands of the inferior glenohumeral ligament (arrowheads).

capsular insertion to the glenoid margin.[49,58] Insertion of the capsule to the glenoid margin is known as type I. Type II capsular insertion refers to insertion at the glenoid neck within 1 cm of the labral base, and type III describes an insertion on the scapula more than 1 cm medial to the labral base.[49] Type III capsular insertions are associated with anterior instability but, in the author's experience, these insertions are a common finding, even in patients with no instability. Correlation of capsular insertion types with clinically significant instability should be viewed with caution in the absence of other signs of instability. In addition, an overdistended capsule at MR arthrography may produce prominent anterior and posterior recesses, falsely simulating a type III insertion and capsular laxity.

The long head of the biceps tendon has an intracapsular portion and an extracapsular portion. The intracapsular portion extends from its insertion at the superior labrum to the bicipital groove.[59,60] The long head of the biceps tendon originates from the superior aspect of the labrum and supraglenoid tubercle, and the triceps tendon from the infraglenoid tubercle inferiorly, constituting additional supportive structures of the glenohumeral joint. The space between the anterior margin of the supraspinatus muscle and the superior margin of the subscapularis muscle is called the rotator cuff interval. The joint capsule covers this space, and contains the long head of the biceps tendon, the coracohumeral ligament, and the SGHL. Ozsoy and colleagues[60] have shown that sectioning the rotator cuff interval in cadaveric shoulders

significantly increases anterior, posterior, and inferior humeral head translation. These investigators concluded that the function of the rotator cuff interval is to limit inferior translation of the glenohumeral joint in the adducted shoulder, and to provide stability against posterior dislocation in flexion or ABER.

The muscles around the shoulder are also important contributors to the stability of the shoulder joint. The rotator cuff muscles and, perhaps to a lesser degree, the long bicipital tendon provide dynamic compression of the humeral head into the glenoid fossa, centering the humeral head and countering the oblique translational forces generated during the act of throwing.[60–63] Another factor contributing to the stability of the glenohumeral joint is scapulothoracic coordination during throwing. This coordination is achieved mainly through synchronization with the latissimus dorsi, pectoralis major, and serratus anterior muscles.[63] There is a 2:1 ratio of glenohumeral to scapulothoracic motion during abduction.[63] Failure of the scapulothoracic coordination may place additional stress on the capsulolabral complex, hence increasing the risk of soft tissue damage. It has been shown that patients with shoulder instability have increased scapulothoracic asymmetry.[62,63]

THE THROWING MECHANISM

To understand the pathophysiology of glenohumeral instability in the throwing athlete, it is important to know the normal joint motion during the act of throwing. With minor differences in various sports, overhead throwing actions all have similar throwing mechanics.[62] There are 6 phases in the overhead throwing motion: windup, early cocking, late cocking, acceleration, deceleration, and follow-through (**Fig. 11**).[62,63] During the windup phase there is minimal stress loading and muscular activity of the shoulder. At the end of this phase the shoulder is in minimal internal rotation and slight abduction (positions 1 and 2, **Fig. 11**). During the second phase of early cocking, the shoulder reaches 90° of abduction and 15° of horizontal abduction (elbow posterior to the coronal plane of the torso) (position 3, **Fig. 11**). During this phase there is early activation of the deltoid muscle and late activation of the rotator cuff muscles, with the exception of the subscapularis muscle. During the third phase of late cocking the shoulder ends in maximum external rotation of 170° to 180°, maintaining 90° to 100° of abduction. The 15° of horizontal abduction changes to 15° of horizontal adduction (position 4, **Fig. 11**). The scapula retracts to facilitate this position and provide a stable base for the humeral head. The combination of ABER forces posterior translation of the humeral head on the glenoid. The activity of the deltoid muscle decreases while the rotator cuff muscles reach their peak. During the terminal portion of the late cocking phase, the subscapularis, latissimus dorsi, pectoralis major, and serratus anterior muscles increase their activity. During the fourth phase of acceleration, abduction is maintained while the shoulder rotates to ball release (position 5, **Fig. 11**). The scapula protracts as the body moves forward and the humeral head recenters in the glenoid fossa, decreasing the stress on the anterior capsule. During the early acceleration phase, the triceps muscle shows marked activity, whereas the latissimus dorsi, pectoralis major, and serratus anterior muscles increase their activity during the late acceleration phase. During the fifth phase of deceleration, the energy not imparted to the ball is dissipated, beginning at the moment of ball release and ending with cessation of humeral rotation to 0°. Abduction is maintained at 100°, and horizontal adduction increases to 35°. All muscle groups contract violently, with eccentric

contraction, allowing the arm to slow down. During this phase, joint loads and compressive forces are high posteriorly and inferiorly through strong contraction of the biceps muscle. During the sixth phase of follow-through, the body moves forward with the arm until the motion ceases. Shoulder rotation decreases to 30°, horizontal adduction increases to 60°, and abduction is maintained at 100° while joint loads decrease, ending in adduction (position 6, **Fig. 11**).

PATHOPHYSIOLOGY AND MR IMAGING MANIFESTATIONS

Instability of the glenohumeral joint is classified according to the etiology or direction of the instability. Based on the etiology, 3 main types of shoulder instability are recognized: traumatic, atraumatic, and microtraumatic.[64–66] Traumatic and atraumatic instability are not frequently seen in overhead-throwing athletes. These athletes usually complain of gradually increasing shoulder pain at some position during the throwing motion, and the symptoms are the consequence of multiple episodes of microtrauma rather than a single episode of injury (traumatic instability) or generalized joint laxity (atraumatic instability).[64] The acronyms TUBS (traumatic, unilateral, Bankart lesion, surgery) and AMBRI (atraumatic, multidirectional, bilateral, rehabilitation, inferior capsular shift) have been used as a simple guide to classification and treatment of shoulder instability (**Box 1**).[65–68] The acronym AIOS (acquired, instability, overstress, surgery) is added to include the microtraumatic instability developing in the throwing athlete.

According to the direction of laxity testing, shoulder instability can also be classified into anterior, posterior, and multidirectional instability (MDI).

TRAUMATIC AND ATRAUMATIC INSTABILITY

Traumatic glenohumeral instability is typically initiated by a specific traumatic event, followed by other episodes of dislocation or subluxation with a unidirectional pattern. In the vast majority

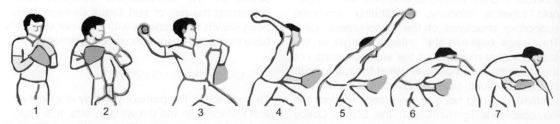

Fig. 11. Phases of throwing mechanism. **1**, neutral; **2**, windup phase; **3**, cocking phase; **4**, acceleration; **5**, late acceleration; **6**, deceleration; **7**, late deceleration.

<table>
<tr><td>

Box 1
Mnemonics of glenohumeral instability

TUBS

Trauma

Unidirectional

Bankart lesion

Surgery

AMBRII

Atraumatic

Multidirectional

Bilateral

Rehabilitation

Inferior capsular shift

Interval closure

AIOS

Acquired

Instability

Overstress

Surgery

</td></tr>
</table>

combination of injuries represents the source of chronic instability, particularly injury involving the IGHL, which is the most important passive stabilizer of the shoulder joint (**Table 2**).

BANKART LESION

Injury to the anteroinferior capsulolabral complex secondary to anteroinferior dislocation is the most frequently recognized labral lesion, called the "Bankart lesion" (**Fig. 12**). The Bankart lesion is commonly associated with an impaction fracture of the posterosuperior aspect of the humeral head, the Hill-Sachs lesion.[71] Although generally common in sports, this type of instability is rarely observed in throwers or overhead athletes but, when present, can cause secondary damage to the rotator cuff as well as the superior and posterior labrum. The classic labral injury described by Bankart is a complete detachment of the anteroinferior labroligamentous complex from the glenoid, associated with rupture of the scapular periosteum.[71] The Bankart lesion represents the most common form of labroligamentous injury in patients with first-time traumatic dislocations of the shoulder.[71,72] Due to the lost contact with the periosteum, the lesion shows no tendency to heal. Surgical treatment is by reattachment of the labroligamentous complex to the glenoid either arthroscopically or during an open procedure (Bankart repair).[71] MR arthrography typically shows a deformed anteroinferior labrum, which is completely separated from the glenoid and

of athletes, traumatic instability occurs in an anteroinferior direction when a sudden force overwhelms the anterior capsular structures while the athlete's arm is in an abducted, externally rotated, and extended position.[65–70] The resulting

Table 2
Bankart lesion and variants

Lesion	Definition
Classic Bankart	Tear of the anterior inferior labrum with capsuloperiosteal stripping
Perthes	Tear of the anterior inferior labrum without capsuloperiosteal stripping
ALPSA	Anterior labrum periosteal sleeve avulsion: anterior labral tear with posterior medial displacement and capsuloperiosteal stripping
HAGL	Humeral avulsion glenohumeral ligaments: avulsion of the humeral insertion of the anterior band of the IGHL
BAGHL	Bony avulsion glenohumeral ligament: same as HAGL with humeral body avulsion
Floating AIGHL	Floating anterior inferior glenohumeral ligament: combined Bankart and HAGL
SLAP	Superior labrum anterior posterior: tear of the superior labrum extending in different directions (10 types described)
POLPSA	Posterior labrocapsular periosteal sleeve avulsion: similar to ALPSA but involves the posterior labrum
GLAD	Glenoid labrum articular cartilage disruption: labral tear with associated avulsion of articular cartilage

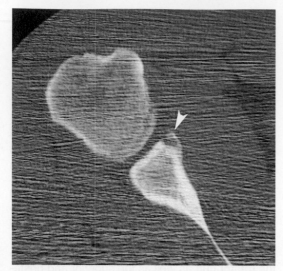

Fig. 12. Noncontrast axial CT shows small osseous fragment of the anteroinferior glenoid consistent with an osseous Bankart lesion (*arrowhead*).

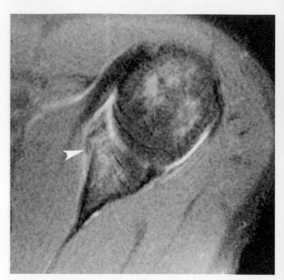

Fig. 13. Osseous Bankart lesion. Axial T1 fat-suppressed image of MR arthrogram shows anteroinferior detached labral tear and associated glenoid fracture fragment (*arrowhead*).

therefore is "floating" in the anterior capsular recess adherent to the anterior band of the IGHL.[71–74]

OSSEOUS BANKART LESION

In an osseous, or bony Bankart lesion (see **Fig. 12**), an osseous fragment of variable size is avulsed from the anteroinferior glenoid together with the labroligamentous complex. The size of the fragment influences treatment. Larger glenoid defects can cause recurrent instability after stabilizing soft tissue procedures such as the Bankart procedure, particularly in contact athletes.[64,65,74] In a study with cadaveric specimens and experimentally created defects of the glenoid rim, the critical fragment size was greater than 7 mm average width.[65–68] The "inverted pear" geometry is the reverse of the normal pear-shaped glenoid, which means that its anteroposterior diameter below the mid-glenoid notch is smaller than that above it.[69] This configuration usually precludes arthroscopic repair, and represents an indication for fragment refixation or bone grafting. MR arthrography is less accurate in depiction of bony Bankart lesions compared with CT or CT arthrography.[69] Smaller osseous fragments can easily be overlooked, particularly if fat suppression is used, whereas glenoid fractures with larger fragments can usually be diagnosed with confidence on MR imaging (**Fig. 13**).

PERTHES LESION

The Perthes lesion (**Fig. 14**) is a variant of the Bankart lesion, which also occurs in patients with

acute anterior instability. In the Perthes lesion, the anteroinferior labroligamentous complex is detached from the glenoid, but differs from the Bankart lesion in that the periosteum remains intact and is stripped anteromedially.[67,73] Therefore, though only loosely attached, the labrum may remain in its normal anatomic position. The integrity of the periosteum allows partial "healing"

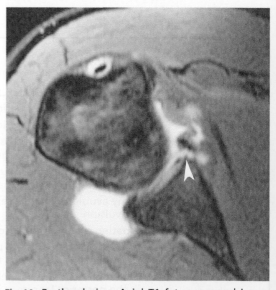

Fig. 14. Perthes lesion. Axial T1 fat-suppressed image of MR arthrogram shows anteroinferior labral tear (*arrowhead*) that remains attached to the glenoid periosteum.

of the labrum, which might also become resynovialized and thus, although incompetent, can look normal on arthroscopic inspection. Because scar tissue may prevent contrast media from entering the labral tear, nondisplaced Perthes lesions can be difficult to detect on MR arthrography as well.[72,73] MR arthrograms obtained in the ABER position have been reported to be more sensitive in the diagnosis of Perthes lesions compared with conventional transverse MR arthrograms.[67] The ABER position can at times help to visualize nondisplaced Perthes lesions by separating the base of the anteroinferior labrum from the glenoid and consecutively allowing the entrance of contrast media.[23] On the other hand, displaced or slightly displaced lesions can be realigned with the glenoid, and therefore be less conspicuous on ABER images than on transverse images obtained in the neutral position.[22,23]

ANTERIOR LABROLIGAMENTOUS PERIOSTEAL SLEEVE AVULSION LESION

The ALPSA lesion (**Fig. 15**) is also called the "medialized Bankart lesion," and is more common in patients with recurrent rather than with first-time traumatic dislocations of the shoulder.[72,74] The ALPSA lesion is an anteroinferior labral avulsion with medial displacement and inferior rotation of the labroligamentous complex together with an intact periosteum in a sleevelike fashion, causing incompetence of the IGHL and secondary anterior instability. The labrum may eventually heal and be resynovialized in this abnormal position.[64]

Transformation of the ALPSA lesion into a Bankart lesion by dissection of the complex from the glenoid followed by anatomic refixation (Bankart repair) has been recommended as the treatment of choice.[64] On MR arthrography, there is medial and inferior displacement of the deformed labroligamentous complex, which is best seen on axial and coronal oblique images. Contrast medium often outlines a crease or cleft between the glenoid and the nodular-shaped fibrous tissue on the glenoid neck, whereas the glenoid edge typically lacks a normal labral structure.[72] Familiarity with these signs can prevent misinterpretation of the ALPSA lesion as an anatomic variant in cases with only slight displacement of the labrum. Posterior labrocapsular sleeve avulsion (POLPSA) is similar to ALPSA, but affects the posterior labrum and is associated with posterior instability (see **Fig. 15**).[64,65]

GLENOLABRAL ARTICULAR DISRUPTION LESION

The glenolabral articular disruption (GLAD) lesion (**Fig. 16**) is a nondisplaced tear of the anteroinferior labrum in combination with an articular cartilage lesion of the anteroinferior quadrant of the glenoid.[75] There is no associated capsular-periosteal stripping. The injury is thought to result from glenohumeral impaction while the arm is abducted and externally rotated. Persistent anterior shoulder pain after a fall onto an outstretched arm is the most common clinical presentation, and arthroscopic debridement is the proposed treatment of choice.[76,77] Because the anterior fibers of the IGHL remain strongly attached to the labrum and

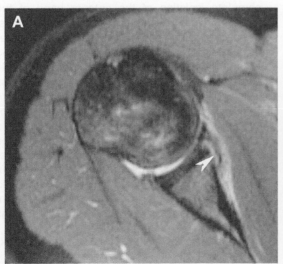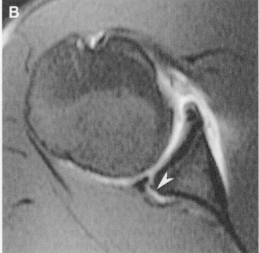

Fig. 15. (*A*) ALPSA lesion. Axial T1 fat-suppressed image of MR arthrogram shows anteroinferior labral tear (*arrowhead*) with stripping of the adjacent glenoid periosteum. (*B*) POLPSA lesion. Axial T1 fat-suppressed image of MR arthrogram shows posterior labrocapsular sleeve avulsion labral tear (*arrowhead*) with stripping of the adjacent posterior glenoid periosteum.

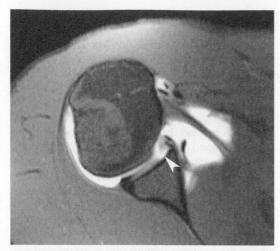

Fig. 16. GLAD lesion. Axial T1 fat-suppressed image of MR arthrogram shows anteroinferior labral tear (*arrowhead*) with full-thickness loss of adjacent cartilage.

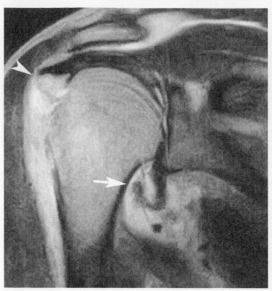

Fig. 17. HAGL lesion. Coronal T2 fat-suppressed oblique image shows detached inferior glenohumeral ligament from humeral attachment (*arrow*) with an avulsed supraspinatus tendon (*arrowhead*).

glenoid, the GLAD lesion is usually not associated with anterior instability. The degree of articular cartilage damage is variable, ranges from fibrillation to deep surface defects with loose fragments of cartilage that remain attached to the anterior labrum, and can be undermined by contrast media on MR arthrography.[75,76,78–80] If the chondral lesion is small and therefore hardly visible on MR imaging, the GLAD lesion can look similar to instability-related labral injuries. It is therefore important to note that the labrum is not displaced, and both the IGHL and periosteum are intact.

HUMERAL AVULSION OF GLENOHUMERAL LIGAMENT LESION

In contrast to the Bankart lesion and its variants, the humeral avulsion of glenohumeral ligament (HAGL) lesion (Fig. 17) does not involve the labro-ligamentous complex at the glenoid, but represents an isolated tear of the IGHL at its humeral insertion following vigorous shoulder dislocation.[79,80] The injury is associated with anterior instability, and represents a pitfall at arthroscopy as well as open shoulder surgery, because it can be overlooked if the area of the humeral neck is not specifically evaluated.[75,78–80] Most patients in whom a HAGL lesion is detected are involved in contact sports, such as rugby, American football, or ice hockey.[76,77,80] Treatment is by surgical re-attachment of the IGHL to its humeral insertion.[81] In subacute cases in which there is no appreciable joint effusion, HAGL lesions can only be confidently diagnosed with MR arthrography. The IGHL avulsed from its humeral attachment is

seen as a J-shaped rather than a U-shaped structure on coronal oblique arthrograms, and contrast extravasation can occur at its insertion site (see Fig. 17). Acute injuries are usually associated with edematous changes of the soft tissues anterior to the humeral neck.[77] Approximately 20% of HAGL lesions occur with avulsion of a bony fragment from the humerus (bony HAGL, BHAGL).[80–84] On rare occasions the HAGL lesion can be associated with a classic Bankart lesion. Due to the complete isolation of the anterior band of the IGHL that results from this combination of injuries, the lesion has been described as the floating anterior inferior glenohumeral ligament (floating AIGHL).[80,85–88] Other associated injuries include subscapularis tears and Hill-Sachs defects, as well as osteochondral lesions.[89–91]

In athletes, the decision whether an arthroscopic or an open procedure should be performed to achieve the most favorable outcome can be difficult.[77,81–84] Criteria in favor of open rather than arthroscopic surgery include involvement in contact sports, presence of a relevant glenoid defect or Hill-Sachs defect, a HAGL lesion, and poor quality of the labroligamentous complex.[80,83–85]

With arthroscopy as the "gold standard," Bankart and Bankart variant lesions are correctly classified with a sensitivity of 77%, a specificity of 91%, and an accuracy of 84%. MR arthrography also has high concordance with arthroscopy for lesions that cannot be assigned to one specific type mentioned earlier.[82,84] All of these "nonclassifiable" lesions with degenerative changes and scar tissue formation are typically observed in patients with chronic anterior instability. On MR arthrography, these injuries are characterized by a swollen inferior glenohumeral ligament complex without distinct depiction of the labrum, IGHL, and scapular periosteum.[80,84–88]

HILL-SACHS DEFECT

The Hill-Sachs defect is a compression injury of the posterolateral humeral head, which develops during anteroinferior dislocation as the relatively large and soft humeral head impacts against the comparatively small and hard glenoid.[89] The incidence of the lesion at arthroscopy varies from 47% to 100% among different series of patients with first-time traumatic dislocations.[84] The depth and size of a Hill-Sachs lesion ranges from shallow chondral defects to deep osteochondral impaction fractures.[75,84] In athletes with hyperlaxity at the time of the first shoulder dislocation, the humeral injury typically is small or absent. Osteochondral Hill-Sachs defects that involve less than one-third of the circumference of the humeral head are regarded as having an excellent prognosis. Larger lesions, especially if oriented with their long axis parallel to the glenoid, can engage the anterior corner of the glenoid in ABER, and lead to repeated subluxations or dislocations.[91] On axial MR images, the Hill-Sachs defect is seen at or slightly above the level of the coracoid process (Fig. 18). False-positive diagnoses can occur due to misinterpretation of a normal anatomic groove at the posterolateral humerus, which is found caudad to that position.[80] In acute or subacute cases with edema of adjacent bone marrow, the impaction injury can easily be detected on fat-suppressed intermediate/T2-weighted or STIR (short τ inversion recovery) images. Chronic lesions, particularly if small, are often better visualized with CT.[91] However, clinically significant osteochondral defects are usually seen by MR and rarely necessitate further imaging.

ATRAUMATIC GLENOHUMERAL INSTABILITY

Atraumatic glenohumeral instability is typically multidirectional, and is seen in individuals with congenital hypermobility syndrome. The diagnosis is based on clinical examination, and typically involves both shoulders.[92–95] The increased baseline laxity of the shoulder in athletes with generalized hypermobility is advantageous for several types of sports, but may increase the risk of long-term injury with damage to intra- and periarticular structures.[1,2] If conservative management fails, MDI is usually treated surgically by inferior capsular shift and closure of the rotator interval.[91] There are no specific findings to diagnose atraumatic glenohumeral instability by MR imaging or MR arthrography.[69] In most nonathletic AMBRI patients, MR arthrography shows an increased capsular volume but no or little substantial alterations of the intra-articular structures. Laxity of the capsule in athletes is often associated with secondary damage to the labrum and the rotator cuff.[93] The labrum may be hypoplastic, torn, or degenerated. There may

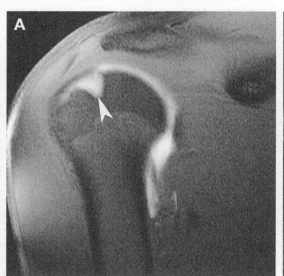
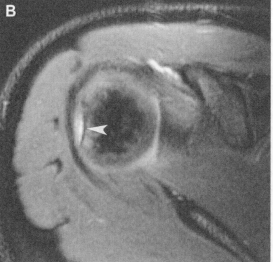

Fig. 18. (A) Axial and (B) coronal oblique T1-weighted images show cortical defect of the posterior superior humeral head consistent with a Hill-Sachs defect (arrowhead).

be associated abnormalities of the biceps anchor and the articular surface of the rotator cuff.[94,95] MR arthrography can help with therapeutic decisions by identification or exclusion of significant intra-articular pathology that might represent an indication for surgical repair in addition to capsular reduction.

MICROTRAUMATIC GLENOHUMERAL INSTABILITY

Microtraumatic glenohumeral instability results from chronic trauma of the capsular structures in athletes who repetitively perform the overhead throwing mechanism. Microinstability is typically seen unilaterally in the dominant shoulder of the athlete. Repetitive ABER can cause microtrauma of the anterior capsule, producing anterior instability. Repetitive overhead activity with abduction, flexion, and internal rotation may cause posterior microinstability as a result of injury to the posterior labroligamentous elements.[4] Structural abnormalities that occur as a result of microtraumatic glenohumeral instability are diagnosed by MR arthrography, and include anterior or posterior capsular laxity, labral injuries, and tears of the rotator cuff caused by secondary impingement.[85]

POSTEROSUPERIOR GLENOID IMPINGEMENT

PSI is a form of internal impingement that represents a common problem in throwers and overhead athletes, presenting with acute or chronic posterior shoulder pain.[4,5,47,48] Impingement occurs between the articular side of the supraspinatus tendon and the posterosuperior edge of the glenoid, evident in ABER.[49] In throwers and overhead athletes, posterosuperior impingement can lead to a typical pattern of injuries, the so-called kissing lesions, which includes abnormalities of the undersurface of the rotator cuff, the posterosuperior labrum, the greater tuberosity, and the superior bony glenoid.[47,48,50–52] The development of PSI has been attributed to repetitive stretching of the anterior capsular structures, particularly the IGHL, with consequent anterior microinstability, which results in anterior subluxation of the humeral head in abduction and external rotation during overhead movements. This development allows excessive contact between the rotator cuff and the posterosuperior glenoid.[47,48] This theory is not universally accepted. Other investigators described a contracture of the posteroinferior capsule and a posterior superior labral anterior to posterior (SLAP) lesion as the essential lesions for the development of PSI in throwers.[3] Although the basic mechanism is still subject to discussion,

the high coincidence of PSI and SLAP lesions is undoubted. There is a huge overlap of clinical symptoms in athletes with SLAP lesions, PSI, or both. Contact between the undersurface of the rotator cuff and the posterosuperior glenoid, as seen on arthroscopy, is not pathologic. PSI should only be diagnosed if this contact is associated with clinical symptoms and abnormalities of the involved anatomic structures.[2,13,51,52] Conservative treatment is usually sufficient in athletes with minor structural abnormalities, whereas surgical debridement and repair in combination with capsular plication are indicated when rotator cuff and labral abnormalities are present.

MR imaging can be used to diagnose PSI and guide therapeutic decisions by delineating the extent of articular damage. Because MR arthrography is more accurate than conventional MR imaging in the detection of partial rotator cuff tears, labral tears, and SLAP lesions, it is regarded as the imaging modality of choice in patients with suspected PSI, which is accompanied by a combination of these abnormalities.[50,95–97] MR arthrography (Fig. 19) shows articular-sided partial tearing of the supraspinatus or infraspinatus tendons. Rotator cuff tendon abnormalities typically involve the posterior part of the supraspinatus tendon. Abnormality of the posterosuperior labrum ranges from degenerative change to tears and detachment, and can be associated with ganglia and SLAP lesions. Osseous abnormalities of the greater tuberosity and the superior glenoid are best seen on fluid-sensitive sequences by fat-suppressed intermediate or T2-weighted images, and include erosions, bone marrow edema, cyst formation, and sclerosis.[50–52] MR arthrograms obtained in the ABER position may show contact between the lesions of the rotator cuff and the superior labrum/glenoid, and might even reveal interposition of the supraspinatus tendon pinched between the glenoid and the greater tuberosity. The ABER position may show subluxation of the humeral head and associated attenuation or tear of the anterior band of the IGHL.[50]

SUPERIOR LABRAL ANTERIOR TO POSTERIOR LESIONS

SLAP lesions of the shoulder are common injuries in athletes, representing tears of the superior glenoid labrum that extend in an anterior to posterior direction.[55,98] Four different types of SLAP lesions have been described in the original classification by Snyder[99]: type 1, degenerative fraying of the superior labrum; type 2, avulsion of the superior labrum and biceps anchor from the glenoid; type 3,

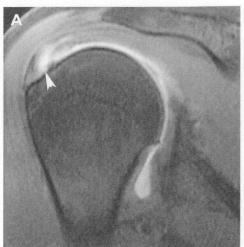 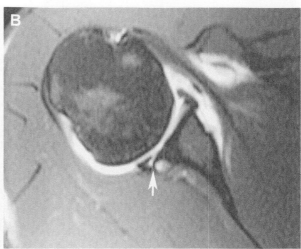

Fig. 19. Coronal T1 (*A*) and axial T1 (*B*) fat-suppressed images of MR arthrogram shows imaging features of posterior superior impingement with undersurface tear of the posterior supraspinatus (*arrowhead*) and tear of the posterior labrum (*arrow*).

bucket-handle tear of the superior labrum with preserved biceps anchor; and type 4, bucket-handle tear of the superior labrum involving the long head of biceps tendon.[99] This classification has been expanded with several further types of lesions, which mainly represent combinations of the most common form, the SLAP type 2 lesion, with other injuries of the labrum, medial glenohumeral ligament, or rotator cuff.[100,101] However, only the Snyder classifications have found wide acceptance, and most institutions categorize these injuries as types 1 to 4 with or without associated lesions. Type 1 and 2 lesions are typically caused by repetitive torsion of the biceps anchor, "the peelback mechanism" in throwers and overhead athletes, whereas type 3 and 4 lesions occur more often after a fall onto an outstretched arm or onto a flexed elbow.[100] Type 2 lesions are frequently observed in athletes with traumatic anterior shoulder instability, in which they develop in association with lesions of the anteroinferior labroligamentous complex (most often a classic Bankart lesion). In these cases, the labroligamentous avulsion can be considered as the main lesion, with the SLAP lesion being an associated injury.[55] Surgical treatment is indicated in all types of SLAP lesions except type 1 lesions, which are usually of no clinical relevance. Because type 2 and 4 lesions impair the stabilizing function of the biceps insertion and therefore can provoke glenohumeral instability, secondary impingement, and rotator cuff lesions, they are commonly treated by refixation. Type 3 bucket-handle tears are usually not surgically reattached but treated by simple debridement.[55,98] MR arthrography has proven to

be better than conventional MR imaging in the identification of SLAP lesions, and has been shown to be reliable in the assessment of stability of the biceps anchor and for the detection of associated injuries.[101] However, its ability to correctly classify the different types of lesions is limited.[100] Most SLAP lesions are best depicted on MR arthrograms oriented in the coronal oblique plane (**Fig. 20**). Increased signal intensity or surface irregularity of the superior labrum can be seen in type 1 lesions, which, however, can only infrequently be diagnosed by MR imaging. Type 2 lesions are characterized by linear extension of contrast media into the superior labrum and the biceps anchor. This most common type of SLAP lesion also represents the most problematic in terms of differential diagnosis. False-positive and false-negative diagnoses of a SLAP type 2 lesion can be caused by misinterpretation of a sublabral recess as a tear. The sublabral recess is typically oriented medially and points at the supraglenoid tubercle. The most important criterion distinguishing the presence of a SLAP type 2 lesion from a sublabral recess is lateral or superior extension of the tear. If the tear extends medially (like a sublabral recess) it often shows irregular margins or a relatively wide separation between the labrum and the glenoid. In individuals with traumatic anterior instability, the type 2 lesion often originates from an anteroinferior tear of the labroligamentous complex that extends cranially into the superior labrum and the biceps anchor.[55] Type 3 lesions are characterized by a vertical and an additional horizontal contrast interface, which separate the avulsed superior labrum as a triangular-shaped fragment from the intact biceps

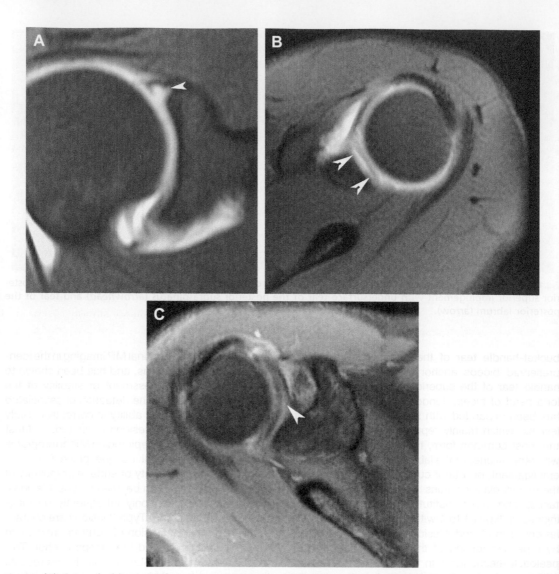

Fig. 20. (*A*) Coronal oblique T1 fat-suppressed image of MR arthrogram demonstrating type 2 superior labral anterior to posterior (SLAP) tear (*arrowhead*). (*B*) Axial T1 fat-suppressed image of MR arthrogram demonstrating bucket-handle tear of the superior labrum: type 3 SLAP labral tear. (*C*) Axial T1 fat-suppressed image of MR arthrogram demonstrating type 4 SLAP tear extending into the biceps tendon (*arrowheads*).

tendon. In Type 4 lesions the horizontal component of the tear additionally extends into the long head of biceps tendon. The bucket-handle fragment is therefore composed of the superior labrum as well as a portion of the tendon, and may be displaced from the superior glenoid.[101]

ANTERIOR INSTABILITY

Traumatic injury is the most common cause of shoulder instability, accounting for approximately 95% of anterior shoulder dislocations.[1–4] The sequelae of traumatic anterior dislocation is related to the age of the patient at the time of initial dislocation and the degree of injury. The patient's

age at the time of injury is inversely related to the recurrence rate. In patients younger than 20 years, recurrent dislocation rates have been reported as high as 90% in the athletic population. The rate of recurrence drops to between 50% and 75% in patients aged 20 to 25 years. In patients older than 40 years, anterior dislocation is associated with lower rates of instability but high rates of rotator cuff tears. The incidence of rotator cuff tears in patients older than 40 years at the time of initial dislocation is 15%, and the incidence climbs to 40% in patients older than 60 years.[1] The recurrence rate is directly related to the degree of injury to the supporting structures. The presence and size of the Bankart tear, the presence and size of osseous lesions including Hill-Sachs defects, osseous Bankart lesions, and glenoid bone loss, and the degree of capsular and rotator cuff pathology all play an important role. Anterior shoulder instability traditionally was treated using open techniques that were based on restoring the capsulolabral anatomy. Over time, understanding of anterior shoulder dislocations and the resulting instability has improved. Significant advances in arthroscopic equipment have allowed use of the arthroscope to address anatomically the various lesions that cause instability. The ideal patient for anterior surgical stabilization has clear unidirectional instability and has failed conservative management.

POSTERIOR INSTABILITY

Compared with anterior instability, posterior shoulder instability is an uncommon entity, accounting for 2% to 10% of instability cases. Fifty percent of cases are thought to occur secondary to trauma. The spectrum of pathology ranges from acute to chronic cases and from recurrent posterior subluxations to locked posterior dislocations. Recurrent posterior subluxations are more common in overhead throwers, tennis players, butterfly and freestyle swimmers, weightlifters, and football linemen. True recurrent posterior dislocations are rare compared with recurrent posterior subluxations. Acute posterior dislocations typically result from a direct blow to the anterior shoulder or from indirect forces with the shoulder in flexion, internal rotation, and adduction. Common indirect causes include electric shock and convulsive seizures. Recurrent posterior subluxation may result from repetitive microtrauma to the posterior capsule without a single traumatic antecedent event. Repetitive microtrauma results in attenuation of the posterior capsular tissue. Overhead throwers, tennis players, and swimmers develop pain associated with laxity of the posterior capsule, and fatigue of the static and dynamic stabilizers. A subset of throwers with glenohumeral internal rotation deficit is thought to experience repetitive microtrauma after ball release, resulting in progressive tearing of the posteroinferior labrum. Mechanical symptoms or pain occur during follow-through, and are common findings.

MULTIDIRECTIONAL INSTABILITY

MDI encompasses symptomatic involuntary subluxation or dislocation of the glenohumeral joint in more than one direction, including the inferior, anterior, or posterior directions. Discrepancies in definition exist, making determination of its true prevalence and comparison of different clinical and research studies difficult. The underlying pathogenesis is multifactorial, including capsular redundancy secondary to congenital soft tissue laxity, significant trauma, or repetitive microtrauma, as seen in throwing athletes and swimmers. Regardless of etiology, management of patients with MDI is primarily nonoperative, and is aimed at strengthening and improving proprioception of the dynamic stabilizers of the glenohumeral joint and periscapular muscles. When nonoperative treatment fails, surgical treatment of the capsular redundancy by imbrication and, when necessary, labral repair, is considered. The etiology of MDI is multifactorial, and current theories focus on anatomic, biomechanical, and neuromuscular abnormalities. Typical pathology observed in patients with multidirectional includes a large, patulous inferior pouch and a wide rotator interval, structures important to inferior stability. The pouch extends anteriorly and posteriorly to varying degrees, creating a global increase in capsular volume that results in overall laxity. In patients with MDI, the capsule has alterations in type and quantity of collagen.

Imaging for patients with clinical MDI is performed to exclude other causes of shoulder pain and instability, and to look for concomitant pathology. Plain radiographs of the shoulder with MDI are typically normal, but they should be evaluated for humeral head defects or glenoid bone defects. In cases of suspected humeral head or glenoid bone deficiency, a CT scan should be obtained. MR imaging using intra-articular contrast is used to detect capsular redundancy and labral injury.

SUMMARY

Sports-related glenohumeral instability is a complex subject. MR imaging has an important role in evaluation of the athlete's shoulder and guiding therapeutic decisions. The radiologist should be familiar with the mechanisms and classification of injuries, as well as the advantages and limitations of imaging techniques. MR arthrography represents the best imaging modality for the assessment of the labrum, glenohumeral ligaments, and capsule of the shoulder in athletes with suspected glenohumeral instability or with idiopathic shoulder pain.

REFERENCES

1. Borsa PA, Laudner KG, Sauers EL. Mobility and stability adaptations in the shoulder of the overhead athlete: a theoretical and evidence-based perspective. Sports Med 2008;38(1):17–36.

2. Chant CB, Litchfield R, Griffin S, et al. Humeral head retroversion in competitive baseball players and its relationship to glenohumeral rotation range of motion. J Orthop Sports Phys Ther 2007;37(9): 514–20.

3. Lugo R, Kung P, Ma CB. Shoulder biomechanics. Eur J Radiol 2008;68(1):16–24.

4. Applegate GR, Hewitt M, Snyder SJ, et al. Chronic labral tears: value of magnetic resonance arthrography in evaluating the glenoid labrum and labral-bicipital complex. Arthroscopy 2004;20:959–63.

5. Pappas AM, Goss TP, Kleinman PK. Symptomatic shoulder instability due to lesions of the glenoid labrum. Am J Sports Med 1983;11:279–88.

6. Coumas JM, Waite RJ, Goss TP, et al. CT and MR evaluation of the labral capsular ligamentous complex of the shoulder. AJR Am J Roentgenol 1992;158:591–7.

7. Garneau RA, Renfrew DL, Moore TE, et al. Glenoid labrum: evaluation with MR imaging. Radiology 1991;179:519–22.

8. Legan JM, Burkhard TK, Goff WB II, et al. Tears of the glenoid labrum: MR imaging of 88 arthroscopically confirmed cases. Radiology 1991;179:241–6.

9. McCauley TR, Pope CF, Jokl P. Normal and abnormal glenoid labrum: assessment with multiplanar gradient-echo MR imaging. Radiology 1992;183:35–7.

10. Gusmer PB, Potter HG, Schatz JA, et al. Labral injuries: accuracy of detection with unenhanced MR imaging of the shoulder. Radiology 1996;200: 519–24.

11. Tirman PFJ, Stauffer AE, Crues JV, et al. Saline magnetic resonance arthrography in the evaluation of glenohumeral instability. Arthroscopy 1993;9: 550–9.

12. Palmer WE, Brown JH, Rosenthal DI. Labral-ligamentous complex of the shoulder: evaluation with MR arthrography. Radiology 1994;1994:645–51.

13. Magee T, Williams D, Mani N. Shoulder MR arthrography: which patient group benefits most? AJR Am J Roentgenol 2004;183:969–74.

14. Roger B, Skaf A, Hooper AW, et al. Imaging findings in the dominant shoulder of throwing athletes: comparison of radiography, arthrography, CT arthrography, and MR arthrography with arthroscopic correlation. AJR Am J Roentgenol 1999;172:1371–80.

15. Tuite MJ, DeSmet AA, Norris MA, et al. MR diagnosis of labral tears of the shoulder: value of T2*-weighted gradient-recalled echo images made in external rotation. AJR Am J Roentgenol 1995;164:941–4.

16. Tuite MJ, Asinger D, Orwin JF. Angled oblique sagittal MR imaging of rotator cuff tears: comparison with standard oblique sagittal images. Skeletal Radiol 2001;30:262–9.

17. Farmer KD, Hughes PM. MR arthrography of the shoulder: fluoroscopically guided technique using a posterior approach. AJR Am J Roentgenol 2002;178:433–4.

18. Depelteau H, Bureau NJ, Cardinal E, et al. Arthrography of the shoulder: a simple fluoroscopically guided approach for targeting the rotator cuff interval. AJR Am J Roentgenol 2004;182:329–32.

19. Catalano OA, Manfredi R, Vanzulli A, et al. MR arthrography of the glenohumeral joint: modified posterior approach without imaging guidance. Radiology 2007;242:550–4.

20. Zwar RB, Read JW, Noakes JB. Sonographically guided glenohumeral joint injection. AJR 2004; 183:48–50.

21. Cicak N, Matasović T, Bajraktarević T. Ultrasonographic guidance of needle placement for shoulder arthrography. J Ultrasound Med 1992;11(4):135–7.

22. Saleem AM, Lee JK, Novak LM. Usefulness of the abduction and external rotation views in shoulder MR arthrography. AJR Am J Roentgenol 2008; 191(4):1024–30.

23. Tirman PFJ, Bost FW, Steinbach LS, et al. MR arthrographic depiction of tears of the rotator cuff: benefit of abduction and external rotation of the arm. Radiology 1994;192:851–6.

24. Song HT, Huh YM, Kim S, et al. Anterior-inferior labral lesions of recurrent shoulder dislocation evaluated by MR arthrography in an adduction internal rotation (ADIR) position. J Magn Reson Imag 2006;23:29–35.

25. Shankman S, Bencardino J, Beltran J. Glenohumeral instability: evaluation using MR arthrography of the shoulder. Skeletal Radiol 1999;28:365–82.

26. Steinbach LS, Palmer WE, Schweitzer ME. Special focus session. MR arthrography. RadioGraphics 2002;5:1223–46.

27. Beltran J, Rosenberg ZS, Chandnani VP, et al. Glenohumeral instability: evaluation with MR arthrography. Radiographics 1997;17:657–73.

28. Sethi PM, Kingston S, Elattrache N. Accuracy of anterior intra-articular injection of the glenohumeral joint. Arthroscopy 2005;21:77–80.

29. Chung CB, Dwek JR, Feng S, et al. MR arthrography of the glenohumeral joint: a tailored approach. AJR Am J Roentgenol 2001;177:217–9.

30. Lee SY, Lee JK. Horizontal component of partial-thickness tears of rotator cuff: imaging characteristics and comparison of ABER view with oblique coronal view at MR arthrography initial results. Radiology 2002;224:470–6.

31. Friedman RJ, Bonutti PM, Genez B. Cine magnetic resonance imaging of the subcoracoid region. Orthopedics 1998;21:545–8.

32. Sans N, Richardi G, Railhac JJ, et al. Kinematic MR imaging of the shoulder: normal patterns. AJR Am J Roentgenol 1996;167:1517–22.

33. Cardinal E, Buckwalter KA, Braunstein EM. Kinematic magnetic resonance imaging of the normal

shoulder: assessment of the labrum and capsule. Can Assoc Radiol J 1996;47:44–50.

34. Beaulieu CF, Hodge DK, Bergman AG, et al. Glenohumeral relationships during physiologic shoulder motion and stress testing: initial experience with open MR imaging and active imaging-plane registration. Radiology 1999;212:699–705.

35. Allmann KH, Uhl M, Gufler H, et al. Cine-MR imaging of the shoulder. Acta Radiol 1997;38:1043–6.

36. Hall FM, Rosenthal DI, Goldberg RP, et al. Morbidity from shoulder arthrography: etiology, incidence, and prevention. AJR Am J Roentgenol 1981;136:59–62.

37. Newberg AH, Munn CS, Robbins AH. Complications of arthrography. Radiology 1985;155:605–6.

38. Perazella MA. Current status of gadolinium toxicity in patients with kidney disease. Clin J Am Soc Nephrol 2009;4(2):461–9.

39. Jung JY, Yoon YC, Yi SK, et al. Comparison study of indirect MR arthrography and direct MR arthrography of the shoulder. Skeletal Radiol 2009;38(7): 659–67.

40. Oh DK, Yoon YC, Kwon JW, et al. Comparison of indirect isotropic MR arthrography and conventional MR arthrography of labral lesions and rotator cuff tears: a prospective study. AJR Am J Roentgenol 2009;192(2):473–9.

41. Neumann CH, Petersen SA, Jahnke AH. MR imaging of the labral–capsular complex: normal variations. AJR Am J Roentgenol 1991;157:1015–21.

42. Park YH, Lee JY, Moon SH, et al. MR arthrography of the labral capsular ligamentous complex in the shoulder: imaging variations and pitfalls. AJR Am J Roentgenol 2000;175:667–72.

43. Williams MM, Snyder SJ, Buford D. The Buford complex—the cordlike middle glenohumeral ligament and absent anterosuperior labrum complex: a normal anatomic capsulolabral variant. Arthroscopy 1994;10:241–7.

44. Tirman PFJ, Feller JF, Palmer WE, et al. The Buford complex—a variation of normal shoulder anatomy. MR arthrographic imaging features. AJR Am J Roentgenol 1996;166:869–73.

45. Tuite MJ, Orwin JF. Anterosuperior labral variants of the shoulder: appearance on gradient-recalled-echo and fast spin-echo MR images. Radiology 1996;199:537–40.

46. Tuite M, Blankenbaker DG, Siefert M, et al. Sublabral foramen and Buford complex: inferior extent of the unattached or absent labrum in 50 patients. Radiology 2002;223:137–42.

47. Smith DK, Chopp TM, Aufdemorte TB, et al. Sublabral recess of the superior glenoid labrum: study of cadavers with conventional non-enhanced MR imaging, MR arthrography, anatomic dissection, and limited histologic examination. Radiology 1996;201:251–6.

48. Yeh L, Kwak S, Kim YS, et al. Anterior labroligamentous structures of the glenohumeral joint: correlation and anatomic dissection in cadavers. AJR Am J Roentgenol 1998;171:1229–36.

49. Beltran J, Bencardino J, Mellado J, et al. MR arthrography of the shoulder: variations and pitfalls. Radiographics 1997;17:1403–12.

50. Tuite MJ, Rutkowski A, Enright T, et al. Width of high signal and extension posterior to biceps tendon as signs of superior labrum anterior to posterior tears on MRI and MR arthrography. AJR Am J Roentgenol 2005;185:1422–8.

51. Beltran J, Bencardino J, Padron M, et al. The middle glenohumeral ligament: normal anatomy, variants and pathology. Skeletal Radiol 2002;31:253–62.

52. Moseley HF, Overgaard B. The anterior capsular mechanism in recurrent anterior dislocation of the shoulder. J Bone Joint Surg 1962;44:913–27.

53. Flannigan B, Kursunoglu-Brahme S, Snyder S, et al. MR arthrography of the shoulder: comparison with conventional MR imaging. AJR Am J Roentgenol 1990;155:829–32.

54. Merila M, Heliö H, Busch LC, et al. The spiral glenohumeral ligament: an open and arthroscopic anatomy study. Arthroscopy 2008;24(11):1271–6.

55. Caspari RB, Beach WR. Arthroscopic anterior shoulder capsulorrhaphy. Sports Med Arthrosc 1993;1(4):237–41.

56. Moore SM, Stehle JH, Rainis EJ, et al. The current anatomical description of the inferior glenohumeral ligament does not correlate with its functional role in positions of external rotation. J Orthop Res 2008;26(12):1598–604.

57. Gagey N, Ravaud E, Lassau JP. Anatomy of the acromial arch: correlation of anatomy and magnetic resonance imaging. Surg Radiol Anat 1993;15(1):63–70.

58. Pouliart N, Somers K, Gagey O. Arthroscopic glenohumeral folds and microscopic glenohumeral ligaments: the fasciculus obliquus is the missing link. J Shoulder Elbow Surg 2008;17(3):418–30.

59. Ilahi OA, Cosculluela PE, Ho DM. Classification of anterosuperior glenoid labrum variants and their association with shoulder pathology. Orthopedics 2008;31(3):226.

60. Ozsoy MH, Bayramoglu A, Demiryurek D, et al. Rotator interval dimensions in different shoulder arthroscopy positions: a cadaveric study. J Shoulder Elbow Surg 2008;17(4):624–30.

61. Ebaugh DD, McClure PW, Karduna AR. Three-dimensional scapulothoracic motion during active and passive arm elevation. Clin Biomech (Bristol, Avon) 2005;20(7):700–9.

62. von Eisenhart-Rothe R, Matsen FA 3rd, Eckstein F, et al. Pathomechanics in atraumatic shoulder instability: scapular positioning correlates with humeral head centering. Clin Orthop Relat Res 2005;(433): 82–9.

63. Hirashima M, Ohtsuki T. Exploring the mechanism of skilled overarm throwing. Exerc Sport Sci Rev 2008;36(4):205–11.

64. Simons P, Joekes E, Nelissen RG, et al. Posterior labrocapsular periosteal sleeve avulsion complicating locked posterior shoulder dislocation. Skeletal Radiol 1998;27:588–90.

65. Yu JS, Ashman CJ, Jones G. The POLPSA lesion: MR imaging findings with arthroscopic correlation in patients with posterior instability. Skeletal Radiol 2002;31:396–9.

66. Oberlander MA, Morgan BE, Visotsky JL. The BHAGL lesion: a new variant of anterior shoulder instability. Arthroscopy 1996;12:627–33.

67. Waldt S, Burkart A, Imhoff AB, et al. Anterior shoulder instability: accuracy of MR arthrography in the classification of anteroinferior labroligamentous injuries. Radiology 2005;237(2):578–83.

68. Hantes ME, Venouziou AI, Liantsis AK, et al. Arthroscopic repair for chronic anterior shoulder instability: a comparative study between patients with Bankart lesion and patients with combined Bankart and superior labral anterior posterior lesions. Am J Sports Med 2000;37(6):1093–8.

69. Lo IK, Parten PM, Burkhart SS. The inverted pear glenoid: an indicator of significant glenoid bone loss. Arthroscopy 2004;20(2):169–74.

70. Ozbaydar M, Elhassan B, Diller D, et al. Results of arthroscopic capsulolabral repair: Bankart lesion versus anterior labroligamentous periosteal sleeve avulsion lesion. Arthroscopy 2008;24(11):1277–83.

71. Loredo R, Longo C, Salonen D, et al. Glenoid labrum: MR imaging with histologic correlation. Radiology 1995;196:33–41.

72. Neviaser TJ. The anterior labroligamentous periosteal sleeve avulsion lesion: a cause of anterior instability of the shoulder. Arthroscopy 1993;9:17–21.

73. Schreinemachers SA, van der Hulst VP, Jaap Willems W, et al. Is a single direct MR arthrography series in ABER position as accurate in detecting anteroinferior labroligamentous lesions as conventional MR arthography? Skeletal Radiol 2009;38(7):675–83.

74. Tirman PFJ, Steinbach LS, Feller JF, et al. Humeral avulsion of the anterior shoulder stabilizing structures after anterior shoulder dislocation: demonstration by MR and MR arthrography. Skeletal Radiol 1996;25:743–8.

75. Sanders TG, Tirman PFJ, Linares R, et al. The glenolabral articular disruption lesion: MR arthrography with arthroscopic correlation. AJR Am J Roentgenol 1999;172:171–5.

76. Tonino PM, Gerber C, Itoi E, et al. Complex shoulder disorders: evaluation and treatment. J Am Acad Orthop Surg 2009;17(3):125–36.

77. Antonio GE, Griffith JF, Yu AB, et al. First-time shoulder dislocation: high prevalence of labral injury and age-related differences revealed by MR arthrography. J Magn Reson Imaging 2007;26(4):983–91.

78. Chung CB, Sorenson S, Dwek JR, et al. Humeral avulsion of the posterior band of the inferior glenohumeral ligament: MR arthrography and clinical correlation in 17 patients. AJR Am J Roentgenol 2004;183:355–9.

79. Parameswaran AD, Provencher MT, Bach BR Jr, et al. Humeral avulsion of the glenohumeral ligament: injury pattern and arthroscopic repair techniques. Orthopedics 2008;31(8):773–9.

80. Warner JJ, Beim GM. Combined Bankart and HAGL lesion associated with anterior shoulder instability. Arthroscopy 1997;13(6):749–52.

81. Mohtadi NG, Vellet AD, Clark ML, et al. A prospective, double-blind comparison of magnetic resonance imaging and arthroscopy in the evaluation of patients presenting with shoulder pain. J Shoulder Elbow Surg 2004;13(3):258–65.

82. Woertler K, Waldt S. MR imaging in sports-related glenohumeral instability. Eur Radiol 2006;16(12):2622–36.

83. Melvin JS, Mackenzie JD, Nacke E, et al. MRI of HAGL lesions: four arthroscopically confirmed cases of false-positive diagnosis. AJR Am J Roentgenol 2008;191(3):730–4.

84. Brophy RH, Marx RG. The treatment of traumatic anterior instability of the shoulder: nonoperative and surgical treatment. Arthroscopy 2009;25(3):298–304.

85. Bennett GE. Shoulder and elbow lesions of the professional baseball pitcher. JAMA 1941;117:510–4.

86. De Maeseneer M, Jaovisidha S, Jacobson JA, et al. The Bennett lesion of the shoulder. J Comput Assist Tomogr 1998;22:31–4.

87. Steinbach LS, Tirman PFJ, Peterfy CA, et al. Shoulder magnetic resonance imaging. Philadelphia: Lippincott-Raven; 1998.

88. Hottya GA, Tirman PFJ, Bost FW, et al. Tear of the posterior shoulder stabilizers after posterior dislocation: MR imaging and MR arthrographic findings with arthroscopic correlation. AJR Am J Roentgenol 1998;171:763–8.

89. Workman TK, Burkhard TK, Resnick D, et al. Hill-Sachs lesion: comparison of detection with MR imaging, radiography, and arthroscopy. Radiology 1992;185:847–52.

90. Jin W, Ryu KN, Park YK, et al. Cystic lesions in the posterosuperior portion of the humeral head on MR arthrography: correlations with gross and histologic findings in cadavers. AJR Am J Roentgenol 2005;184:1211–5.

91. Richards RD, Sartoris DJ, Pathria MN, et al. Hill-Sachs lesion and normal humeral groove: MR

imaging features allowing their differentiation. Radiology 1994;190:665–8.

92. Jobe CM. Posterior superior glenoid impingement: expanded spectrum. Arthroscopy 1995;11: 530–6.

93. Walch G, Boileau P, Noel E, et al. Impingement of the deep surface of the supraspinatus tendon on the posterosuperior glenoid rim: an arthroscopic study. Shoulder Elbow Surg 1992;1:238–45.

94. Liu SH, Boynton E. Posterior superior impingement of the rotator cuff on the glenoid rim as a cause of shoulder pain in the overhead athlete. Arthroscopy 1993;9:697–9.

95. Tirman PFJ, Bost F, Garvin GJ, et al. Posterosuperior glenoid impingement of the shoulder: findings at MR imaging and MR arthrography with arthroscopic correlation. Radiology 1994;193:431–6.

96. Weishaupt D, Zanetti M, Nyffeler RW, et al. Posterior glenoid rim deficiency in recurrent (atraumatic) posterior shoulder instability. Skeletal Radiol 2000; 29:204–10.

97. Tirman PFJ, Feller JF, Janzen DL, et al. Association of glenoid labral cysts with labral tears and glenohumeral instability: radiologic findings and clinical significance. Radiology 1994;190:653–8.

98. Longo C, Loredo R, Yu J, et al. Pictorial essay. MRI of the glenoid labrum with gross anatomic correlation. J Comput Assist Tomogr 1996;20(3): 487–95.

99. Snyder S, Karzel R, Del Pizzo W, et al. SLAP lesions of the shoulder. Arthroscopy 1990;6:274–9.

100. Neri BR, Vollmer EA, Kvitne RS. Isolated type II superior labral anterior posterior lesions: age-related outcome of arthroscopic fixation. Am J Sports Med 2009;37(5): 937–42.

101. Bedi A, Allen AA. Superior labral lesions anterior to posterior-evaluation and arthroscopic management. Clin Sports Med 2008;27(4):607–30.

Overuse and Traumatic Injuries of the Elbow

Catherine L. Hayter, MBBS, Bruno M. Giuffre, MBBS, FRANZCR*

KEYWORDS
- Elbow joint • MR imaging • Injuries
- Ligaments • Elbow anatomy

The elbow is one of the more commonly injured joints in recreational and professional sports. The role for MR imaging is increasing for evaluating athletes with elbow pain, especially those who present with nonlocalizable symptoms or an acute injury superimposed on chronic injuries or tendinopathy. Extensive literature is available on this problem, particularly in the orthopedic and sports medicine fields. The goal of this article is to provide a current, referenced overview of the key problems for the generalist radiologist.

ANATOMY
Bony and Articular

The elbow is composed of the ulnohumeral, radiocapitellar, and proximal radioulnar joints, which are all located within a single synovial-lined capsule. It is one of the most congruent joints in the body, allowing for two types of motion: 150° flexion from full extension and 160° of axial rotation.[1]

The elbow is stabilized by osseous and soft tissue structures. Osseous structures account for a significant proportion of elbow joint stability, but only at the extremes of flexion and extension.[2] The most important bony stabilizer in extension is the articulation between the trochlea and the sigmoid notch of the olecranon.[3] During the extremes of flexion, the coronoid process of the ulna inserts in the coronoid fossa of the distal humerus, contributing to stability. The two most important ligamentous stabilizers are the anterior bundle of the medial collateral ligament and the ulnar band of the lateral collateral ligament.[4]

Together, these two key ligaments sling symmetrically in the frontal plane to aid valgus and varus stability.[5] Dynamic stabilizers include the surrounding muscles, particularly those arising from the common flexor and extensor tendons.

The shape of the bony surfaces is complex and normal anatomy accounts for two commonly encountered "pseudolesions" on MR imaging that may be mistaken for pathology. The trochlea articulates with greater sigmoid (or trochlear) notch of the ulna. Separated by a slight ridge, the capitellum articulates with the radial head. Hyaline articular cartilage covers nearly the full circumference of the trochlea (330°), whereas only the anterior 180° of the capitellum is covered by articular cartilage (**Fig. 1**A and B). This disparity contributes to the pseudodefect of the capitellum (discussed later).

The surface of the trochlear notch of the ulna is also complex, with articular cartilage covering the internal surface in a varied "figure-of-eight" pattern.[6] At the junction between the anterior and posterior facets an interruption to the articular surface occurs, which can mimic an intraarticular body or a cartilage defect (**Fig. 2**A and B).

Medial (Ulnar) Collateral Ligament Complex

The medial collateral ligament (MCL) complex consists of three distinct parts: the anterior, posterior, and transverse or oblique bundles (**Fig. 3**).

The anterior bundle (A-MCL) is the strongest ligament in the elbow and the largest component of the medial collateral ligament complex.[3] It arises from the anterior inferior surface of the

The authors report no conflict of interest. No financial supports were provided in the writing of this article.
Department of Radiology, Royal North Shore Hospital, University of Sydney, Reserve Road, St. Leonards, Sydney NSW 2065, Australia
* Corresponding author.
E-mail address: bgiuffre@nsccahs.health.nsw.gov.au (B.M. Giuffre).

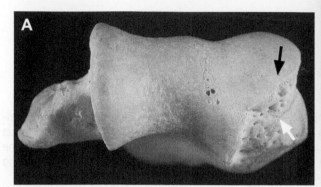

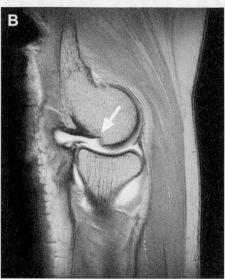

Fig. 1. Pseudodefect of the capitellum. Inferior view of the distal humerus (A) shows that hyaline cartilage covers nearly the full circumference of the trochlea (left). In contrast, only the anterior 180° of the capitellum (right) is covered by articular cartilage (black arrow). The posterior bare area (white arrow) contributes to the pseudodefect of the capitellum. On sagittal MRI (B) the capitellar pseudodefect (white arrow) is located posteriorly and should be not be confused with an osteochondral lesion.

medial humeral epicondyle, passes deep to the origin of the common flexor tendon, and inserts on the sublime tubercle on the medial aspect of the coronoid process of the ulna. The A-MCL is itself composed of anterior and posterior bands, which are taut in complementary parts of the flexion arc, so that the A-MCL is taut from 0° to

120° of flexion and is the primary stabilizer against valgus instability.[4,7] The A-MCL is best seen on coronal MR images (Fig. 4A).

The A-MCL is also well seen in sagittal MR images, and this can be a useful additional view to help assess this important structure (Fig. 4B–D). However, a normal invagination of synovium

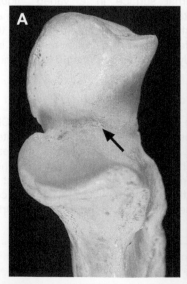

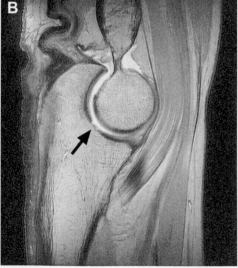

Fig. 2. Trochlear groove and trochlear ridge. Anterior view of the trochlear notch of the ulna (A) shows that articular cartilage covers the internal surface in a "figure-of-eight" pattern. An interruption to the articular surface is present at the junction between the anterior and posterior parts, known as the trochlear ridge (black arrow). On sagittal MRI (B), this normal pattern should not be mistaken for a cartilage defect.

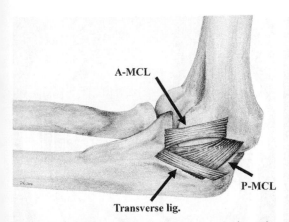

Fig. 3. The medial collateral ligament complex. The medial collateral ligament complex consists of the anterior bundle (A-MCL), posterior bundle (P-MCL), and oblique or transverse bundle. The A-MCL runs from the medial humeral epicondyle to the sublime tubercle on the coronoid process of the ulna and is the primary stabilizer against valgus instability.

occurs at the proximal aspect of the A-MCL, which may create signal hyperintensity adjacent to its humeral origin, and should not be misinterpreted as an undersurface partial-thickness tear.[8]

The posterior bundle of the MCL runs from the posterior surface of the medial humeral epicondyle to the posteromedial olecranon. It is more a fan-shaped thickening of the posterior capsule of the elbow joint than a distinct ligamentous structure.[3,4] The posterior bundle is a secondary stabilizer of the elbow joint against valgus and internal rotatory stress, but only at 120° of elbow flexion.[9] It is taut in flexion and therefore difficult to assess on MR imaging when the elbow is extended.[8] The oblique (transverse) bundle connects the anterior and posterior bundles along the medial olecranon. Because it is a variable structure with negligible role in joint stability, it is not routinely evaluated on MR imaging.[4,10]

Lateral (Radial) Collateral Ligament Complex

The lateral collateral ligament (LCL) complex consists of the lateral ulnar collateral, annular, and radial collateral ligaments (**Fig. 5**). The lateral collateral ligament complex is less well defined than the MCL and its appearance can vary considerably among individuals.[4]

The lateral ulnar collateral ligament (LUCL) arises from the posteroinferior aspect of the lateral humeral epicondyle, courses along the posterolateral margin of the radial head, and inserts on the supinator crest of the ulna.[11] The LUCL is one of the most important ligamentous stabilizers against varus and rotatory stress.[12] It is taut in extension

and, like the A-MCL, is best seen on coronal MR images. Because it is obliquely oriented, it must be followed from anterior to posterior on sequential images (**Fig. 6**A and B).

The annular ligament is a thick band that attaches to the sigmoid notch anteriorly and posteriorly. It encircles the radial head and stabilizes the proximal radioulnar joint.[13] The radial collateral ligament (RCL) originates from a facet just anterior to the LUCL component, from the center of the lateral epicondyle, runs deep to the common extensor tendon, and blends with the fibers of the annular ligament anteriorly. Unlike the MCL, the RCL is taut throughout flexion.[14]

The interaction of the RCL, LUCL, and annular ligaments in varus stability is complex and remains contentious.[15] Recent anatomic studies have shown that although variations can occur in the morphology of the LUCL (cordlike throughout or cordlike proximally and more membranous distally), the more functionally important part is the proximal section. This finding has implications in imaging. Demonstration of the humeral attachment is very important in lateral ligament imaging. In general, the coronal plane is the best plane to show the RCL and LUCL. Occasionally the sagittal plane may be more useful for showing the proximal attachment and the axial plane may be helpful for assessing the distal attachment.

Muscular and Tendinous Structures of the Elbow

The musculature of the elbow is divided into medial, lateral, anterior, and posterior compartments. The common flexor and extensor tendons are responsible for most musculotendinous pathology of the elbow, and localizing pathology to an individual muscle is often not necessary.

The medial muscle group includes the pronator teres and the four superficial flexors: the flexor carpi radialis, palmaris longus, flexor carpi ulnaris, and flexor digitorum superficialis. These muscles flex the wrist and pronate the forearm. The flexor carpi radialis, palmaris longus, flexor carpi ulnaris, humeroulnar head of flexor digitorum superficialis, and part of pronator teres arise from the medial epicondyle by way of the common flexor tendon. The common flexor tendon is best assessed on coronal MR images.

The lateral muscle group consists of three components: the superficial group, the common extensors, and the supinator muscle. They function to extend the wrist and supinate the forearm. The superficial group includes the brachioradialis and extensor carpi radialis longus, which arise from the supracondylar ridge proximal to the

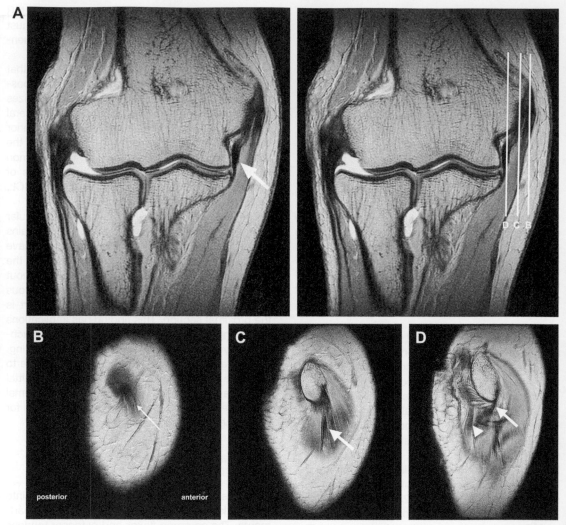

Fig. 4. Anterior bundle of the medial collateral ligament (A-MCL). The A-MCL (*white arrow*) is best assessed on the coronal view, as seen on this coronal fast-spin echo image (*A*). The sagittal view (*B–D*) is a helpful additional view to assess the A-MCL (*white arrow*), which lies deep to the common flexor tendon (*thin white arrow*) and anterior to the ulnar nerve (*white arrowhead*).

common extensor origin. The common extensor group is composed of the extensor carpi radialis brevis, extensor digitorum, extensor digiti minimi, and extensor carpi ulnaris. These muscles arise from the lateral epicondyle by way of the common extensor tendon. The most lateral muscle in the superficial group is the extensor carpi radialis brevis. It lies immediately deep to the extensor carpi radialis longus and is the most frequently involved tendon in common extensor pathology. The common extensor tendon is also best assessed on coronal MR images.

The anterior compartment is comprised of the brachialis and biceps muscles, which both function to flex the elbow. The biceps muscle is superficial to the brachialis muscle. Its tendon passes through the cubital fossa to insert on the posterior

aspect of the radial tuberosity. The distal biceps tendon has no tendon sheath. The bicipital aponeurosis or lacertus fibrosis is the continuation of the fascia surrounding the distal biceps muscle. It arises from the distal biceps tendon and courses medially over the median nerve and radial artery to blend with the deep fascia of the forearm, eventually fusing with the periosteum of the ulna.[1] The bicipitoradial bursa separates the distal biceps tendon from the anterior aspect of the radial tuberosity. The distal biceps tendon is best evaluated on axial images or on the flexed abducted supinated (FABS) view.[16] The brachialis tendon insertion is also best seen axially and on the FABS view.[17]

The posterior compartment is composed of the triceps, anconeus, and variably present anconeus

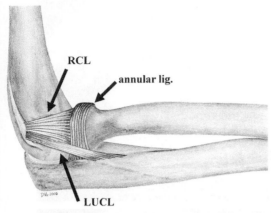

Fig. 5. The lateral collateral ligament complex. The lateral collateral ligament complex consists of the lateral ulnar collateral ligament (LUCL), radial collateral ligament (RCL), and annular ligament. The LUCL runs from the lateral epicondyle and inserts on the supinator crest of the ulna and is the most important stabilizer against varus instability.

epitrochlearis muscles. The medial, lateral, and long heads of triceps blend to form a single musculotendinous unit that inserts into the tip of the olecranon and is separated from the olecranon by the deep olecranon bursa. The triceps tendon is best assessed on sagittal MR images.[18]

Nerves Around the Elbow

The usual course of the nerves at the elbow has been well documented and discussed from the radiologic viewpoint.[19,20] A clear understanding of the nerve anatomy remains essential. Apart from compression of the ulnar and radial nerves at their respective tunnels at the elbow, nerve compression syndromes of the elbow are rare. Passage of the nerves through their respective muscle/fascial planes is best appreciated in the axial plane (Fig. 7).

At the elbow, the ulnar nerve passes from the posterior compartment of the upper arm into the cubital tunnel, where it lies within a groove in the posterior aspect of the medial epicondyle. The cubital tunnel retinaculum forms the roof of the cubital tunnel. The ulnar nerve runs from the tip of the medial epicondyle to the olecranon process and margin of the triceps fascia. After traveling through the cubital tunnel, the nerve passes along the medial aspect of the elbow, medial to the posterior bundle of the MCL, and then passes between the humeral and ulnar heads of flexor carpi ulnaris to enter the anterior compartment of the forearm. At the elbow, the ulnar nerve innervates the flexor carpi ulnaris and medial flexor digitorum profundus.

The radial nerve travels along the lateral aspect of the elbow joint, supplying the medial and lateral heads of triceps and brachioradialis muscles. Deep to the fascia of the brachioradialis muscle at the level of the radiocapitellar joint, the radial nerve divides into its motor branch, the posterior interosseous nerve (PIN), and its sensory branch, the superficial radial nerve. The PIN passes

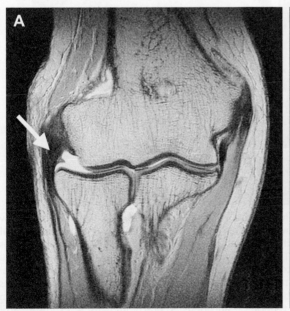

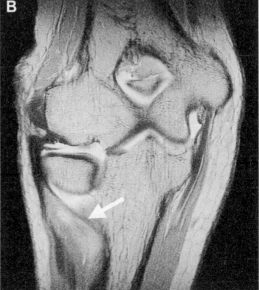

Fig. 6. The lateral ulnar collateral ligament (LUCL). The LUCL (white arrow) is best assessed on coronal MR images. As it passes obliquely in the coronal plane, it must be followed from anterior (A) to posterior (B) on a series of images.

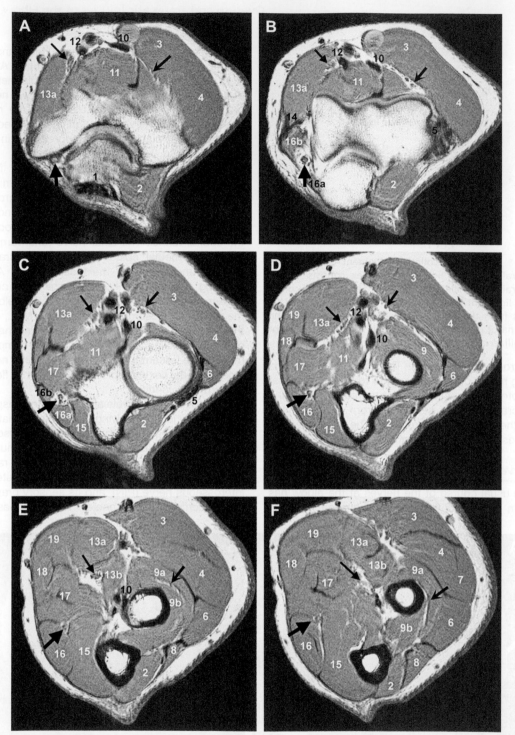

Fig. 7. Course of the nerves around the elbow joint. Selected axial MR images from proximal to distal (*A–F*) show the relationship of the major nerves around the elbow. The ulnar nerve (*black arrow*) runs within the cubital tunnel, passes along the medial aspect of the elbow, then travels between the two heads of flexor carpi ulnaris to enter the anterior compartment of the forearm. The radial nerve (*pointed black arrow*) travels along the lateral aspect of the elbow joint, and gives off the posterior interosseous nerve, which travels in part of the radial tunnel between the two heads of supinator to the posterior forearm. The median nerve (*thin black arrow*) passes anterior to the elbow joint and lies medial to the biceps tendon and brachial artery. It enters the forearm between the two heads of pronator teres. **1**, triceps tendon; **2**, anconeus; **3**, brachioradialis; **4**, extensor carpi radialis longus; **5**, common extensor tendon; **6**, extensor digitorum; **7**, extensor carpi radialis brevis; **8**, extensor carpi ulnaris; **9**, supinator (**9a**, superficial head; **9b**, deep head); **10**, biceps tendon; **11**, brachialis; **12**, brachial artery and vein; **13**, pronator teres (**13a**, humeral head; **13b**, ulnar head); **14**, common flexor tendon; **15**, flexor digitorum profundus; **16**, flexor carpi ulnaris (**16a**, ulnar head; **16b**, humeral head); **17**, flexor digitorum superficialis; **18**, palmaris longus; **19**, flexor carpi radialis.

inferiorly within the radial tunnel, which begins at the level of the capitellum and extends to the lower border of the supinator muscle. It is bound medially by the brachialis muscle and anterolaterally by the brachioradialis and extensor carpi radialis longus muscles. The PIN passes beneath a fibrous arch formed by the proximal edge of the superficial head of the supinator muscle, the arcade of Frohse, and supplies motor branches to the extensor compartment of the forearm.[21]

The median nerve courses distally within the anterior compartment of the arm superficial to the brachialis muscle. At the elbow it passes beneath the bicipital aponeurosis into the antecubital fossa, where it lies medial to the biceps tendon and brachial artery. It then passes between the superficial and deep heads of the pronator teres muscle and runs down the forearm in the plane between the flexor digitorum superficialis and flexor digitorum profundus. The median nerve proper supplies motor branches to the flexor compartment of the forearm.

IMAGING TECHNIQUE

Many competing issues exist in optimally showing the pathoanatomy of the elbow on MR imaging. The need to make the patient comfortable during imaging this eccentrically placed joint and keep the study short to minimize movement artifact competes with the goal of optimizing spatial and contrast resolution. This issue provides some challenges to dictating an "ideal" elbow sequence choice. Ultimately, the local conditions of magnet and coil availability, time constraints, and radiologist preference often determine the specifics.

In general, the elbow is best imaged when patients are supine with the arm at the side, the elbow fully extended, and the forearm supinated. This position optimizes visualization of the collateral ligaments and common flexor and extensor origins in the coronal plane. For large patients or scanner/coil combinations that do not allow off-center imaging, patients can be positioned in the prone position with the arm overhead. However, although this positioning improves image quality, it is uncomfortable for the patient, increasing the chance of motion artifact. This position also often results in forearm pronation, making ligamentous assessment more difficult.

The use of surface coils is essential to provide adequate soft tissue detail. Thin sections (4 mm) and high in-plane resolution (field of view 12–14 cm and matrix 256 × 256 or higher) are essential for optimal demonstration of the pathology at the elbow. High-resolution three-dimensional gradient echo sequences can be useful in evaluating the

ligaments and tendons. These sequences, which are sensitive to magnetic susceptibility effects, can be very useful for assessing small bony intraarticular bodies, but are not advisable in the presence of metal in postoperative patients. Fat-suppression techniques are useful to show areas of edema and fluid collections. Because the elbow is at the margin of the magnet bore, fast inversion recovery techniques occasionally may be preferred over frequency-selective techniques for fat suppression.

MR arthrography has been advocated to increase sensitivity in detecting partial thickness ligamentous tears.[22,23] It can also help assess for possible chondral loose bodies and the presence of a chondral flap in osteochondritis that may require surgical repair. It is however an invasive technique and makes the examination more time consuming and costly. The distension provided post arthrography may also prevent the capsule and ligaments being visualized in the "native" state, leading to potential loss of useful information.[24]

Imaging should be performed in the axial, sagittal, and coronal planes. The decision whether to use an oblique coronal sequence to show the distal portion of the LUCL has received considerable attention in the literature.[25,26] In general, the use of thin sections (≤4 mm) in the bicondylar coronal plane is perfectly adequate for LUCL demonstration.

Additional positioning and planes of scan, such as the FABS view, can help assess specific clinical problems, particularly the distal attachments of the anterior and posterior tendons (biceps, brachialis, and triceps).[16,17] The FABS view is obtained with the patient positioned prone with the shoulder abducted, elbow flexed, and forearm supinated. This position flexes the biceps muscle and pulls the tendon taut. It also directs the radial tuberosity medially, allowing a longitudinal view of the distal biceps tendon in one section and clearly showing its insertion on the radial tuberosity.[16]

BONY AND OSTEOCHONDRAL INJURIES
Fractures

MR imaging can be useful for detecting occult fractures or bone bruises that may be associated with acute trauma. Subtle radial head fractures and fractures of the supra/epicondylar regions in children and adolescents can be readily diagnosed on MR imaging.[27] Particular patterns of fracture may suggest a particular type of injury. Avulsion of the sublime tubercle of the ulna is associated with acute valgus stress to the MCL. If identified on radiographs, MR imaging is useful to determine if the MCL is intact.[28,29] Similarly, an injury such as an avulsed fragment from the supinator crest of the ulna may be a warning that a swollen elbow is more than a simple sprain (**Fig. 8**A and B). Subluxation or dislocation of the elbow can be associated with fractures of the coronoid and radial head. The small flake fracture of the coronoid is not an avulsion fracture, but represents a shear fracture and is typically pathognomonic of a prior episode of subluxation or dislocation.[30]

Chronic elbow overload may be associated with stress fracture of the mid one third of the olecranon process. This injury has been described in gymnasts, javelin throwers, and baseball pitchers from valgus extension overload and repetitive abutment of the olecranon on the olecranon fossa.[31,32] MR imaging may detect changes of stress fractures before they are detected on plain radiographs.

Osteochondral Injuries and Osteochondritis Dissecans of the Capitellum

An acute valgus force to the elbow is one of the most common mechanisms of elbow joint injury and may result in osteochondral injury from impaction and shear forces applied to the articular surfaces. The capitellar articular surface impacts on the radius to produce a chondral or osteochondral injury, which is seen on MR imaging as irregularity of the chondral surface, disruption of the subchondral bone plate, or the presence of

a fracture line. This pattern of injury must be distinguished from the "pseudodefect" of the capitellum.[33] The more anteroinferior location of the lesion, the presence of bone marrow edema and a joint effusion helps confirm the true nature of the osteochondral injury (**Fig. 9**A and B).[33,34]

Similarly, osteochondritis dissecans in the elbow classically involves the anterior aspect of the capitellum. It usually occurs in men between the ages of 12 and 15 years when the capitellar epiphysis is almost completely ossified. Most patients have a history of repetitive overuse of the elbow, such as young male baseball players or young female gymnasts, and usually present without a specific episode of injury.[35,36] Although osteochondritis dissecans can be asymptomatic, with instability or synovitis, pain and mechanical symptoms may ensue. Patients present with pain, tenderness, and swelling over the lateral aspect of the elbow. Radiographs may be normal initially, and in these cases MR imaging is a useful imaging modality.

Early osteochondritis shows focal low-signal intensity in the anterior capitellum on T1-weighted images with or without high signal on T2-weighted images.[37] Some flattening of the subchondral bone plate may be present. More severe lesions show a discrete fragment either in situ or loose in the joint. MR imaging is helpful to document the size of the lesion, assess the overlying cartilage for surface defects, determine the viability of the donor site, and assess for the presence of intraarticular loose bodies. An unstable osteochondritis dissecans

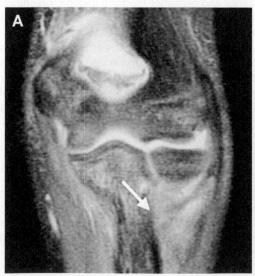
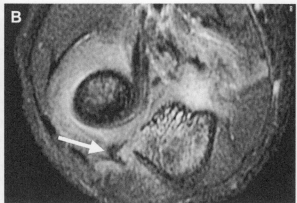

Fig. 8. Avulsion of the supinator crest of the elbow in a 14-year–old boy who fell backward onto an outstretched arm and complained of a swollen elbow. Radiographs suggested a missed dislocation. Coronal fat-saturated fast-spin echo (FSE) (*A*) and axial fat-saturated FSE (*B*) images confirmed an avulsion of the lateral ulnar collateral ligament (*white arrow*) from the supinator crest of the ulna.

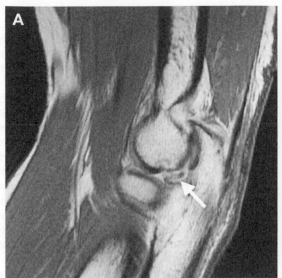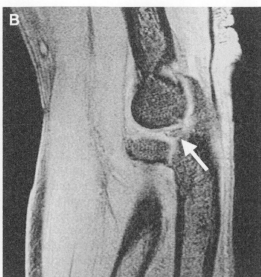

Fig. 9. Acute osteochondral injury of the capitellum in a 60-year-old man who sustained an acute elbow injury 2 months previously and presented with episodic locking. Sagittal fast-spin echo proton density image (*A*) shows the typical anteroinferior location of a traumatic osteochondral lesion (*white arrow*). Sagittal three-dimensional gradient echo image (*B*) more clearly delineates the associated intraarticular loose body.

fragment shows linear high signal on T2-weighted images along the interface between the fragment and the capitellum, which is believed to represent fluid or granulation tissue (**Fig. 10**A and B).[38,39]

Little Leaguer's Elbow

The medial epicondyle apophysis is one of the first sites to ossify in the elbow, appearing at approximately 6 years of age, but is the last to fuse. Before apophyseal fusion, valgus stress to the elbow is imparted to the physis rather than to the MCL.[40] A Salter Harris 1 fracture through the medial epicondyle apophysis is often referred to as *little leaguer's elbow*. If subtle on plain radiographs, MR imaging may be used to image the physis, which is best evaluated on coronal fat-saturated gradient echo images. Chronic

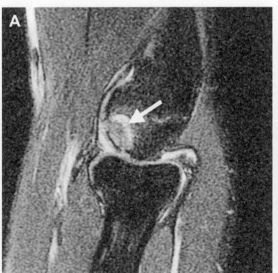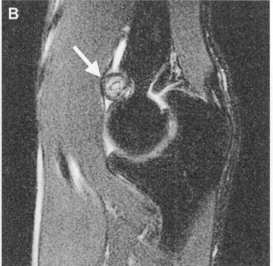

Fig. 10. Osteochondritis dissecans of the capitellum in a 19-year-old man who has a long history of lateral elbow pain. Sagittal fat-saturated fast-spin echo proton density images (*A*) show osteochondritis dissecans with an unstable fragment outlined by a linear high signal (*white arrow*). In the medial aspect of the joint (*B*) a loose cartilage body (*thin white arrow*) is seen lying within the coronoid fossa.

valgus stress may manifest as physeal widening, adjacent soft tissue edema, or fragmentation and resorption of the medial epicondyle ossification center.[41,42] If untreated, fracture through the growth plate can result in deformity or nonunion of the epicondyle.[24]

LIGAMENTOUS INJURIES AND INSTABILITY
Medial Collateral Ligament Injury and Medial Elbow Instability

The MCL is the most commonly injured ligament in the elbow. MCL tears may occur after acute valgus stress or acute elbow dislocation. More commonly, however, MCL tears result from chronic repetitive stress to the elbow elicited by sporting activities involving overhead throwing, such as baseball, tennis, volleyball, and javelin throwing.[43,44] During the late cocking and acceleration phases of throwing, enormous valgus stress is placed on the elbow joint, which may exceed the strength of the A-MCL, the primary stabilizer against valgus stress.[45]

Although complete tears usually produce signs of valgus instability, partial tears may be difficult to detect on clinical examination.[46] Partial tears can be asymptomatic with everyday activities but often generate pain on valgus loading, particularly if repetitive. Medial elbow instability must be differentiated from other causes of medial elbow pain in the athlete, such as medial epicondylitis, flexor–pronator tendon tears, valgus extension overload syndrome, and ulnar neuropathy.[47] The anterior bundle and the humeral and ulnar insertions of the MCL are poorly visualized at arthroscopy,

further emphasizing the important role of MR imaging in diagnosing ligamentous injury.[46,48]

Acute injury to the A-MCL most commonly involves the humeral insertion and may be accompanied by an avulsion fracture of the medial epicondyle.[49] The mid substance of the ligament and ulnar attachment are less commonly involved.[50] An acute tear is seen as high-signal intensity and discontinuity of some or all of the fibers (Fig. 11A and B). In the case of complete rupture, total discontinuity of ligamentous fibers with redundancy and possible ligamentous retraction occurs. Hematoma associated with acute ligamentous disruption may impinge on the ulnar nerve, causing ulnar nerve symptoms.[42] In adolescent and juvenile athletes, occasionally the periosteum is stripped from the ulna as part of this ligamentous injury (Fig. 12A and B).

Partial-thickness tears of the A-MCL may also occur. A characteristic lesion that has been described is a partial-thickness undersurface tear of the A-MCL with avulsion of the ulnar attachment of the deep fibers.[23,51] This lesion has been described as a T sign on MR or CT arthrography, because of tracking of fluid beneath the deep portion of the A-MCL (Fig. 13).[23]

However, as with many tendon abnormalities, the clinical context is important to consider. The presence of a recess at the ulnar attachment of the A-MCL has been shown in up to 50% of patients,[52] and therefore this finding in isolation should not be overinterpreted in asymptomatic patients.

Chronic A-MCL pathology is commonly seen in throwing athletes who sustain repetitive valgus

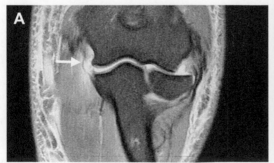
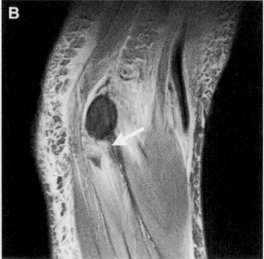

Fig. 11. Complete tear in the anterior bundle of the medial collateral ligament. Coronal fat-saturated fast-spin echo (FSE) (A) and sagittal fat-saturated FSE (B) images show complete rupture of the proximal medial collateral ligament (white arrow).

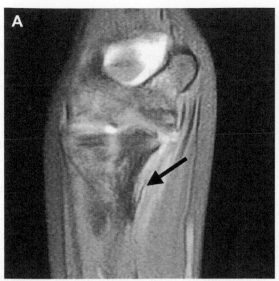
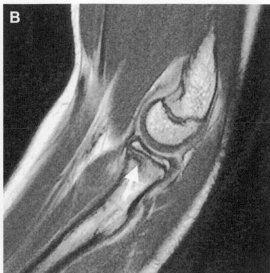

Fig. 12. Anterior bundle of the medial collateral ligament (A-MCL) injury with periosteal stripping in a 13-year-old girl. Coronal fat-saturated fast-spin echo (FSE) image (*A*) shows injury to the distal insertion of the A-MCL with stripping of the periosteum from the ulnar attachment (*black arrow*). Sagittal FSE image (*B*) shows associated compression fracture of the radial neck (*white arrow*) secondary to lateral load injury.

stresses at the elbow. In chronic injury, diffuse increase in signal intensity and thickening of the ligament may occur from micro tears and remodeling.[42] Secondary signs of chronic valgus overload may be seen, as discussed later. Concomitant flexor tendinopathy is common.[8] An acute on chronic pattern may manifest as a remodeled ligament with focally increased signal intensity and adjacent soft tissue edema.[24]

Valgus Extension Overload Syndrome (Posteromedial Impingement)

Chronic A-MCL injury is often associated with valgus extension overload or posteromedial impingement.[53] In this condition the A-MCL is intact but is attenuated from repetitive microtrauma. Shear forces at the posteromedial olecranon eventually cause formation of posteromedial olecranon osteophytes. During elbow extension, these osteophytes impinge on the olecranon fossa, resulting in a decreased range of movement and pain. They may also become detached, forming intraarticular loose bodies.[54] Valgus laxity places excessive strain on the medial soft tissues of the elbow and may also result in common flexor tendinosis and ulnar neuropathy.[55]

If the patient has a clinical history of flexion deformity or a flexion deformity is present on sagittal MR images, posteromedial impingement should be considered. Images should be carefully evaluated for the presence of MCL attenuation and redundancy, osteophytes on the posteromedial olecranon, and intraarticular loose bodies.[24,55]

Radiocapitellar Overload Syndrome

Rupture or attenuation of the MCL also results in increased compressive forces applied to the lateral joint, with the radiocapitellar joint eventually

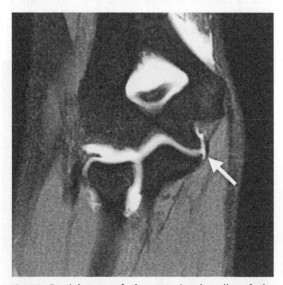

Fig. 13. Partial tear of the anterior bundle of the medial collateral ligament (A-MCL) in a 15-year-old girl who presented with pain on throwing. Coronal fat-saturated fast-spin echo MR arthrogram showed a partial tear of the A-MCL (*white arrow*). The appearance has been described as a "T sign" on MR arthrography because of fluid tracking beneath the deep portion of the A-MCL. Partial ligamentous tear was confirmed at surgery and repaired.

acting as a static resistor of valgus instability. This condition may result in osteochondral injuries of the capitellum and radial head from repeated abutment of the radial head against the capitellum (**Fig. 14**A and B).[56] Lateral epicondylitis may also develop secondary to chronic valgus instability.

Lateral Collateral Ligament Injury and Posterolateral Rotatory Instability

LCL injury is unusual because varus stress to the elbow in sport is less common. However, LCL tears are important in the development of posterolateral rotatory instability of the elbow because of loss of the primary stabilizer of the elbow against varus stress.[11] Posterolateral rotatory instability (PLRI) is believed to result from a tear of the LUCL.[11] In children, this usually follows an acute traumatic dislocation, but in adults most tears are caused by varus extension injury to the elbow without dislocation,[57] such as after a fall onto an outstretched hand with the forearm supinated. Occasionally disruption of the LUCL may follow overaggressive release of the common extensor tendon origin for the treatment of lateral epicondylitis.[26]

O'Driscoll and colleagues[7] have described a process of progressive injury to the elbow, which proceeds in a circle from the lateral to the medial side of the joint in three stages (**Fig. 15**). Stage 1 of this kinematic pattern of injury is characterized by rotatory subluxation of the ulnohumeral joint

due to an incompetent LUCL, resulting in PLRI. When the elbow is extended with the forearm in supination (as occurs in MR Imaging with arm by the side), the forearm pivots around the medial soft tissue restraints, causing posterolateral subluxation of the radial head with respect to the capitellum.[11,30] The annular ligament remains intact so the radioulnar joint does not dislocate (**Fig. 16**).

Patients with PLRI may present with lateral elbow pain, clicking, locking, instability and dislocation. On examination there is a positive "lateral pivot shift test."[11] While the lateral pivot shift test is an accurate clinical test of PLRI, clinical assessment may not be possible without general anesthesia, as the examination is hampered by patient apprehension and guarding.[11] Plain radiographs are commonly non diagnostic. MR Imaging is therefore the most sensitive test for detecting LUCL pathology in these patients.[58]

Most tears of the LUCL are full thickness tears which involve the humeral origin of the ligament.[11,58] On MR Imaging there is signal hyperintensity, discontinuity and surrounding soft tissue edema (**Fig. 17**A). As with the MCL, a chronically torn and remodeled LUCL will exhibit thickening and abnormal increased signal. In the presence of LUCL injury, sagittal MR images should be examined for secondary signs of PLRI, such as an inability to maintain full extension during the examination and posterior subluxation of the radial head on the sagittal MR images.[42] The bone

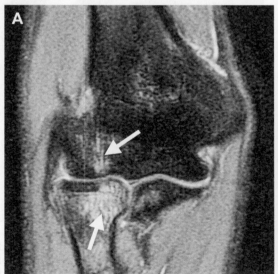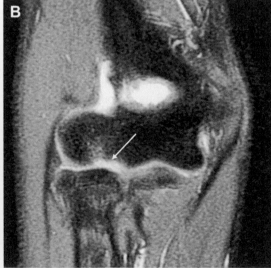

Fig. 14. Radiocapitellar overload syndrome caused by deficient medial collateral ligament (MCL) in a 17-year-old man who presented with a 2-month history of elbow pain on extension. Coronal fat-saturated fast-spin echo images (*A, B*) show edema (*white arrow*) in the radial head and capitellum with associated cartilage damage (*thin white arrow*) resulting from increased compressive forces applied to the lateral joint from rupture of the MCL.

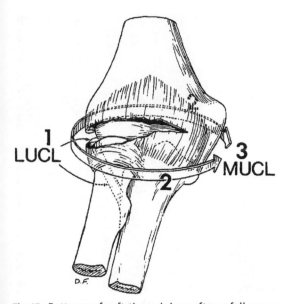

Fig. 15. Patterns of soft tissue injury after a fall on an outstretched hand. Soft tissue injury proceeds in a circle from lateral to medial in three stages. In stage **1** there is disruption of the LUCL. In stage **2** there is disruption of the LCL complex and the anterior and posterior capsule. In stage **3** there is partial or complete disruption of the MCL. (*From* O'Driscoll SW, Morrey BF, Korinek S, et al. Elbow subluxation and dislocation. A spectrum of instability. Clin Orthop Rel Res 1992;280:194; with permission.)

edema pattern of high signal in the posterior capitellum and anterior radial head should also raise the suspicion of PLRI (**Fig. 17**B).

In stage 2 injury as described by O'Driscoll and colleagues (**Fig. 16**), there is more severe stress with rupture of the LCL complex and disruption of the anterior and posterior capsule. This results in a perched dislocation, with the coronoid process perched on the trochlea (**Fig. 18**A and B). Although the A-MCL is intact, the patient will maintain valgus stability after reduction. With associated rupture of the MCL (stage 3) the only remaining stabilizers are the muscles and bony structures of the joint. This renders the elbow grossly unstable.[7,11]

ENTHESOPATHIES AND TENDON INJURIES
Lateral Epicondylitis ("Tennis Elbow")

Tendinosis of the common extensor origin is known as lateral epicondylitis or "tennis elbow." It is associated with repetitive and excessive use of the wrist extensors and is commonly seen in people partaking in sports with overhead arm motion.[59] Lateral epicondylitis is a common condition, developing in over 50% of tennis players at some time or another.[60] It is however, more common in non athletes, mostly presenting between ages 40 and 60 years, and is often seen in workers whose job involves repetitive rotatory

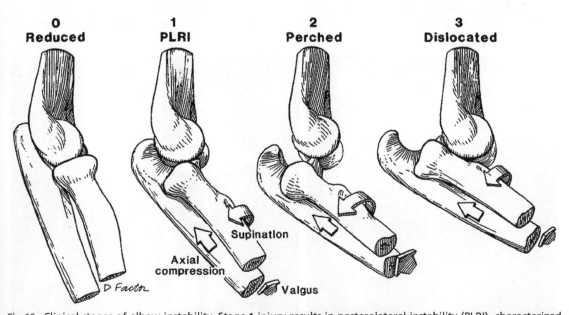

Fig. 16. Clinical stages of elbow instability. Stage **1** injury results in posterolateral instability (PLRI), characterized by posterolateral subluxation of the radial head with respect to the capitellum. Stage **2** injury results in a perched dislocation. In stage **3** injury, the medial, lateral, anterior, and posterior stabilizers are completely disrupted, rendering the elbow grossly unstable and liable to dislocation. (*From* O'Driscoll SW, Morrey BF, Korinek S, et al. Elbow subluxation and dislocation. A spectrum of instability. Clin Orthop Rel Res 1992;280:195; with permission.)

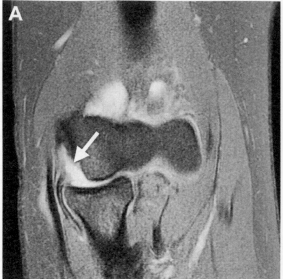
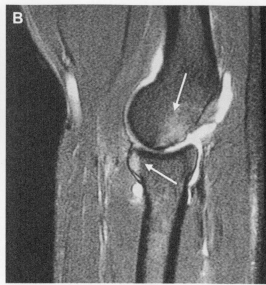

Fig. 17. Lateral ulnar collateral ligament (LUCL) tear resulting in posterolateral instability in a 25-year-old man who presented after acute trauma. Coronal fat-saturated fast-spin echo (FSE) image (A) shows tear of the proximal attachment of the LUCL (*white arrow*). Sagittal fat-saturated FSE image (B) shows bone edema pattern in the posterior capitellum and anterior radial head (*thin white arrows*) and raises the suspicion of associated posterolateral instability.

forearm movements such as carpenters and cleaners.[61]

Patients present with chronic lateral elbow pain, exacerbated by activities that require extension of the wrist. On examination there is point tenderness in the region of the common extensor tendon origin. The role of MR Imaging is not usually to establish the diagnosis of lateral epicondylitis, but to exclude other causes of lateral elbow pain in individuals who fail to respond to conservative management. The degree of the MR evident changes also helps guide decisions regarding surgical management of this condition. Patients without a definite tendon tear on MR Imaging will

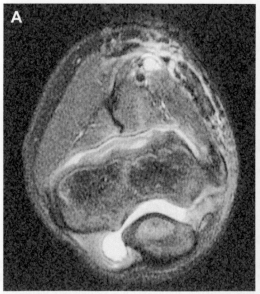
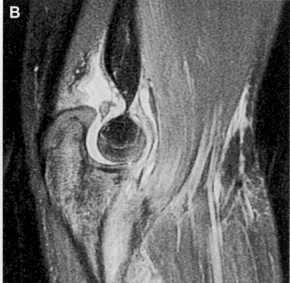

Fig. 18. Stage 2 injury with perched dislocation in a 14-year-old boy who fell backward onto outstretched arm. MRI confirmed injury to the lateral ulnar collateral ligament (see Fig. 8). Axial (A) and sagittal (B) fat-saturated fast-spin echo images show features of stage 2 injury with perched dislocation.

respond poorly to surgical management and will tend to be managed conservatively.[62]

In lateral epicondylitis the common extensor tendon origin is thickened with increased signal intensity on T2 weighted images. The extensor carpi radialis brevis is almost always the most severely affected tendon (**Fig. 19**A and B).[63,64] In the setting of lateral epicondylitis, the LCL should be carefully evaluated for the presence of an associated tear. Most patients who have moderate to severe lateral epicondylitis show partial- or full-thickness tears of the LUCL.[65] If the ligamentous injury is not recognized and the patient undergoes extensor tendon release, surgery may further destabilize the elbow and worsen the patient's symptoms (**Fig. 20**A and B).[55]

In the absence of MR evidence of lateral epicondylitis, other reasonably common entities to consider include partial tear of the distal biceps tendon and, less commonly, posterior interosseous nerve entrapment. These conditions may mimic the symptoms of lateral epicondylitis and may be a differential for the patient presenting with lateral elbow pain and tenderness.[66]

Medial Epicondylitis (Golfer's Elbow)

Medial epicondylitis of pitchers/golfer's elbow is caused by tendinosis at the origin of the common flexor tendon. Medial epicondylitis is much less common than lateral epicondylitis[67] and is almost exclusively seen in athletes who participate in activities that involve repetitive valgus and flexion forces at the elbow, such as golfers, tennis players, swimmers, pitchers, and javelin throwers.

Patients present with chronic medial elbow pain with symptoms exacerbated by activities requiring flexion of the wrist and pronation of the forearm. On examination, patients experience pain on palpation over the anterior aspect of the medial epicondyle. Patients presenting with medial elbow pain often have a confusing clinical picture. Medial elbow pain and point tenderness may be caused by medial epicondylitis, MCL injury or insufficiency, ulnar nerve injury, or medial elbow intraarticular pathology.[8] Even the experienced clinician may have difficulty distinguishing between these causes, making imaging crucial in diagnosing medial epicondylitis.

MR imaging can confirm the diagnosis, assess for associated MCL injury, and facilitate surgical planning by identifying degeneration and tears of the common flexor tendon. MR imaging shows thickening and increased signal intensity at the origin of the common flexor tendon.[68] The origins of the flexor carpi radialis and pronator teres are most commonly involved. Medial epicondylitis may be associated with injury to the MCL and the ligament must be carefully assessed in cases of suspected medial epicondylitis.[69] Ulnar neuropathy is also commonly associated with medial epicondylitis; the ulnar nerve and the surrounding fat planes should be evaluated on axial MR images.[70]

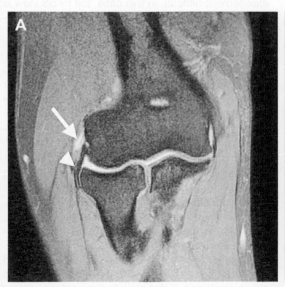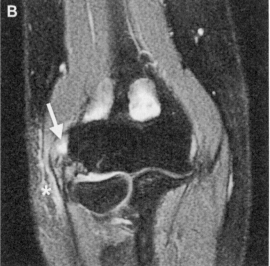

Fig. 19. Lateral epicondylitis with extensor carpi radialis brevis (ECRB) tear. Coronal fat-saturated fast-spin echo (FSE) image (*A*) from a 42-year-old man shows small tear of the ECRB component of the common extensor tendon (*white arrow*) with intact lateral collateral ligament (*white arrowhead*). Coronal fat-saturated FSE image (*B*) in a 40-year-old woman shows a tear in the ECRB (*white arrow*) with more extensive edema in the adjacent soft tissues (*white star*).

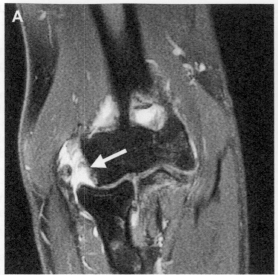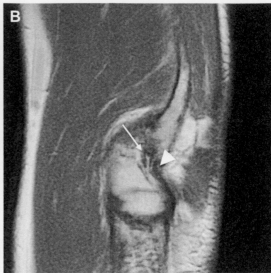

Fig. 20. Lateral epicondylitis with lateral collateral ligament tear. Coronal (*A*) fat-saturated fast-spin echo (FSE) and sagittal (*B*) FSE images in a 55-year-old man show large tear of the common extensor tendon (*white arrow*) with associated tear of the radial collateral ligament (*thin white arrow*) and partial tear of the lateral ulnar collateral ligament (*white arrowhead*).

Biceps Tendinopathy and Biceps Tendon Injuries

Insertional biceps tendinopathy is typically seen in sports that use weight training. Similar to medial and lateral epicondylitis, the tendon shows increased signal intensity with or without accompanying tendon tear. Associated distension of the bicipitoradial bursa may be present, which can contribute to compression of the radial nerve.[71]

Rupture of the distal biceps tendon is uncommon compared with proximal tendon ruptures, accounting for 3% of all biceps tendon injuries.[72] It most commonly occurs in men between 40 and 60 years of age and is almost always the result of a single traumatic event whereby a sudden extension force is applied to the arm with the elbow in mid flexion.[73] Patients present with the feeling of a "pop" or acute pain in the antecubital fossa. If the bicipital aponeurosis is torn, the tendon will retract proximally into the arm and the condition is usually obvious clinically, presenting as a mass in the antecubital fossa with weakness of elbow flexion and forearm supination. A partially torn or torn but nonretracted tendon may, however, be difficult to diagnose clinically, necessitating examination with ultrasound or MR imaging. Partial tears of the distal biceps tendon may present with poorly defined lateral elbow pain with resisted supination.

Most of distal biceps tendon tears occur in the inserting few centimeters of the distal tendon. With a complete rupture of the tendon, the low-signal intensity tendon is absent at its insertion site on the radial tuberosity, with soft tissue edema in the

antecubital fossa.[74] In the case of partial tendon tear, increased signal intensity is present within an abnormally thick or thin biceps tendon.[74,75] Biceps tendon tears may be associated with secondary findings of tendon rupture, such as bone marrow edema within the radial tuberosity and fluid in the bicipitoradial bursa. Some partial tendon tears may be obvious on the axial images. On the sagittal images, however, the obliquity of the tendon may make assessment difficult. In this case, the FABS view is useful for showing the biceps tendon and its attachment in a single image (**Fig. 21**).

Triceps Tendinopathy and Triceps Rupture

Triceps tendinosis is an unusual cause of posterior elbow pain, but may be seen in association with sports that involve rapid or forceful extension of the triceps, such as javelin throwing, baseball, bench-pressing in weight training, and gymnastics.[76] Abnormal signal intensity may be seen at the insertion of the triceps tendon, with or without thickening of the tendon. Triceps tendinosis is frequently associated with other chronic posterior elbow disorders, such as stress reaction of the olecranon process, olecranon osteophytes, loose bodies in the olecranon fossa, and olecranon bursitis.[77]

Rupture of the triceps tendon is a rare injury and is almost always caused by a single traumatic event, such as a direct blow to the posterior elbow or a forceful contraction of the triceps muscle with the elbow flexed.[78–80] Ruptures are mostly seen in association with stress sports, such as football and weight lifting. Triceps ruptures most

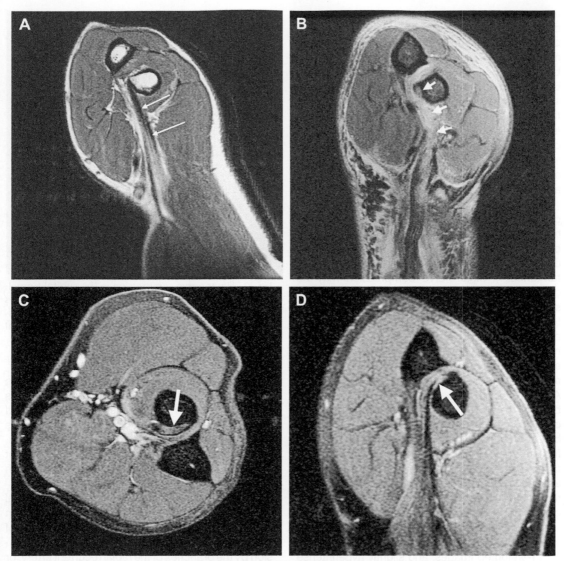

Fig. 21. Distal biceps tendon injuries. Flexed abducted supinated (FABS) fast-spin echo (FSE) image (*A*) shows the normal distal biceps insertion (*thin white arrow*) in a 49-year-old man. FABS fat-saturated FSE image (*B*) in a 71-year-old man shows complete rupture of the distal biceps tendon with tendon retraction (*short white arrows*). In a 58-year-old man, the axial view (*C*) shows a partial tear of the distal biceps tendon (*white arrow*); however, this is better seen on the FABS view (*D*).

commonly occur at the insertion site. Partial ruptures are characterized by a small fluid-filled defect within the distal triceps tendon. Complete rupture shows a large fluid-filled gap between the distal triceps tendon and the olecranon process, with variable tendon retraction.[81]

NEUROPATHIES

The radial, median, and ulnar nerves are vulnerable to compression as they pass through their myofascial or fibroosseous tunnels at the elbow. Compression neuropathies may mimic ligamentous or tendinous pathology clinically, presenting with localized elbow pain. Imaging of the nerve is most useful to help confirm the level of compression (seen as a change in the nerve's caliber or signal, or apparent through distal muscle denervation or atrophy) and to investigate a possible specific cause of the compression (such as a space-occupying mass). Usually, no specific cause is found and the imaging is a useful means to exclude a remediable cause.

Ulnar Nerve and Cubital Tunnel Syndrome

The ulnar nerve may be injured by an isolated traumatic event, compressed at the elbow within the cubital tunnel, or secondarily involved through other medial joint pathology. Ulnar neuropathy commonly occurs in association with MCL injury, medial epicondylitis, and flexor-pronator strain. Up to 40% of athletes with MCL injury[82] and 60% of patients with medial epicondylitis[83] have symptoms of ulnar neuropathy. Compression of the ulnar nerve at the elbow is referred to as *cubital tunnel syndrome*. Patients present with aching pain on the medial aspect of the elbow and proximal forearm with or without sensory symptoms along the ulnar border of the hand and ulnar one and half digits.

At the elbow joint, the ulnar nerve may be compressed by the snapping action of the medial head of the triceps muscle during elbow flexion,[84] between the humeral and ulnar heads of the flexor carpi ulnaris,[67] or more commonly, within the cubital tunnel.[85] Ulnar nerve compression may be caused by a cubitus valgus deformity of the elbow, synovitis, medial trochlear osteophytes, hematoma in the setting of MCL rupture, ganglia, loose bodies, muscle hypertrophy, or a thickened retinaculum.[55] The cubital retinaculum is congenitally absent in up to 10% of the population or may be replaced by the anconeus epitrochlearis muscle.[85] Absence of the retinaculum results in hypermobility of the nerve and may result in subluxation or dislocation of the nerve. The nerve may also be spontaneously compressed during elbow flexion when the cubital tunnel retinaculum is taut.[85] When the retinaculum is replaced by the anconeus epitrochlearis muscle, the capacity of the cubital tunnel is greatly reduced, which may contribute to nerve compression (**Fig. 22**).[86]

The ulnar nerve is best seen on axial images and should be of uniform signal, isointense to muscle on T1-weighted images, and slightly hyperintense to muscle on T2-weighted images. The nerve is superficially located at the elbow and is almost always surrounded by a ring of fat. Thickening of the nerve proximal to the point of compression and increased signal intensity may occur. In more chronic cases, changes of denervation and atrophy in the adjacent flexor carpi ulnaris and flexor digitorum profundus muscles may be seen (**Fig. 23**A and B).[87]

Radial Nerve and Radial Tunnel Syndrome

Compression of the radial nerve at the elbow presents clinically as radial tunnel syndrome, a syndrome most commonly seen in sports or occupations requiring repetitive rotatory movements of the forearm. Patients present with pain in the radial aspect of the forearm with localized pain to palpation just distal to the lateral

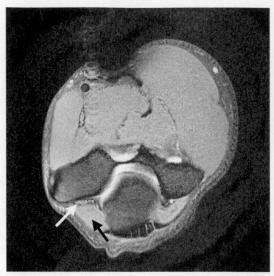

Fig. 22. Ulnar nerve compression in the cubital tunnel. Axial fast-spin echo image in a 38-year-old man shows the anconeus epitrochlearis (*black arrow*), compressing the ulnar nerve (*white arrow*) in the cubital tunnel.

epicondyle. Numbness in the distribution of the radial nerve and weakness of wrist extensors may be present.[88] In the absence of sensory and motor symptoms, localized pain and tenderness may mimic the presentation of lateral epicondylitis. Radial tunnel syndrome is therefore an important differential diagnosis in patients presenting with lateral elbow pain.[64]

Compression of the radial nerve within the radial tunnel may be caused by radial head subluxation or a Monteggia fracture, synovitis, or thickening of the anterior capsule of the elbow joint, and compression by the branches of the radial recurrent artery, or by mass lesions such as ganglia.[19,21,88] Compression of the posterior interosseous nerve (PIN) is referred to as deep radial nerve syndrome or supinator syndrome.[20] The PIN may be compressed as it passes beneath the arcade of Frohse or between the two layers of the supinator muscle.[21,89,90] Although the radial nerve and PIN are difficult to identify at the elbow, MR imaging may be useful to detect space-occupying lesions (**Fig. 24**A and B) that may be responsible for nerve compression and to detect secondary changes of denervation in the extensor muscles of the forearm.[91]

Entrapment of the PIN is seen in up to 5% of patients who have lateral epicondylitis.[76] The symptoms of PIN compression may also mimic those of lateral epicondylitis. The fat planes around the PIN should therefore be evaluated in all patients presenting with lateral joint pain and symptoms suggesting lateral epicondylitis.[92]

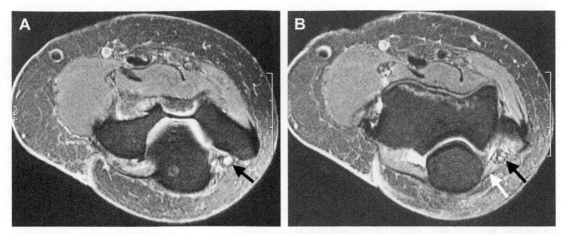

Fig. 23. Ulnar neuritis with distal denervation. Axial fat-saturated fast-spin echo images (*A, B*) show ulnar neuritis with high signal in the ulnar nerve (*black arrow*) and associated high signal in the flexor digitorum profundus (*white arrow*) secondary to denervation. (*Courtesy of* Dr. Tony Peduto, Castlereagh Imaging, Westmead.)

Median Nerve and Pronator Syndrome

Median nerve entrapment at the elbow results in the pronator syndrome.[20,93] It is most commonly seen in sports that involve repetitive pronation and supination of the forearm. Patients present with pain in the volar aspect of the forearm with or without sensory symptoms in the radial two and a half digits, and weakness of the thenar muscles. Symptoms are exacerbated by resisted pronation of the forearm.[19,94,95]

Compression of the median nerve can occur at multiple sites. At the elbow, the most frequent site of compression is at the pronator teres muscle where the nerve may be compressed by a fibrous band as it runs between the superficial and deep heads of the pronator teres muscle. The next most common site of compression is by a fibrous arch formed by the proximal margin of the flexor digitorum superficialis muscle. The median nerve may also be compressed at the elbow by a thick bicipital aponeurosis or a scarred lacertus

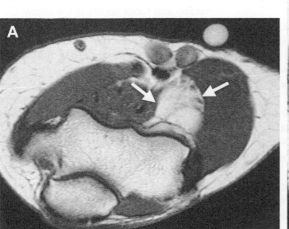

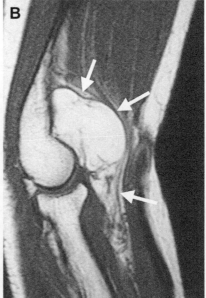

Fig. 24. Radial nerve compression. Sagittal (*A*) and axial (*B*) fast-spin echo images show a lipoma (*white arrow*) compressing the radial nerve, close to the origin of the posterior interosseous nerve. (*Courtesy of* Dr. Tony Peduto, Castlereagh Imaging, Westmead.)

fibrosis.[19,94,95] Although the median nerve is difficult to identify at the elbow because of the minimal amount of perifascicular fat, MR imaging may be useful to detect space-occupying lesions or secondary changes of denervation in the pronator teres muscle.[91]

SUMMARY

MR imaging of the elbow is a useful and important investigation in sports injuries of the elbow. Recreational and professional sporting persons can injure their elbow in many different ways, and a good clinical evaluation helps to direct the MR imaging examination. The most common injuries are lateral epicondylitis, MCL injury, and distal biceps tendon injury. Nerve compression syndromes often require investigation, but the goal of imaging is mainly to exclude a space-occupying lesion and occasionally to show distal muscle denervation. Acute or chronic ligamentous injuries of the A-MCL and LUCL are associated with well-recognized clinical instability syndromes. MR images should be carefully examined for secondary signs that may indicate an instability syndrome of the elbow.

ACKNOWLEDGMENTS

Grateful acknowledgment is made to Dr. Dzung Vu, anatomist and artist, for assistance with **Figs. 3** and **5**, and to Dr. Jeff Hughes, orthopaedic surgeon, and Dr. Ken Crichton, sports physician, for their clinical input.

REFERENCES

1. Morrey B. Anatomy of the elbow joint. In: Morrey B, editor. The elbow and its disorders. Philadelphia: Saunders; 1993. p. 16–52.
2. Morrey BF, An KN. Articular and ligamentous contributions to the stability of the elbow joint. Am J Sports Med 1983;11:315–9.
3. Regan WD, Korinek SL, Morrey BF, et al. Biomechanical study of ligaments around the elbow joint. Clin Orthop Rel Res 1991;271:170–9.
4. Morrey BF, An KN. Functional anatomy of ligaments of the elbow. Clin Orthop Rel Res 1985;201:84–90.
5. O'Driscoll SW, Horii E, Morrey B, et al. Anatomy of the ulnar part of the lateral collateral ligament of the elbow. Clin Anat 1992;5:296–303.
6. Rosenberg ZS, Beltran J, Cheung Y, et al. MR imaging of the elbow: normal variant and potential diagnostic pitfalls of the trochlear groove and cubital tunnel. Am J Roentgenol 1995;164:415–8.
7. O'Driscoll SW, Morrey BF, Korinek S, et al. Elbow subluxation and dislocation—a spectrum of instability. Clin Orthop Rel Res 1992;280:186–97.
8. Gaary EA, Potter HG, Altchek DW. Medial elbow pain the throwing athlete: MR imaging evaluation. Am J Roentgenol 1997;168:795–800.
9. Floris S, Olsen BS, Dalstra M, et al. The medial collateral ligament of the elbow joint: anatomy and kinematics. J Shoulder Elbow Surg 1998;7:345–51.
10. Callaway GH, Field LD, Deng XH, et al. Biomechanical evaluation of the medial collateral ligament of the elbow. J Bone Joint Surg Am 1997;79A:1223–31.
11. O'Driscoll SW, Bell DF, Morrey BF. Posterolateral rotatory instability of the elbow. J Bone Joint Surg Am 1991;73A:440–6.
12. Olsen BS, Vaesel MT, Sojbjerg JO, et al. Lateral collateral ligament of the elbow joint: anatomy and kinematics. J Shoulder Elbow Surg 1996;5:103–12.
13. Dunning CE, Zarzour ZDS, Patterson SD, et al. Ligamentous stabilizers against posterolateral rotatory instability of the elbow. J Bone Joint Surg Am 2001;83A:1823–8.
14. Morrey B, Sanchez-Sotelo J. The elbow and its disorders. Philadelphia: Saunders Elsevier; 2009.
15. Takigawa N, Ryu J, Kish VL, et al. Functional anatomy of the lateral collateral ligament complex of the elbow: morphology and strain. J Hand Surg Br 2005;30B:143–7.
16. Giuffre BM, Moss MJ. Optimal positioning for MR imaging of the distal biceps brachii tendon: flexed abducted supinated view. Am J Roentgenol 2004; 182:944–6.
17. Sanal HT, Chen L, Negrao P, et al. Distal attachment of the brachialis muscle: anatomic and MR imaging study in cadavers. Am J Roentgenol 2009;192: 468–72.
18. Belentani C, Pastore D, Wangwinyuvirat M, et al. Triceps brachii tendon: anatomic-MR imaging study in cadavers with histologic correlation. Skeletal Radiol 2009;38:171–5.
19. Posner MA. Compressive neuropathies of the median and radial nerves at the elbow. Clin Sports Med 1990;9:343–63.
20. Andreisek G, Crook DW, Burg D, et al. Peripheral neuropathies of the median, radial, and ulnar nerves: MR imaging features. Radiographics 2006; 26:1267–87.
21. Spinner M. The arcade of Frohse and its relationship to posterior interosseous nerve paralysis. J Bone Joint Surg Br 1968;50:809–12.
22. Nakanishi K, Masatomi T, Ochi T, et al. MR arthrography of elbow: evaluation of the ulnar collateral ligament of elbow. Skeletal Radiol 1996;25:629–34.
23. Schwartz ML, Alzahrani S, Morwessel RM, et al. Ulnar collateral ligament injury in the throwing athlete—evaluation with saline-enhanced MR arthrography. Radiology 1995;197:297–9.
24. Kaplan LJ, Potter HG. MR imaging of ligament injuries to the elbow. Magn Reson Imaging Clin N Am 2004;12:221–32.

25. Carrino JA, Morrison WB, Zou KH, et al. Lateral ulnar collateral ligament of the elbow: optimization of evaluation with two-dimensional MR imaging. Radiology 2001;218:118–25.

26. Cotten A, Jacobson J, Brossmann J, et al. Collateral ligaments of the elbow: conventional MR imaging and MR arthrography with coronal oblique plane and elbow flexion. Radiology 1997;204:806–12.

27. Tuite MJ, Kijowski R. Sports-related injuries of the elbow: an approach to MRI interpretation. Clin Sports Med 2006;25:387–408.

28. Glajchen N, Schwartz ML, Andrews JR, et al. Avulsion fracture of the sublime tubercle of the ulna: a newly recognized injury in the throwing athlete. Am J Roentgenol 1998;170:627–8.

29. Salvo JP, Rizio L, Zvijac JE, et al. Avulsion fracture of the ulnar sublime tubercle in overhead throwing athletes. Am J Sports Med 2002;30:426–31.

30. O'Driscoll SW. Classification and evaluation of recurrent instability of the elbow. Clin Orthop Rel Res 2000;370:34–43.

31. Hulkko A, Orava S, Nikula P. Stress fractures of the olecranon in javelin throwers. Int J Sports Med 1986;7:210–3.

32. Maffulli N, Chan D, Aldridge MJ. Overuse injuries of the olecranon in young gymnasts. J Bone Joint Surg Br 1992;74:305–8.

33. Rosenberg ZS, Beltran J, Cheung YY. Psuedodefect of the capitellum—potential MR imaging pitfall. Radiology 1994;191:821–3.

34. Faber KJ. Coronal shear fractures of the distal humerus: the capitellum and trochlea. Hand Clin 2004;20:455–64.

35. Omer GE Jr. Primary articular osteochondroses. Clin Orthop Relat Res 1981;158:33–40.

36. Brown R, Blazina ME, Kerlan RK, et al. Osteochondritis of the capitellum. J Sports Med 1974;2: 27–46.

37. Takahara M, Shundo M, Kondo M, et al. Early detection of osteochondritis dissecans of the capitellum in young baseball players—report of three cases. J Bone Joint Surg Am 1998;80A:892–7.

38. Kijowski R, De Smet AA. MRI findings of osteochondritis dissecans of the capitellum with surgical correlation. Am J Roentgenol 2005;185:1453–9.

39. Peiss J, Adam G, Casser R, et al. Gadopentetate dimeglumine enhanced MR imaging of osteonecrosis and osteochondritis dissecans of the elbow—initial experience. Skeletal Radiol 1995;24:17–20.

40. Resnick D, Goergen T. Growth plate injuries about the elbow. In: Resnick D, Goergen T, editors. Diagnosis of bone and joint disorders. Philadelphia: WB Saunders; 2002. p. 2742–6.

41. Sugimoto H, Ohsawa T. Ulnar collateral ligament in the growing elbow—MR imaging of normal development and throwing injuries. Radiology 1994;192: 417–22.

42. Potter HG. Imaging of posttraumatic and soft tissue dysfunction of the elbow. Clin Orthop Rel Res 2000; 370:9–18.

43. Ciccotti MG, Jobe FW. Medial collateral ligament instability and ulnar neuritis in the athlete's elbow. Instr Course Lect 1999;48:383–91.

44. Jobe FW, Nuber G. Throwing injuries of the elbow. Clin Sports Med 1986;5:621–36.

45. Hang YS, Lippert FG III, Spolek GA, et al. Biomechanical study of the pitching elbow. Int Orthop 1979;3:217–23.

46. Timmerman LA, Schwartz ML, Andrews JR. Preoperative evaluation of the ulnar collateral ligament by magnetic resonance imaging and computed tomography arthrography. Evaluation in 25 baseball players with surgical confirmation. Am J Sports Med 1994;22:26–31 [discussion: 32].

47. Cain EL, Dugas JR, Andrews JR. Ulnar nerve injury in the throwing athlete. Sports Med Arthroscopy Rev 2003;11:40–6.

48. Field LD, Savoie FH. The arthroscopic evaluation and management of elbow trauma and instability. Oper Tech Sports Med 1998;6:22–8.

49. Bennett J, Tullos H. Acute injuries to the elbow. In: Nicholas J, Hershman E, editors. The upper extremity in sports medicine. St Louis (MO): Mosby; 1990. p. 326–7.

50. Potter HG, Ho ST, Altchek DW. Magnetic resonance imaging of the elbow. Semin Musculoskelet Radiol 2004;8:5–16.

51. Timmerman LA, Andrews JR. Undersurface tear of the ulnar collateral ligament in baseball players. A newly recognized lesion. Am J Sports Med 1994;22:33–6.

52. Munshi M, Pretterklieber ML, Chung CB, et al. Anterior bundle of ulnar collateral ligament: evaluation of anatomic relationships by using MR imaging, MR arthrography, and gross anatomic and histologic analysis. Radiology 2004;231:797–803.

53. Ouellette H, Bredella M, Labis J, et al. MR imaging of the elbow in baseball pitchers. Skeletal Radiol 2008; 37:115–21.

54. Wilson FD, Andrews JR, Blackburn TA, et al. Valgus extension overload in the pitching elbow. Am J Sports Med 1983;11:83–8.

55. Kijowski R, Tuite M, Sanford M. Magnetic resonance imaging of the elbow. Part II: abnormalities of the ligaments, tendons, and nerves. Skeletal Radiol 2005;34:1–18.

56. Anderson J, Read J. Atlas of imaging in sports medicine. Sydney: McGraw-Hill; 2008.

57. Nestor BJ, Odriscoll SW, Morrey BF. Ligamentous reconstruction for posterolateral rotatory instability of the elbow. J Bone Joint Surg Am 1992;74A:1235–41.

58. Potter HG, Weiland AJ, Schatz JA, et al. Posterolateral rotatory instability of the elbow: usefulness of MR imaging in diagnosis. Radiology 1997;204: 185–9.

59. Frostick SP, Mohammad M, Ritchie DA. Sport injuries of the elbow. Br J Sports Med 1999;33: 301–11.

60. Maylack FH. Epidemiology of tennis, squash, and racquetball injuries. Clin Sports Med 1988;7:233–43.

61. Coonrad RW, Hooper WR. Tennis elbow: its course, natural history, conservative and surgical management. J Bone Joint Surg Am 1973;55:1177–82.

62. Aoki M, Wada T, Isogai S, et al. Magnetic resonance imaging findings of refractory tennis elbows and their relationship to surgical treatment. J Shoulder Elbow Surg 2005;14:172–7.

63. Morris M, Jobe FW, Perry J, et al. Electromyographic analysis of elbow function in tennis players. Am J Sports Med 1989;17:241–7.

64. Nirschl RP, Pettrone FA. Tennis elbow. The surgical treatment of lateral epicondylitis. J Bone Joint Surg Am 1979;61:832–9.

65. Bredella MA, Tirman PFJ, Fritz RC, et al. MR imaging findings of lateral ulnar collateral ligament abnormalities in patients with lateral epicondylitis. Am J Roentgenol 1999;173:1379–82.

66. Nirschl RP, Ashman ES. Elbow tendinopathy: tennis elbow. Clin Sports Med 2003;22:813–36.

67. Campbell WW, Pridgeon RM, Sahni SK. Entrapment neuropathy of the ulnar nerve at its point of exit from the flexor carpi ulnaris muscle. Muscle Nerve 1988; 11:467–70.

68. Martin CE, Schweitzer ME. MR imaging of epicondylitis. Skeletal Radiol 1998;27:133–8.

69. Ollivierre CO, Nirschl RP, Pettrone FA. Resection and repair for medial tennis elbow. A prospective analysis. Am J Sports Med 1995;23:214–21.

70. Nirschl RP. Elbow tendinosis/tennis elbow. Clin Sports Med 1992;11:851–70.

71. Skaf AY, Boutin RD, Dantas RWM, et al. Bicipitoradial bursitis: MR imaging findings in eight patients and anatomic data from contrast material opacification of bursae followed by routine radiography and MR imaging in cadavers. Radiology 1999;212:111–6.

72. Agins HJ, Chess JL, Hoekstra DV, et al. Rupture of the distal insertion of the biceps brachii tendon. Clin Orthop Rel Res 1988;234:34–8.

73. Friedmann E. Rupture of distal biceps brachii tendon—report on 13 cases. JAMA 1963;184:60–3.

74. Falchook FS, Zlatkin MB, Erbacher GE, et al. Rupture of the distal biceps tendon—evaluation with MR imaging. Radiology 1994;190:659–63.

75. Williams BD, Schweitzer ME, Weishaupt D, et al. Partial tears of the distal biceps tendon: MR appearance and associated clinical findings. Skeletal Radiol 2001;30:560–4.

76. Safran MR. Elbow injuries in athletes—a review. Clin Orthop Rel Res 1995;310:257–77.

77. Herzog RJ. Magnetic Resonance Imaging of the elbow. Magn Reson Q 1993;9:188–210.

78. Anderson KJ, Lecocq JF. Rupture of the triceps tendon. J Bone Joint Surg Am 1957;39:444–6.

79. Bach BR Jr, Warren RF, Wickiewicz TL. Triceps rupture. A case report and literature review. Am J Sports Med 1987;15:285–9.

80. Sollender JL, Rayan GM, Barden GA. Triceps tendon rupture in weight lifters. J Shoulder Elbow Surg 1998;7:151–3.

81. Gaines ST, Durbin RA, Marsalka DS. The use of magnetic resonance imaging in the diagnosis of triceps tendon ruptures. Contemp Orthop 1990;20:607–11.

82. Chen FS, Rokito AS, Jobe FW. Medial elbow problems in the overhead-throwing athlete. J Am Acad Orthop Surg 2001;9:99–113.

83. Teitz CC, Garrett WE Jr, Miniaci A, et al. Tendon problems in athletic individuals. Instr Course Lect 1997;46:569–82.

84. Hayashi Y, Kojima T, Kohno T. A case of cubital tunnel syndrome caused by the snapping of the medial head of the triceps brachii muscle. J Hand Surg Am 1984;9:96–9.

85. O'Driscoll SW, Horii E, Carmichael SW, et al. The cubital tunnel and ulnar neuropathy. J Bone Joint Surg Br 1991;73:613–7.

86. Dahners LE, Wood FM. Anconeus epitrochlearis, a rare cause of cubital tunnel syndrome: a case report. J Hand Surg Am 1984;9:579–80.

87. Britz GW, Haynor DR, Kuntz C, et al. Ulnar nerve entrapment at the elbow: correlation of magnetic resonance imaging, clinical, electrodiagnostic, and intraoperative findings. Neurosurgery 1996;38: 458–65 [discussion: 465].

88. Lister GD, Belsole RB, Kleinert HE. The radial tunnel syndrome. J Hand Surg Am 1979;4:52–9.

89. Spinner M, Freundlich BD, Teicher J. Posterior interosseous nerve palsy as a complication of Monteggia fractures in children. Clin Orthop Relat Res 1968;58:141–5.

90. Spinner RJ, Lins RE, Collins AJ, et al. Posterior interosseous nerve compression due to an enlarged bicipital bursa confirmed by MR IMAGING. J Hand Surg Br 1993;18:753–6.

91. Rosenberg ZS, Beltran J, Cheung YY, et al. The elbow: MR features of nerve disorders. Radiology 1993;188:235–40.

92. Jobe FW, Ciccotti MG. Lateral and medial epicondylitis of the elbow. J Am Acad Orthop Surg 1994;2:1–8.

93. Rosenberg ZS, Bencardino J, Beltran J. MR features of nerve disorders at the elbow. Magn Reson Imaging Clin N Am 1997;5:545–65.

94. Hartz CR, Linscheid RL, Gramse RR, et al. The pronator teres syndrome: compressive neuropathy of the median nerve. J Bone Joint Surg Am 1981; 63:885–90.

95. Johnson RK, Spinner M, Shrewsbury MM. Median nerve entrapment syndrome in the proximal forearm. J Hand Surg Am 1979;4:48–51.

MR Imaging of Traumatic and Overuse Injuries of the Wrist and Hand in Athletes

David A. Lisle, MBBS, FRANZCR[a,b,c,*],
Gary J. Shepherd, MBBS, FRANZCR[d],
Gregory A. Cowderoy, MBBS, FRANZCR[e],
Paul T. O'Connell, MBBS, FRANZCR[f]

KEYWORDS
- Hand • MR imaging • Sports injuries
- Sports medicine • Trauma • Wrist

Injuries to the wrist and hand are common in athletes, comprising 3% to 9% of all athletic injuries.[1] Many of the injuries caused by athletic activities may also be seen in work-related and occupational health settings. Most bony injuries of the wrist and hand are diagnosed with clinical assessment and plain radiographs. The accuracy of radiographic assessment may be enhanced with various stress maneuvers to assess for carpal instability. Multidetector row CT may assist in surgical planning for complex injuries, such as comminuted fractures of the distal radius. Scintigraphy has been used to diagnose radiographically occult fractures in situations where an immediate diagnosis is required. The ability of MR imaging to image accurately the bony cortex and bone marrow makes it an ideal modality for the diagnosis of radiographically occult bony injuries.[2]

As with bony disorders, traumatic and overuse injuries of tendons, ligaments, and nerves are often diagnosed and managed adequately with clinical assessment alone. In most situations, a plain radiograph is performed to exclude associated or unexpected skeletal pathology. Clinical assessment may be supplemented by simple clinical tests, such as nerve conduction studies. Increasingly, however, more sophisticated imaging is being used to diagnose soft tissue pathology of the wrist and hand. Musculoskeletal ultrasound and MR imaging provide accurate imaging of most of the tendons, ligaments, nerves, and arteries of the wrist and hand. Musculoskeletal ultrasound has been employed in many applications, particularly in those parts of the world where this modality has been used to a high standard for many years.[3] Major limitations of musculoskeletal ultrasound include the difficulty of imaging accurately some of the intrinsic structures of the wrist, including the triangular fibrocartilage complex (TFCC), as well as its inability to image bone bruises and other subtle bony pathology. With the use of high-resolution coils and appropriate imaging sequences, MR imaging is able to image most of the relevant structures, including small intrinsic finger ligaments and pulleys.

[a] Division of Medical Imaging, University of Queensland Medical School, Herston, Brisbane Q 4029, Australia
[b] Queensland Diagnostic Imaging, 259 Wickham Terrace, Brisbane Q 4000, Australia
[c] The Royal Chidlren's Hospital, Brisbane, Australia
[d] Qscan Radiology Clinics, PO Box 222, RBH Post Office, Herston, Brisbane Q 4029, Australia
[e] Radiology Department, Queensland Diagnostic Imaging, Brisbane Private Hospital, 259 Wickham Terrace, Brisbane Q 4000, Queensland, Australia
[f] Queensland Diagnostic Imaging, St Andrews Hospital, Brisbane, Australia
* Corresponding author. 17 Ayr Street, Riccarton, Christchurch 8011, New Zealand.
E-mail address: dlisle97@gmail.com (D.A. Lisle).

Magn Reson Imaging Clin N Am 17 (2009) 639–654
doi:10.1016/j.mric.2009.06.007

OCCULT FRACTURES AND BONE BRUISES

Approximately one sixth of scaphoid fractures are radiographically occult at the time of initial presentation.[4] Other carpal fractures may also be difficult to diagnose radiographically. The usefulness of MR imaging in occult wrist fractures, including cortical fractures and bone bruises, has been described.[4] A recent study comparing multidetector row CT and MR imaging for the assessment of occult scaphoid fractures demonstrated multidetector row CT to have a higher sensitivity for the detection of cortical fractures, whereas MR imaging was superior at diagnosing trabecular injury.[5] MR imaging is able to diagnose occult scaphoid fractures with a high degree of accuracy, including 100% negative predictive value in the immature skeleton (**Fig. 1**).[2] Other radiographically occult sports-related wrist fractures, such as hook of hamate fracture caused by striking the ground with a golf club, may also be diagnosed on MR imaging (**Fig. 2**). A fracture is seen on MR imaging as a low-signal line extending across the bone on all sequences,[2] accompanied by marrow edema. MR imaging examination of the wrist to screen for radiographically occult scaphoid fractures at the time of initial presentation has been shown to be a cost-effective protocol.[6] This may be especially true in elite athletes, for whom an immediate diagnosis is paramount.

Also known by the term *bone contusion*, a bone bruise consists of injury to trabeculae without other evidence of fracture.[7] Unable to be diagnosed radiographically or with CT, bone bruises are seen on MR imaging as areas of increased

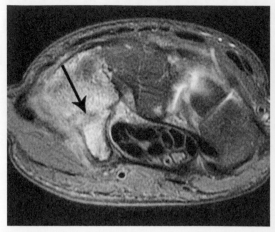

Fig. 2. Hook of hamate fracture. Axial fat-saturated T2-weighted sequence shows a fracture line through the base of the hook of the hamate (*arrow*) with marrow edema of the hook and body of the hamate.

marrow signal on fluid-weighted, fat-suppressed sequences (**Fig. 3**).

STRESS FRACTURES

Stress fracture, also known by the term *fatigue fracture*, occurs when repetitive stress is applied to normal bone. Repetitive stress, sometimes accompanied by muscle fatigue, leads to a pathologic continuum of microdamage that exceeds bony repair, leading to eventual structural failure and fracture.[8] More common in weight-bearing parts of the skeleton, stress fractures have also been

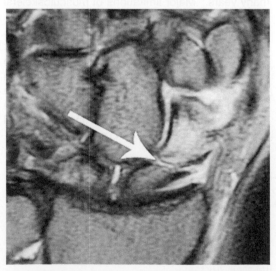

Fig. 1. Scaphoid fracture. Coronal fat-saturated T2-weighted sequence shows a fracture line through the waist of the scaphoid (*arrow*) with marrow edema in the proximal pole.

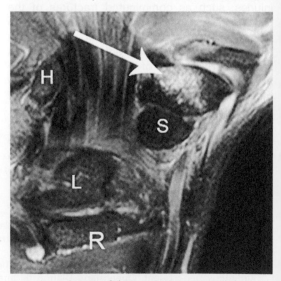

Fig. 3. Bone bruise of the trapezium. Coronal short tau inversion recovery (STIR) sequence in a 44-year-old male with persistent wrist pain after a fall shows focal marrow edema in the trapezium (*arrow*). Note normal marrow signal in the hook of hamate (H), lunate (L), scaphoid (S), and radius (R).

reported in the upper limb, including the wrist and hand. Stress fracture of the scaphoid is described in activities that involve repeated dorsiflexion of the wrist, including shot putting and gymnastics.[9] Other much less commonly reported sites of stress fractures include the hook of hamate in racquet sports,[10] the pisiform in volleyball,[11] the triquetrum in break dancing,[12] the second metacarpal in tennis,[13] and the fifth metacarpal in a softball pitcher.[14] MR imaging is as accurate as scintigraphy at demonstrating stress fractures.[15] MR imaging findings of an early stress reaction include marrow edema and periosteal fluid. This may progress to a stress fracture, which is seen on MR imaging as a low-signal line or cortical breach.[15] MR imaging may be used to grade stress injuries and to assist in the management of these injuries in elite athletes, with tailoring of the required duration of cessation of inciting activity.[16]

A particular type of stress injury, epiphysiolysis, may be seen affecting the distal radius in adolescent gymnasts.[15] This injury, which may be bilateral, is thought to be due to repeated compressive forces causing stress fracture of the distal radial growth plate or metaphyseal failure.[17] MR imaging findings in distal radial epiphysiolysis include widening of the growth plate, extending of physeal cartilage tongues into the metaphysis, and bruising of metaphyseal bone (**Fig. 4**).[17]

OSTEONECROSIS OF THE WRIST

Osteonecrosis not associated with a fracture may affect the lunate, scaphoid, and, less commonly,

the capitate and hook of hamate. These bones are at risk of developing osteonecrosis because of the relatively limited nature of their vascularity.[18] Osteonecrosis of the lunate, also known as Kienböck disease, most commonly affects young male manual workers.[19] Plain radiographs are usually adequate for diagnosis, staging, and treatment planning, though MR imaging may be useful in early cases.[19] MR imaging in Kienböck disease shows reduced signal in the lunate on T1- and T2-weighted images,[18] with fragmentation and collapse seen in advanced cases (**Fig. 5**). Preiser disease refers to osteonecrosis of the scaphoid in the absence of a scaphoid fracture. Preiser disease may be due to repetitive microtrauma or as a complication of drug therapy.[2] MR imaging is the method of choice for the diagnosis of Preiser disease.[2] Two patterns of osteonecrosis as defined by MR imaging are described.[20] Type I cases show MR imaging signal abnormality involving the whole of the scaphoid. Type II cases show MR imaging signal changes limited to 50% or less of the scaphoid, and generally have a better prognosis. MR imaging signal changes range from ischemia in early cases, with low signal on T1 and patchy high signal on T2, to frank necrosis in more established cases, producing reduced signal on all sequences (**Fig. 6**).

BONY IMPACTION (ABUTMENT) SYNDROMES

Impaction syndromes may occur secondary to trauma or surgery, or result from activities that lead to excessive carpal loading. Various anatomic variants predispose to the development of these syndromes. Impaction syndromes are usually

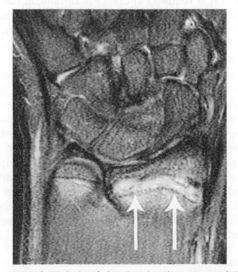

Fig. 4. Epiphysiolysis of the distal radius. Coronal STIR sequence in a 14-year-old gymnast with persistent wrist pain worsened by activity shows increased signal, widening, and irregularity of the distal radial growth plate (*arrows*).

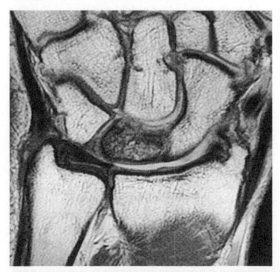

Fig. 5. Avascular necrosis of the lunate (Kienböck disease). Coronal proton density sequence shows abnormal low signal throughout the marrow of the lunate with irregularity of the cortical margins.

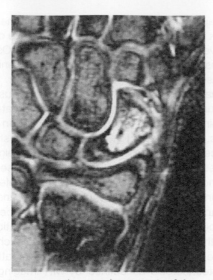

Fig. 6. Nontraumatic avascular necrosis of the scaphoid (Preiser disease). Coronal STIR sequence shows abnormal high signal throughout the marrow of the scaphoid with irregularity of the cortical surface of the proximal pole.

diagnosed with clinical assessment and plain radiography. MR imaging may also be useful to confirm the diagnosis as well to document specific findings in relation to cartilage and bone marrow changes and to associated injuries of the TFCC and other structures.

Ulnar impaction syndrome, also known as ulnocarpal abutment, is a degenerative condition of the ulnar side of the wrist. Ulnar variance, which refers to the relative lengths of the distal articular surfaces of the radius and ulna, is independent of the length of the ulnar styloid process.[21] Positive ulnar variance exists where the distal ulnar articular surface projects distal to the radius. Positive ulnar variance predisposes patients to ulnar impaction syndrome and may be congenital in nature or secondary to malunion of a distal radial fracture.[22]

Ulnar styloid impaction is caused by an excessively long ulnar styloid process or a nonunited styloid process impacting on the proximal triquetrum.[23] Ulnar impingement syndrome occurs in association with a short ulna (negative ulnar variance). Ulnar shortening may be congenital or due to previous surgery or trauma.[24] The shortened ulna produces a painful pseudarthrosis with the distal radius. Hamatolunate impaction occurs uncommonly where a second articular facet at the distal ulnar surface of the lunate articulates with the hamate.[25] MR imaging findings in these impaction syndromes are similar and include cartilage irregularity, bone marrow edema, subchondral irregularity, and cystic change of the impacting bony surfaces (**Fig. 7**).[26]

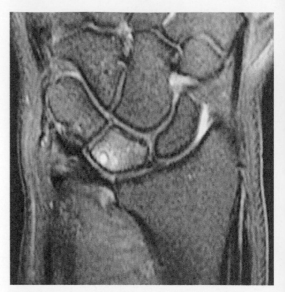

Fig. 7. Ulnar impaction (abutment) syndrome. Coronal STIR shows marrow edema in the lunate with cyst formation deep to the proximal cortical surface.

TENDON TEARS

Tendon tears may be open, due to lacerations, or closed. Tendon tears more commonly involve the extensor tendons and extensor mechanism of the fingers than the flexor tendons.[27]

Open Tendon Tears

Most open tendon tears are diagnosed and managed clinically, with no need for imaging assessment beyond plain radiographs. Where imaging is required in complex or difficult cases, ultrasound provides a reliable, noninvasive method for delineating the anatomy of tendon tears. MR imaging may also be used to demonstrate the site of tendon tear and to localize the torn tendon ends. A full-thickness tendon tear is seen on MR imaging as a gap in the tendon with fraying and irregularity of the torn tendon ends (**Fig. 8**).[27] Varying degrees of tendon retraction may be encountered. The complexity and interconnectedness of the extensor mechanism of the fingers often prevents retraction.[28] MR imaging may also be useful for the diagnosis of partial tendon tears.[29] Partial tendon tears are seen on MR imaging as focal areas of increased signal within the tendon on T1-weighted images associated with irregularity of the tendon outline.[27]

Closed Tendon Tears

Closed tendon injuries are usually the result of impaction causing sudden forced stretching of a tendon. Such injuries may also be due to repetitive direct trauma.

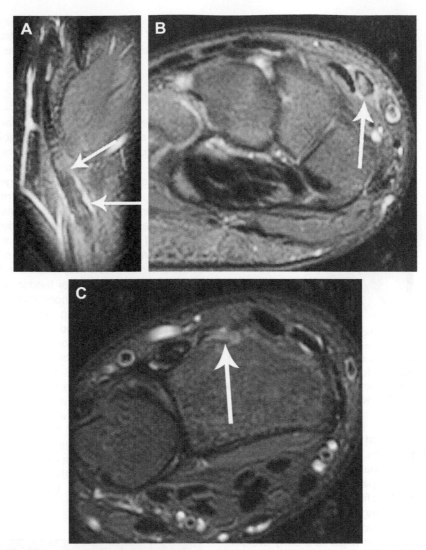

Fig. 8. Tear of the extensor pollicis longus tendon in a 24-year-old male who injured his wrist in a jet-ski accident. (*A*) Oblique coronal STIR sequence shows thickening and irregularity of the extensor pollicis longus tendon with some fluid in the tendon sheath (*arrows*). (*B*) Axial fat-saturated T2-weighted sequence shows thickening and high signal of the distal torn end of the extensor pollicis longus tendon at the level of the wrist joint (*arrow*). (*C*) A more proximal transverse fat-saturated T2-weighted sequence at the level of the distal radius shows the empty third extensor compartment (*arrow*). The proximal torn tendon is retracted into the forearm (not shown).

Jersey finger

The most common closed flexor tendon injury is avulsion of the flexor digitorum profundus. Isolated avulsion of the flexor digitorum superficialis may occur, but is rare.[27] Jersey finger most commonly involves the ring finger and occurs in rugby players as the result of grasping an opponent's clothing. This causes forcible hyperextension of the distal interphalangeal joint resulting in avulsion of the flexor digitorum profundus insertion, with loss of active flexion of the distal interphalangeal joint (**Fig. 9**).[30] Flexor digitorum profundus avulsion is classified into four types, depending on bony involvement and retraction:[30]

Type I: retraction of the flexor digitorum profundus tendon into the palm

Type II: retraction to the proximal interphalangeal (PIP) joint

Type III: avulsed bone fragment held in place distally by the A4 pulley

Type IV: Type III bone avulsion with simultaneous avulsion of the tendon from the bone fragment

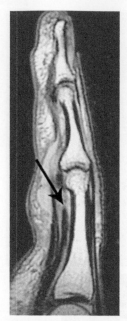

Fig. 9. Tear of the flexor digitorum profundus tendon in the ring finger of a 26-year-old rugby player. Sagittal proton density sequence shows complete avulsion of the flexor digitorum profundus tendon from the base of the distal phalanx. The torn tendon end (*arrow*) is retracted proximally to the level of the A2 pulley.

Mallet finger

Mallet finger is the most common closed extensor tendon injury in athletes. It most commonly occurs in sports that involve ball catching, including softball, baseball, basketball, and netball. Impact of the ball on the tip of the finger causes forced flexion of the distal interphalangeal joint, resulting in avulsion of the terminal extensor tendon. The most common injury in mallet finger is a bony avulsion at the tendon insertion. In cases where the bone fragment is large, there may be volar subluxation of the distal interphalangeal joint. Less commonly, the bone is intact and the tendon itself is ruptured. This type of injury may require imaging with ultrasound or MR imaging to confirm the diagnosis.

Boutonnière injury

Lateral volar dislocation of the PIP joint, acute flexion injury of the PIP joint, or a direct blow to the middle phalanx of an extended finger may result in rupture of the central slip of the extensor tendon at or near to its insertion at the base of the middle phalanx.[31] Central slip disruption may be difficult to recognize in the early acute phase as extension of the PIP joint may be maintained by the lateral bands.[27] With unrecognized injuries the lateral bands displace in a lateral, volar direction resulting in the boutonnière deformity[32] with flexion of the PIP joint and extension of the distal

interphalangeal joint. MR imaging may be particularly useful for the diagnosis of central slip tear in early acute cases, where clinical assessment is difficult.[27]

Extensor (Dorsal) Hood Injury

At the level of the metacarpophalangeal (MCP) joints, the extensor tendons are stabilized by the extensor (dorsal) hood. The extensor hood is composed of fibrous sagittal bands and more distal transverse bands. Each sagittal band is a thin fibrous sheet that extends from the volar plate around the MCP joints to insert into the extensor tendon. More distally, intrinsic extensor muscles of the hand contribute transverse fibers to the extensor hood. Tearing of the sagittal bands of the extensor hood may result in subluxation or dislocation of the extensor tendon at the level of the MCP joint. Extensor hood injuries may occur from a direct blow forcing the finger into flexion, or with forced flexion and ulnar deviation of the finger.[31] The most common site of extensor hood injury is a tear of the radial sagittal band of the middle finger, though any finger may be affected.[31] Injury to the extensor hood may also occur as a result of repetitive trauma in boxers.[33] MR imaging is able to accurately demonstrate extensor hood injuries.[34] Findings on transverse MR images include irregularity, focal discontinuity, and focal thickening of the extensor hood components, especially the sagittal bands, plus subluxation or dislocation of the extensor tendon (Fig. 10).[27]

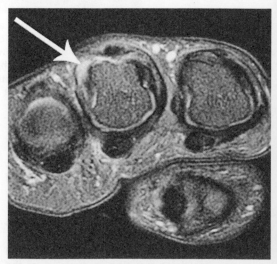

Fig. 10. Dorsal (extensor) hood injury. Axial fat-saturated T2-weighted sequence through the MCP joint of the middle finger shows high signal and discontinuity of the ulnar sagittal band (*arrow*) of the dorsal hood.

Flexor Pulley Injuries

The synovial sheaths surrounding the flexor tunnels in the fingers are bound down by a series of fibrous pulleys. There are five transverse or annular pulleys, numbered from proximal to distal A1 to A5, and three cruciform pulleys. The cruciform pulleys, numbered C1 to C3, consist of criss-crossing fibers. The pulleys are distributed from the MCP joint to the distal interphalangeal joint. The major function of the pulleys is to stabilize the flexor tendons, avoiding displacement or bowstringing during finger flexion.[35] The cruciform pulleys permit deformation of the tendon sheath during flexion without tendon impingement.[27] The A2 pulley, located at the proximal third of the proximal phalanx, and the A4 pulley, located at the midshaft of the middle phalanx, are the broadest and most functionally significant of the pulleys.

Flexor pulley injuries occur in sports that result in forced extension of a flexed finger, most typically in rock climbers.[32] Pulley ruptures related to rock climbing most commonly involve the ring and middle fingers.[35] Injuries typically begin at the A2 pulley, followed by the A3 and A4 pulleys.[32] MR imaging is an accurate technique for the diagnosis of pulley rupture. Disrupted pulleys may be directly visualized on transverse MR images, with thickening, irregularity, and increased signal in the position of the pulley (**Fig. 11**).[27] More commonly, the diagnosis of pulley rupture is made on sagittal images of the flexed finger by visualization of an increased gap between the tendon and the phalanges, commonly referred to as bowstringing.[32] The degree of bowstringing correlates with the underlying injury.[35] In complete tears of the A2 pulley, bowstringing extends from the PIP joint to the base of the proximal phalanx. Bowstringing that does not reach to the base of the proximal phalanx indicates an incomplete tear of the A2 pulley.

TENDON PATHOLOGY RELATED TO OVERUSE

Sports-related overuse syndromes affecting the wrist and hand tendons are common, particularly in sports that involve club or racquet use, such as tennis and golf, and in sports that involve repeated loading and stresses on the wrist, such as rowing and gymnastics.[33] When discussing tendon pathology, it is important to use the correct terminology. Inflammation of tendon synovial sheaths may occur due to repetitive stress and is termed tenosynovitis or tenovaginitis.[28] It is now realized that most tendon pathology related to overuse is degenerative in nature, and not inflammatory. Evidence for this includes histologic studies of chronically symptomatic tendons that show predominantly degenerative changes and little or no inflammation.[36] The term tendinitis, which implies inflammation, has been used incorrectly in the literature to describe painful tendon pathology. The term tendinosis may be used to describe a degenerative pathology of tendon. Tendinopathy is probably a more appropriate term to refer to a symptomatic primary tendon disorder,

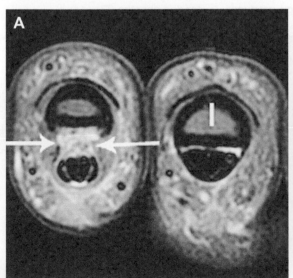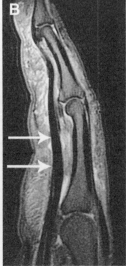

Fig. 11. Tear of the A2 pulley in the middle finger of a 28-year-old rock climber. (A) Axial STIR sequence shows high signal and discontinuity of the A2 pulley (arrows) and a gap between the flexor tendons and the proximal phalanx. Compare this appearance with the normal index finger (I). (B) Sagittal fat-saturated T2-weighted sequence shows bowstringing of the flexor tendon (arrows).

as this makes no assumption as to the underlying pathologic process.[36]

MR imaging findings in tendinopathy and tenosynovitis include tendon thickening and irregularity, areas of high signal within the tendon substance, fluid in the tendon sheath, thickening of the tendon sheath, and edema in surrounding soft tissue planes.[37] The most common sites of tendon pathology due to overuse are the first (abductor pollicis longus and extensor pollicis brevis) and sixth (extensor carpi ulnaris [ECU]) extensor compartments. First-compartment tenosynovitis and tendinopathy, also known as de Quervain tenosynovitis, is commonly seen in rowers, players of racquet sports, and weight trainers.[33] De Quervain tenosynovitis is also a common workplace-related repetitive-stress injury.[38] Sixth-compartment overuse may be encountered in sports requiring repetitive wrist use,[26] such as rowing and tennis. ECU tendinopathy may also be associated with other ulnar-sided wrist pathology, including tears of the TFCC. Subluxation or dislocation of the ECU tendon out of the ulnar groove may be associated with tendinopathy and is usually the result of trauma-producing volar flexion and ulnar deviation of the wrist in golfers, weightlifters, and rodeo riders.[33] Dislocation of ECU is best seen on transverse MR images. These must be performed with the wrist in supination, as in the neutral position or pronation, the dislocated ECU tendon may be normally located in the ulnar groove (**Fig. 12**).

Flexor tendinopathies also occur in golfers and players of racquet sports,[11] and most commonly involve the flexor carpi radialis and the flexor carpi ulnaris. Flexor carpi radialis pathology produces the typical MR imaging findings of tendon swelling and signal change with fluid distension of the tendon sheath. There is no synovial sheath around the flexor carpi ulnaris. Calcific tendinopathy of the flexor carpi ulnaris may be seen just proximal to the insertion of the tendon into the pisiform.[11]

Intersection (Crossover) Syndromes

Two main extensor tendon crossover points have been identified. The more proximal of these, also known as the intersection, is formed by the first extensor compartment tendons crossing superficial to the second extensor compartment. The intersection lies about 4 to 8 cm proximal to the distal radius. The more distal crossover is where the third extensor compartment (extensor pollicis longus) crosses superficial to the second extensor compartment, just distal to the radius. Tendinopathies may occur at these crossover points. Tendinopathy and peritendinitis at the proximal crossover, known as intersection syndrome, occurs in sports that cause overuse and friction, such as rowing, canoe paddling, racquet sports, horseback riding, and skiing.[37] Adventitial bursitis may develop and produce palpable swelling, as well as tenderness and crepitus. The most typical MR imaging finding in intersection syndrome is peritendinous edema surrounding the first and second extensor compartments (**Fig. 13**).[39] A less common intersection tenosynovitis may be seen at the distal crossover. The typical MR imaging appearance of this entity is fluid distending the second and third extensor compartment tendon sheaths (**Fig. 14**).[40]

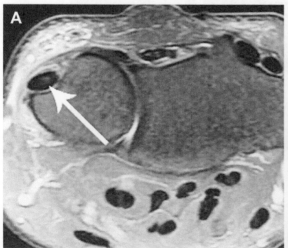 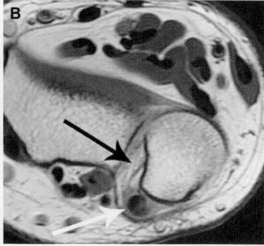

Fig. 12. Tendinopathy and dislocation of the extensor ECU tendon in a 19-year-old tennis player with persistent ulnar-sided wrist pain. (*A*) Axial fat-saturated T2-weighted sequence with the hand pronated shows thickening and increased signal of the ECU tendon (*arrow*). (*B*) Axial proton density sequence with the hand supinated shows dislocation of the ECU tendon (*white arrow*) from the ulnar groove (*black arrow*).

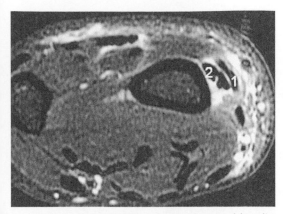

Fig. 13. Intersection syndrome in a 28-year-old cyclist with pain and crepitus in the distal forearm. Axial fat-saturated T2-weighted sequence at the level of the crossover of the first (1) and second (2) extensor compartments shows abnormal high signal in the adjacent soft tissues.

WRIST LIGAMENTS

Wrist stability is maintained by a series of intrinsic and extrinsic ligamentous structures. The most important of the intrinsic structures are the scapholunate ligament (SLL), the lunotriquetral ligament (LTL), and the TFCC. A complex partly ligamentous structure partly composed of fibrocartilage, the TFCC will be considered in this section. The extrinsic ligaments are a series of capsular thickenings that originate in the forearm and insert into the carpal bones. Injury to these intrinsic and extrinsic structures can cause debilitating pain and instability following an injury to the wrist.

The SLL is a C-shaped structure with dorsal and volar transverse fibers plus a central portion. The central portion is composed of fibrocartilage and is best seen on coronal MR images as a delta-shaped structure of intermediate signal.[41] The dorsal band and the thinner, weaker volar band are best seen on transverse images as linear, low-signal structures.[41] The LTL is also C-shaped with dorsal and volar bands and a thin membranous intermediate band. The volar band of LTL is stronger and thicker than the dorsal and intermediate bands. The extrinsic ligaments may be divided into volar and dorsal components. The volar extrinsic ligaments are thicker and stronger than the dorsal and are the major stabilizers during wrist motion.[37]

Acute injuries of the intrinsic and extrinsic wrist ligaments are often diagnosed with a combination of clinical assessment and radiographs. Radiographs may include a variety of stress views to assess for carpal instability. MR imaging may be used in the acute setting to delineate injuries in elite athletes or in complex difficult injuries. More commonly, MR imaging is used to assess patients with wrist pain that fails to resolve following trauma, or patients with chronic pain that may be accentuated by activity. The most commonly encountered wrist ligament injury is tearing of the SLL. SLL injury results from excessive wrist extension and ulnar deviation and is common in any activity that may result in a fall.[1] Traumatic tears of the SLL may be partial or full thickness and may involve the central ligament or either of the bony attachments, more commonly the scaphoid attachment.[41] Tears of the LTL are much less common and may be traumatic or degenerative.

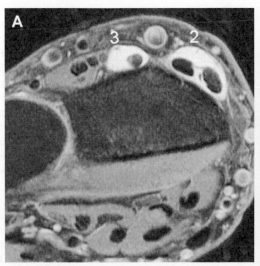

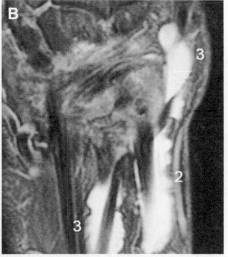

Fig. 14. Distal crossover tenosynovitis. Axial (A) and coronal (B) STIR sequences at the level of the crossover of the second (2) and third (3) extensor compartments show fluid distending the tendon sheaths.

A traumatic tear of the LTL typically results from a fall on a dorsiflexed wrist that forces the forearm into pronation.[26] LTL tears may also be caused by injury sustained in palmar flexion or extreme dorsiflexion in weightlifters and gymnasts.[41]

The reported accuracy of MR imaging in diagnosing intrinsic ligament injuries is variable. Sensitivity and specificity of MR imaging for the diagnosis of SLL tears varies from 50% to 93% and 35% to 89% respectively.[41] Reported sensitivity and specificity for the detection of LTL tears with MR imaging are 40% to 100% and 33% to 100% respectively.[26] The literature on this topic, however, is sometimes difficult to interpret. Some studies assess the performance of MR imaging in a clinical setting, while others use cadaveric wrists.[42] Furthermore, studies vary as to technique, with some investigators using standard MR imaging while others perform MR arthrography. MR arthrography has been reported as superior to standard MR imaging in the diagnosis of wrist ligament tears.[43]

MR imaging signs of ligament rupture include nonvisualization of the ligament; fraying, thinning, and irregularity; and fluid signal traversing the ligament on T2-weighted images.[26,41] Widening of the space between scaphoid and lunate with fraying or elongation of the SLL ligament may also be seen (**Fig. 15**). Widening of the space between the lunate and triquetrum tends not to occur with LTL tear, though loss of normal alignment or "step-off" of the lunotriquetral joint may be seen. (**Fig. 16**).[26] Other signs of carpal instability may also be seen on MR imaging. Tear of the SLL may lead to dorsal intercalated segmental

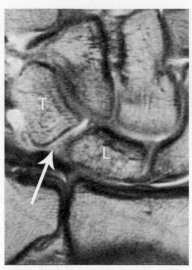

Fig. 16. Tear of the LTL. Coronal proton density sequence shows discontinuity of the LTL (*arrow*) with loss of normal alignment of triquetrum (T) and lunate (L).

instability with increased angle between the axes of scaphoid and lunate (normal range 30–60°) on sagittal scans. Volar intercalated segmental instability with reduced angle between the axes of scaphoid and lunate may be seen in association with LTL tears. However, tears of the intrinsic ligaments alone are usually not sufficient to produce instability. Carpal instability is usually related to combined tears of intrinsic and extrinsic ligaments.[44] MR imaging may also demonstrate extrinsic ligament injuries with torn ligament fibers separated by fluid.[41]

The presence of a ganglion may be a useful sign of chronic intrinsic ligament tear. True ganglia are thin-walled cysts containing viscous mucous fluid. Synovial cysts are the result of joint disruption with herniation of the synovial lining. Up to 30% of wrist ganglia are in fact due to ligament tears with synovial herniation.[45] Such ganglia are most commonly seen arising from the dorsal fibers of SLL (**Fig. 17**). Ganglion formation may also be seen in association with extrinsic ligament disruption.[41] However, wrist ganglia may be found in up to 50% of asymptomatic volunteers.[46] It is therefore important to correlate the presence of a ganglion on MR imaging with clinical findings and to exclude other diagnoses before proceeding to surgical excision.

Triangular Fibrocartilage Complex Tear

The TFCC is a complex structure that functions as a major stabilizer of the distal radioulnar joint and as a cushion for the ulnar carpus.[26] The TFCC is composed of multiple closely related structures: the central fibrocartilage disc, the dorsal and volar

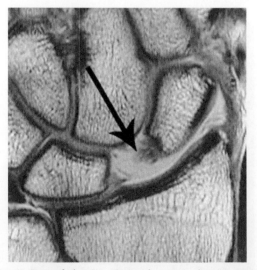

Fig. 15. Tear of the SLL. Coronal proton density sequence shows widening of the gap between the scaphoid and lunate. Torn fibers of the SLL are shown (*arrow*).

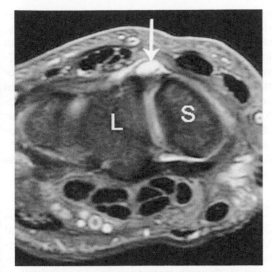

Fig. 17. Ganglion of the SLL. Axial STIR sequence at the level of the scaphoid (S) and lunate (L) shows a ganglion (*arrow*) on the dorsal surface of the SLL.

radioulnar ligaments, the ulnolunate and ulnotriquetral ligaments, the ECU tendon sheath, and the meniscal homolog. The TFCC, seen on coronal MR images as a low-signal biconcave structure, extends from the distal radius between the carpus and the distal ulna to insert into the ulnar styloid. This insertion is complex and includes attachments to the fovea at the base of the ulnar styloid as well as the tip of the process.[41] Occasionally, the ulnar insertion of the TFCC may appear as a solid low-signal structure spanning the ulnar styloid process without differentiation into bands.[37] Degenerative thinning and perforation of the central portion of the TFCC may be seen

as part of the aging process and may be difficult to interpret in elderly patients.[41]

Tears of the TFCC may be classified as traumatic or degenerative.[47] There are no specific MR imaging signs to differentiate traumatic from degenerative tears, though other factors, such as clinical history, age of patient, and the presence of associated injuries, may be relevant.[37] Acute traumatic tear of the TFCC may be the result of a fall causing rotational stress to the wrist. TFCC injury causing ulnar-sided wrist pain may also result from repetitive stress in participants of a variety of activities, including gymnastics, racquet sports, hockey, golf, boxing, waterskiing, and pole vaulting.[33] Traumatic tears of the TFCC may involve the radial or ulnar insertions, or the central disc. Avulsion of the radial insertion of the TFCC may be associated with a radial fracture.[37] Tears of the ulnar attachments, also known as peripheral or distal tears, may be associated with fractures of the ulnar styloid process.[37] MR imaging signs of full-thickness TFCC tears include abnormal fluid signal that traverses the TFCC from the radiocarpal joint to the distal radioulnar joint (Fig. 18). The presence of fluid in the distal radioulnar joint is a nonspecific sign that may be seen in other causes of distal radioulnar joint pathology.[48] Partial-thickness TFCC tears are best seen on coronal T2-weighted images, with fluid signal extending to only one articular surface, usually the proximal.[37] MR imaging is a highly accurate technique for the diagnosis of TFCC tears with reported sensitivity and specificity of up to 100% and 93% respectively.[41] Lower accuracy has been reported for the diagnosis of peripheral (ulnar-sided) TFCC tears.[49] Bone marrow

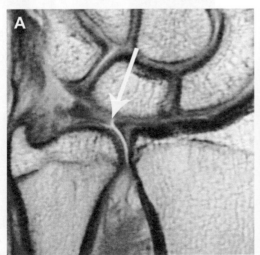
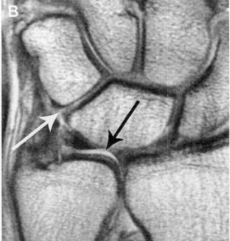

Fig. 18. Central tear of the TFCC in two athletes. (*A*) Coronal proton density sequence shows a small central defect in the TFCC (*arrow*). (*B*) Coronal proton density sequence shows a large central defect in the TFCC (*black arrow*). Note an associated tear of the LTL (*white arrow*).

edema of the dorsal aspect of the distal ulna deep to the ECU tendon may be a useful secondary sign on MR imaging of peripheral TFCC tears (**Fig. 19**).[50]

INJURIES OF THE JOINTS OF THE HAND

Most fractures and dislocations of finger and thumb joints can be diagnosed and managed with clinical and radiographic assessment only. More sophisticated imaging may be required where injuries fail to settle, or in specific situations, such as suspected tear of the ulnar collateral ligament (UCL) of the first MCP joint. The radial and ulnar collateral ligaments and the volar plate are the supporting structures of the PIP and MCP joints. The collateral ligaments are best seen on coronal MR images as thin low-signal bands on each side of the joint. The volar plate is best seen on sagittal MR images as a triangular low-signal structure. The flexor tendons and extensor mechanism contribute to the stability of the joints.

Dislocation of the MCP joint is uncommon and is usually treated conservatively. Irreducibility of a dislocation may be caused by interposition of the volar plate in the joint[51] and this may be shown with MR imaging. The PIP joint is the most commonly injured joint in the hand. Dislocation of the PIP joint may be the result of a "sideways" force, either abduction or adduction, or may be due to hyperextension or rotation. An abducting or adducting force tends to injure the collateral ligaments, with volar plate avulsion encountered in more serious injuries. MR signs of collateral ligament rupture include ligament discontinuity, detachment from bone, and thickening and increased signal within the ligament on T2-weighted images (**Fig. 20**).[27] Hyperextension or rotation-type injuries tend to involve the volar plate with disruption of the collateral ligaments and fractures seen in more severe cases. MR signs of volar plate injury include contour irregularity and heterogeneous signal on T1- and T2-weighted images.[27] A gap between the base of the volar plate and the underlying bone indicates avulsion (**Fig. 21**).

Skier's (Gamekeeper's) Thumb

Skier's thumb refers to a tear of the UCL of the first MCP joint. This injury is caused by violent abduction of the thumb[52] and was historically encountered in Scottish gamekeepers, who used their thumbs to break the necks of animals by pushing forcibly on the backs of the animal's head.[32] Today the injury is known as skier's thumb. Rupture of the UCL of the first MCP joint accounts for 6% of all skiing injuries[52] and is caused by a fall while holding a ski pole, with forcible abduction and extension of the thumb.

Four separate muscles form the thenar eminence and operate the first MCP joint. One of these muscles, the adductor pollicis, inserts with the first palmar interosseous muscle to the base of the proximal phalanx of the thumb. The aponeurosis of the adductor pollicis covers the UCL.[53] The spectrum of UCL injuries encompasses

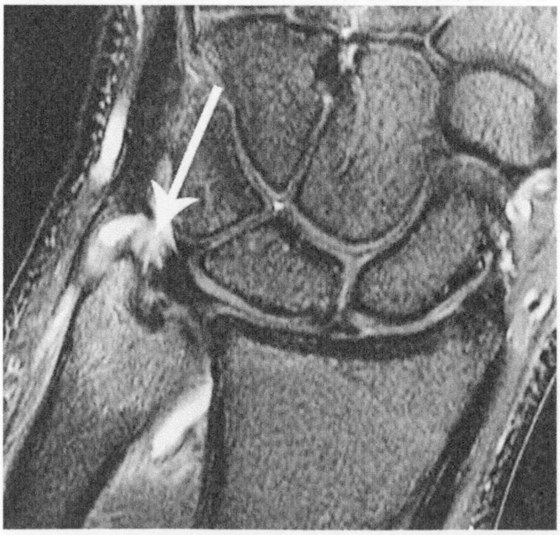

Fig. 19. Peripheral tear of the TFCC. Coronal fat-saturated T2-weighted sequence shows a peripheral (ulnar-sided) tear of the TFCC (*arrow*). Note associated bone marrow edema in the distal ulna and fluid in the distal radioulnar joint.

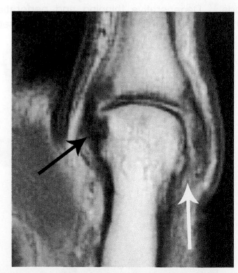

Fig. 20. Tear of the radial collateral ligament of the thumb. Coronal proton density sequence of the MCP joint of the thumb shows detachment of the proximal end of the radial collateral ligament (*white arrow*). The UCL is intact (*black arrow*).

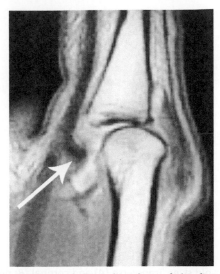

Fig. 21. Avulsion of the volar plate of the first MCP joint in a 23-year-old female who suffered a hyperextension injury of the thumb. Sagittal proton density sequence of the first MCP joint shows the volar plate (*arrow*) separated from the base of the proximal phalanx.

ligament strain, partial tear, and full-thickness tear (Fig. 22).[53] Full-thickness tears may be nondisplaced or displaced. Tears of the UCL usually involve the distal insertion of the ligament at the base of the proximal phalanx[33] and bony avulsion may be seen in 12% of injuries.[53] When a bony avulsion is present, the degree of displacement can be assessed radiographically. In displaced

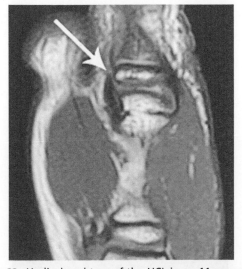

Fig. 22. Undisplaced tear of the UCL in an 11-year-old boy who suffered an abduction and hyperextension injury of the thumb while playing rugby. Coronal T1-weighted sequence of the first MCP joint shows an undisplaced tear of the distal insertion of the UCL (*arrow*).

rupture of the UCL, there may be proximal retraction and subsequent displacement of the torn ligament superficial to the adductor aponeurosis. This is known as the Stener lesion[52] and implies an unstable injury requiring surgical repair. A Stener lesion may be diagnosed with ultrasound or MR imaging. MR signs of an undisplaced tear of the UCL are similar to those of other collateral ligament injuries as described above. With a Stener lesion, the torn ligament appears as a rounded or stumplike low-signal structure projecting superficial to the adductor aponeurosis (Fig. 23).[27,32]

NERVE PATHOLOGY RELATED TO OVERUSE

Carpal tunnel syndrome (CTS) is the most common entrapment neuropathy in the upper limb. CTS has a wide variety of local and systemic causes, including inflammatory arthropathies, amyloidosis, and diabetes.[54] In the athlete, CTS may be caused by fractures and dislocations, or by overuse tenosynovitis of the flexor tendons. It is also well known that peripheral nerve function may be disrupted by mechanical overload[38] and CTS is encountered in sports associated with repetitive flexion and extension of the wrist. These sports include swimming, bodybuilding, and wheelchair athletics.[37] Transient CTS is encountered in sports that result in vibration and repetitive direct force, such as long-distance cycling[55] and Enduro motorcycling.[56]

The ulnar nerve at the wrist passes through the Guyon canal. In the proximal canal, the ulnar nerve lies between the pisiform and the ulnar artery. Distal to the pisiform, the ulnar nerve divides into a deep motor branch and a superficial, predominantly sensory, branch. These ulnar nerve branches are closely related to the hook of the hamate. Injury to the ulnar nerve may be seen in athletes as a complication of fracture of the hook of the hamate or pisiform. Ulnar neuropathy is also seen in athletes taking part in racquet sports, martial arts, cycling, and similar activities involving repetitive or continuous pressure to the ulnar wrist.[11] Cycling is a particularly common cause of ulnar neuropathy. The term *handlebar palsy* refers to a compression syndrome of the deep motor branch of the ulnar nerve and is particularly common in downhill mountain biking.[57]

The combination of history, physical examination, and simple clinical tests, such as the Phalen and Tinel tests, is usually sufficient for the diagnosis of peripheral nerve disorders.[58] Furthermore, most sports-related nerve palsies are transient and are relieved by simple maneuvers, such as wearing padded gloves or changing the shape of handlebars. MR imaging is rarely required, though

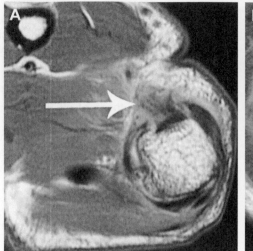
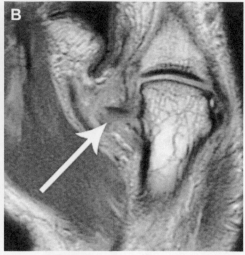

Fig. 23. Displaced tear of the UCL with Stener lesion in a 24-year-old skier. Transverse (*A*) and coronal (*B*) proton density sequences show the torn UCL projecting horizontally (*arrows*).

has a role when symptoms are persistent. MR imaging is able to diagnose correctly most space-occupying lesions within the carpal tunnel or Guyon canal, including tenosynovitis, ganglia, and accessory muscles. MR imaging findings of CTS due to repetitive trauma include flattening of the median nerve within the flexor retinaculum, swelling of the median nerve proximal to the flexor retinaculum, anterior bowing of the flexor retinaculum, thickening and irregularity of the flexor retinaculum, and increased signal of the median nerve on T2-weighted images.[59]

ARTERIAL PATHOLOGY RELATED TO OVERUSE

Irreversible damage of the radial or ulnar arteries may be caused by a variety of occupational or sporting activities that involve use of the palm as a hammer.[60] The ulnar artery is most commonly affected. The term *hypothenar hammer syndrome* (HHS) refers to damage to the ulnar artery caused by repetitive trauma.[61] HHS may be seen in occupations where the ulnar side of the palm is used to hammer or push hard objects[61] or where there is repeated vibration and trauma, such as operating a jackhammer. HHS is also encountered in athletes engaged in such activities as handball, baseball, tennis, break-dancing, and golf.[11] Damage to the arterial wall may result in aneurysm formation or thrombosis. Distal embolization causing occlusion of digital arteries may also be encountered. The athlete with HHS may present with sudden, intermittent, or gradual onset of ischemic symptoms in the fingers of the affected hand.[61] Compression of the ulnar nerve by an aneurysm

may cause numbness of the ring and little fingers. Angiographic features of HHS include tortuosity of the ulnar artery giving a corkscrew configuration, saccular or fusiform aneurysm formation, occlusion of the ulnar artery due to thrombosis, and occlusion of digital arteries due to emboli.[11,61] Contrast material–enhanced MR angiography of the hand is a relatively noninvasive examination that produces comparable accuracy to conventional angiography (**Fig. 24**).[62]

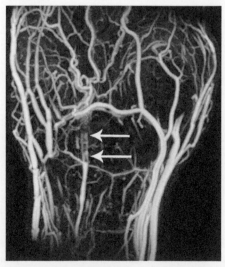

Fig. 24. HHS in a 35-year-old manual worker with intermittent pain and paresthesia in the ring and little fingers. Contrast material–enhanced MR angiography of the hand shows thrombosis of the distal ulnar artery (*arrows*).

SUMMARY

Traumatic and overuse injuries of the hand and wrist are common in athletes. Increasingly, MR imaging is being used to complement clinical and radiographic assessment in the diagnosis and management of these injuries. MR imaging is able to image accurately the bones, tendons, ligaments, nerves, and other small structures of the hand and wrist. This article provides an overview of traumatic and overuse injuries of the hand and wrist in athletes and a review of the MR imaging appearances.

REFERENCES

1. Rettig AC. Athletic injuries of the wrist and hand. Part I: traumatic injuries of the wrist. Am J Sports Med 2003;31:1038–48.
2. Karantanas A, Dailiana Z, Malizos K. The role of MR imaging in scaphoid disorders. Eur Radiol 2007;17:2860–71.
3. Nazarian LN. The top 10 reasons musculoskeletal sonography is an important complementary or alternative technique to MRI. AJR Am J Roentgenol 2008;190:1621–6.
4. Hunter JC, Escobedo EM, Wilson AJ, et al. MR imaging of clinically suspected scaphoid fractures. AJR Am J Roentgenol 1997;168:1287–93.
5. Memarsadeghi M, Breitenseher MJ, Schaefer-Prokop C, et al. Occult scaphoid fractures: comparison of multidetector CT and MR imaging—initial experience. Radiology 2006;240:169–76.
6. Dorsay TA, Major NM, Helms CA. Cost-effectiveness of immediate MR imaging versus traditional follow-up for revealing radiographically occult scaphoid fractures. AJR Am J Roentgenol 2001;177:1257–63.
7. Rangger C, Kathrein A, Freund MC, et al. Bone bruise of the knee: histology and cryosections in 5 cases. Acta Orthop Scand 1998;69:291–4.
8. Anderson MW, Greenspan A. Stress fractures. Radiology 1996;199:1–12.
9. Hanks GA, Kalenak A, Bowman LS, et al. Stress fractures of the carpal scaphoid. J Bone Joint Surg Am 1989;71:938–41.
10. Guha AR, Marynissen H. Stress fracture of the hook of the hamate. Br J Sports Med 2002;36:224–5.
11. Blum AG, Zabel JP, Kohlmann R, et al. Pathologic conditions of the hypothenar eminence: evaluation with multidetector CT and MR imaging. Radiographics 2006;26:1021–44.
12. Lohman M, Kivisaari L, Partio EK. Stress reaction in the carpal bones caused by breakdancing. Emerg Radiol 2003;10:102–4.
13. Waninger KN, Lombardo JA. Stress fracture of index metacarpal in an adolescent tennis player. Clin J Sport Med 1995;5:63–6.
14. Jowett AD, Brukner PD. Fifth metacarpal stress fracture in a female softball pitcher. Clin J Sport Med 1997;7:220–1.
15. Anderson MW. Imaging of upper extremity stress fractures in the athlete. Clin Sports Med 2006;25:489–504.
16. Arendt EA, Griffiths HJ. The use of MR imaging in the assessment and clinical management of stress reactions of bone in high-performance athletes. Clin Sports Med 1997;16:291–306.
17. Shih C, Chang CY, Penn IW, et al. Chronically stressed wrists in adolescent gymnasts: MR imaging appearance. Radiology 1995;195:855–9.
18. Botte MJ, Pacelli LL, Gelberman RH. Vascularity and osteonecrosis of the wrist. Orthop Clin North Am 2004;35:405–21.
19. Schuind F, Eslami S, Ledoux P. Kienbock's disease. J Bone Joint Surg Br 2008;90:133–9.
20. Kalainov DM, Cohen MS, Hendrix RW, et al. Preiser's disease: identification of two patterns. J Hand Surg 2003;28A:767–78.
21. Cerezal L, del Pinal F, Abascal F, et al. Imaging findings in ulnar-sided wrist impaction syndromes. Radiographics 2002;22:105–21.
22. Friedman SL, Palmer AK. The ulnar impaction syndrome. Hand Clin 1991;7:295–310.
23. Topper SM, Wood MB, Ruby LK. Ulnar styloid impaction syndrome. J Hand Surg 1997;22A:699–704.
24. Bell MJ, Hill RJ, McMurtry RY. Ulnar impingement syndrome. J Bone Joint Surg Br 1985;67:126–9.
25. Viegas SF, Patterson RM, Hokanson JA, et al. Wrist anatomy: incidence, distribution, and correlation of anatomic variations, tears and arthrosis. J Hand Surg Am 1993;18:463–75.
26. Coggins CA. Imaging of ulnar-sided wrist pain. Clin Sports Med 2006;25:505–26.
27. Clavero JA, Alomar X, Monill JM, et al. MR imaging of ligament and tendon injuries of the fingers. Radiographics 2002;22:237–56.
28. Clavero JA, Golano P, Farinas O, et al. Extensor mechanism of the fingers: MR imaging—anatomic correlation. Radiographics 2003;23:593–611.
29. Rubin DA, Kneeland JB, Kitay GS, et al. Flexor tendon tears in the hand: use of MR imaging to diagnose degree of injury in cadaver model. AJR Am J Roentgenol 1996;166:615–20.
30. Leddy JP, Packer JW. Avulsion of the profundus tendon insertion in athletes. J Hand Surg Am 1977;2:66–9.
31. Aronowitz ER, Leddy JP. Closed tendon injuries of the hand and wrist in athletes. Clin Sports Med 1998;17:449–67.
32. Peterson JJ, Bancroft LW. Injuries of the fingers and thumb in the athlete. Clin Sports Med 2006;25:527–42.

33. Rettig AC. Athletic injuries of the wrist and hand. Part II: overuse injuries of the wrist and traumatic injuries to the hand. Am J Sports Med 2004;32: 262–72.

34. Drape J-L, Dubert T, Silbermann O, et al. Acute trauma of the extensor hood of the metacarpophalangeal joint: MR imaging evaluation. Radiology 1994;192:469–76.

35. Klauser A, Frauscher F, Bodner G, et al. Finger pulley injuries in extreme rock climbers: depiction with dynamic US. Radiology 2002;222:755–61.

36. Rees JD, Wilson AM, Wolman RL. Current concepts in the management of tendon disorders. Rheumatology (Oxford) 2006;45:508–21.

37. Bencardino JT, Rosenberg ZS. Sports-related injuries of the wrist: an approach to MRI interpretation. Clin Sports Med 2006;25:409–32.

38. van Tulder M, Malmivaara A, Koes B. Repetitive strain injury. Lancet 2007;369:1815–22.

39. Costa CR, Morrison WB, Carrino JA. MRI features of intersection syndrome of the forearm. AJR Am J Roentgenol 2003;181:1245–9.

40. Parellada AJ, Gopez AG, Morrison WB, et al. Distal intersection tenosynovitis of the wrist: a lesser known extensor tendinopathy with characteristic MR imaging features. Skeletal Radiol 2007;36:203–8.

41. Connell D, Page P, Wright W, et al. Magnetic resonance imaging of the wrist ligaments. Australas Radiol 2001;45:411–22.

42. Schmid MR, Schertler T, Pfirrmann CW, et al. Interosseous ligament tears of the wrist: comparison of multi-detector row CT arthrography and MR imaging. Radiology 2005;237:1008–13.

43. Scheck RJ, Kubitzek C, Hierner R, et al. The scapholunate interosseous ligament in MR arthrography of the wrist: correlation with non-enhanced MRI and wrist arthrography. Skeletal Radiol 1997;26:263–71.

44. Theumann NH, Etechami G, Duvoisin B, et al. Association between extrinsic and intrinsic carpal ligament injuries at MR arthrography and carpal instability at radiography: initial observations. Radiology 2006;238:950–7.

45. El-Noueam K, Schweitzer ME, Blasbalg R, et al. Is a subset of wrist ganglia the sequela of internal derangements of the wrist joint? MR imaging findings. Radiology 1999;212:537–40.

46. Lowden CM, Attiah M, Garvin G, et al. The prevalence of wrist ganglia in an asymptomatic population: magnetic resonance evaluation. J Hand Surg Br 2005;30:302–6.

47. Palmer AK, Werner FW. The triangular fibrocartilage complex of the wrist—anatomy and function. J Hand Surg Am 1981;6:153–62.

48. Steinbach LS, Smith DK. MRI of the wrist. Clin Imaging 2000;24:298–322.

49. Haims AH, Schweitzer ME, Morrison WB, et al. Limitations of MR imaging in the diagnosis of peripheral tears of the triangular fibrocartilage of the wrist. AJR Am J Roentgenol 2002;178:419–22.

50. Zoga A, Morrison W, Mamelak J, et al. Subtendinous bone marrow at the extensor carpi ulnaris as a harbinger of triangular fibrocartilage tear. (Abstract SSM21–05). In: Programs and abstracts of the 91st Radiological Society of North America. Chicago: 2005.

51. Kahler DM, McCue FC III. Metacarpophalangeal and proximal interphalangeal joint injuries of the hand, including the thumb. Clin Sports Med 1992;11:57–76.

52. Spaeth HJ, Abrams RA, Bock GW, et al. Gamekeeper thumb: differentiation of nondisplaced and displaced tears of the ulnar collateral ligament with MR imaging. Radiology 1993;188:553–6.

53. Ebrahim FS, Maeseneer MD, Jager T, et al. US diagnosis of UCL tears of the thumb and Stener lesions: technique, pattern-based approach, and differential diagnosis. Radiographics 2006;26:1007–20.

54. Aroori S, Spence RA. Carpal tunnel syndrome. Ulster Med J 2008;77:6–17.

55. Akuthota V, Plastaras C, Lindberg K, et al. The effect of long-distance bicycling on ulnar and median nerves: an electrophysiologic evaluation of cyclist palsy. Am J Sports Med 2005;33:1224–30.

56. Sabeti-Aschraf M, Serek M, Pachtner T, et al. The Enduro motorcyclist's wrist and other overuse injuries in competitive Enduro motorcyclists: a prospective study. Scand J Med Sci Sports 2008;18:582–90.

57. Capitani D, Beer S. Handlebar palsy—a compression syndrome of the deep terminal (motor) branch of the ulnar nerve in biking. J Neurol 2002;249:1441–5.

58. Lisle DA, Johnstone SA. Usefulness of muscle denervation as an MRI sign of peripheral nerve pathology. Australas Radiol 2007;51:516–26.

59. Hochman MG, Zilberfarb JL. Nerves in a pinch: imaging of nerve compression syndromes. Radiol Clin North Am 2004;42:221–45.

60. McCready RA, Bryant MA, Divelbiss JL. Combined thenar and hypothenar hammer syndrome: case report and review of the literature. J Vasc Surg 2008;48:741–4.

61. Ablett CT, Hackett LA. Hypothenar hammer syndrome: case reports and brief review. Clin Med Res 2008;6:3–8.

62. Connell DA, Koulouris G, Thorn DA, et al. Contrast-enhanced MR angiography of the hand. Radiographics 2002;22:583–99.

Imaging of Groin Pain

Peter J. MacMahon, MD, MRCPI[a,*], Brian A. Hogan, MB, FFRRCSI[b],
Martin J. Shelly, MD, MRCPI[a],
Stephen J. Eustace, MD, MSc, MB, FFRRCSI[a,b,c,d,e],
Eoin C. Kavanagh, MD, MB, FFRRCSI[a,b]

KEYWORDS

- Groin • MR imaging • Athletic pubalgia
- Tendon • Ligament

Groin pain is typically an overuse injury due to excessive athletic activity, accounting for approximately 2% to 18% of all sports injuries.[1–3] A study of soccer players in 1999 demonstrated that 8% of players had an episode of groin pain over a 1-year period.[4] A report from 1974 found that nearly two-thirds of soccer players had a history of groin injury during their careers.[5] Indeed, any sport that is associated with rapid changes in speed and direction, or kicking activity in particular, has higher rates of groin injury. Such sports include ice hockey, American football, Australian Rules football, fencing, track and field events, and soccer.[6–8]

Even though injuries to the groin are relatively common, it can be a diagnostic challenge to elucidate the etiology. Patients typically complain of pain over the prepubic, inguinal, and proximal adductor regions that may be referred to the scrotum and perineum.[9] Tenderness on physical examination commonly localizes to the pubic symphysis, pubic tubercle, mid-inguinal region, or adductor longus insertion. In addition, there may be pain on resisted adduction of the hips.[10] Although groin injuries may be acute, they typically have an insidious onset over weeks to months.

The underlying processes that lead to a groin injury are complicated, varied, and incompletely understood. The commonest reported potential causes of overuse injuries of the groin are listed in **Box 1**. Perhaps not surprisingly, there are numerous treatment options for patients with groin pain, ranging from conservative to invasive. Due to

the difficulty in obtaining an accurate diagnosis, patient management and outcomes have historically been unpredictable.[8,11,12]

In clinical practice, the term "athletic pubalgia" is a general term used to describe exertional pubic or groin pain.[13] Most investigators have concluded that the commonest causes of groin pain are adductor longus injury, common adductor-rectus abdominis dysfunction, osteitis pubis, and sportsman's hernia.[9,14–16] This article reviews the anatomy, etiology, and imaging appearances of the commonest causes of athletic pubalgia.

ANATOMY

The pubic symphysis is composed of the paired pubic bones and the intervening fibrocartilaginous articular disc.[17] The medial articular surface of the pubis is grooved and lined by hyaline cartilage. It is thought that the ridged nature of the pubis protects the joint from shear forces.[9] The main function of the fibrocartilaginous disc is to absorb and dissipate axial and shear forces experienced at the pubic symphysis.[18] A thin physiologic cleft (also called the primary cleft) can be located superiorly within the fibrocartilaginous disc (**Fig. 1**).[19] The pubic tubercle arises from the lateral aspect of the pubic crest, a bony projection over the anterior surface of the pubic body. The pubic symphysis does not have a true joint capsule, as the joint does not have a synovial lining.[9,20,21] Surrounding ligaments and tendons provide the majority of the soft tissue support. A thin superior

[a] Department of Radiology, Mater Misericordiae University Hospital, Eccles Street, Dublin 7, Ireland
[b] Department of Radiology, Santry Sports Surgery Clinic, Santry Demense, Dublin 9, Ireland
[c] University College Dublin, Belfield, Dublin 4, Ireland
[d] Institute of Radiological Sciences, University College Dublin, Dublin, Ireland
[e] Department of Radiology, Cappagh National Orthopedic Hospital, Finglas, Dublin 11, Ireland
* Corresponding author.
E-mail address: petermacmahon@yahoo.com (P.J. MacMahon).

Magn Reson Imaging Clin N Am 17 (2009) 655–666
doi:10.1016/j.mric.2009.06.013

pubic ligament bridges the pubic tubercles, which is partly formed from posterior rectus abdominis muscle fascia. The arcuate (inferior pubic) ligament is an important stabilizing structure that forms a strong fibrous arch along the inferior margin of the symphyseal joint. The arcuate ligament blends with the subjacent fibrocartilage disc.[9] A thin anterior pubic ligament also attaches to the underlying articular disc and blends with interconnecting connective tissue anteriorly formed from tendons and ligaments (see **Fig. 1**).

The rectus abdominis muscle acts as a stabilizer of the anterior abdominal wall, originating lateral to the pubic symphysis along the pubic crest. The adductor longus tendon acts to allow thigh adduction and to stabilize the anterior pelvis during the swing phase of the gait.[22] The adductor longus originates just inferior and in line with the rectus abdominis origin along the most anterior aspect of the pubis and just inferior to the pubic crest. The adductor longus tendon is usually entirely tendinous anteriorly, with an accessory muscular origin posterolaterally in 25% of patients.[17,22]

The rectus abdominis and adductor longus muscles are antagonists during rotation and extension of the waist. Of note, the origins of the rectus abdominis and the adductor longus tendons merge anterior to the pubis to form a common structure that is firmly adherent to the prepubic surface.[9,23] The adjacent gracilis and adductor brevis tendons are variably fused with each other and adductor longus as they arise from the inferior pubic body, anterior pubic ligament, and arcuate ligament.[24] Further to this, the rectus abdominis muscle and sheath extends across the anterior pubic surface to interdigitate with the tendon fibers that give origin to the adductor muscle compartment, resulting in the formation of a common adductor-rectus abdominis origin. The obturator externus muscle arises from the anterior surface of the pubis and external surface of the obturator membrane, and can act as an adductor of the hip in addition to causing external rotation. This muscle can therefore be reliably distinguished from the other adductor muscles as the structure arising anterior to the obturator foramen and adjacent portions of the pubic bone.

An anatomic reference book from 1904 refers to interlacing fibers anterior to the pubic symphysis composed predominately of the rectus abdominis and external oblique tendons.[25] Reference is also made to how this tissue is composed of tendons from the "superficial adductors of the thigh." There are additional elements contributing to this prepubic tissue. An infolding of the inferior margin of the external oblique aponeurosis forms the inguinal ligament. Recent cadaveric study has demonstrated that, similar to other apes, humans have a continuation of the inguinal ligament into the lateral aspect of this prepubic connective tissue.[26] In addition, the medial aspect of the external oblique aponeurosis splits in two to form the superficial inguinal ring, the medial crus of

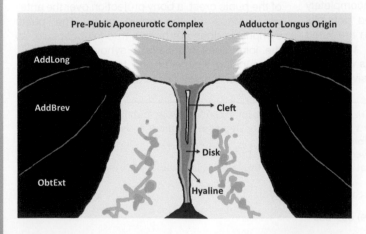

Fig. 1. An axial section through the pubic symphysis below the level of the pubic crest, demonstrating the adductor origin from the prepubic aponeurotic complex (P-PAC). The P-PAC is continuous with the underlying fibrocartilage of the symphysis. AddLong, adductor longus muscle; AddBrev, adductor brevis muscle; ObtExt, obturator externus muscle.

which inserts adjacent to the pubic tubercle and merges with prepubic connective tissue.[25] It has been traditionally taught that the conjoint tendon forms the roof and medial third of the posterior wall of the inguinal canal and inserts onto the pubic crest. Recent research, however, has demonstrated that the concept of a "conjoint" tendon is a rare entity during fresh dissection.[27] The internal oblique and transversus abdominis aponeuroses (which form the posterior wall of the inguinal canal) are typically not conjoined as they insert onto the pubis, but are in fact only closely apposed. It is believed that in previous studies using formalin-preserved cadavers, the two aponeuroses dehydrated and resulted in tissue toughening, thereby producing an apparent conjoint tendon.[27] Further to this, during fresh dissection the most common finding is that the internal oblique and transversus abdominis aponeuroses (the so-called conjoint tendon) actually insert onto the anterior sheath of the lateral aspect of the rectus abdominis, above the pubic crest, with an insertion onto the pubic crest being a rare finding. Hence, the structures that compose the posterior wall of the inguinal canal are reliant on the origin of the rectus abdominis for their integrity. The transversus abdominis and internal oblique muscles also contribute to pubic symphysis stability by increasing apposition of the pubic bodies during gait.[28] Sagittal cross-sectional anatomic studies along the axis of the rectus sheath and adductor tendons have demonstrated a condensation of triangular fibrocartilage inferior to the pubic crest, which likely acts as the main anchor point for the overlying connective tissue and its components (the adductor longus in particular). This condensation of fibrocartilaginous tissue is continuous with the underlying periosteum, anterior pubic ligament, and articular disc.[23] Indeed, it is difficult to define and separate the fibrocartilage disc as an entity distinct from the overlying connective tissue.[19]

In summary, the anterior aspect of the pubis acts as a common origin for important muscular structures around the pubic symphysis. Tissue in this prepubic region not only interconnects the adductor tendons and rectus abdominis, but also integrates with the parasymphyseal support ligaments and elements of the inguinal canal. In addition, there appears to be a fibrocartilaginous component to this prepubic tissue continuous with the articular disc. This complex structure acts as a central anchor point, and is formed by interconnecting fibers of the adductors, rectus abdominis, external oblique, inguinal ligament, anterior pubic ligament, arcuate ligament, and fibrocartilaginous disc, and will be referred to as the prepubic aponeurotic complex (P-PAC) (see

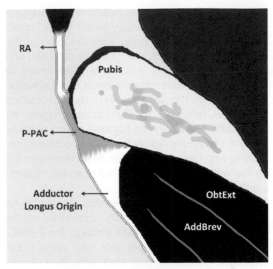

Fig. 2. A sagittal section through the pubis lateral to the symphysis. This schema demonstrates that the rectus abdominis (RA) and adductors are continuous anterior to the pubis through the prepubic aponeurotic complex (P-PAC). AddBrev, adductor brevis muscle; ObtExt, obturator externus muscle.

Figs. 1–3). This complex is crucial to the understanding of the mechanism of groin injuries and thus formulating an accurate diagnosis. For example, proximal adductor tendon injuries involving the P-PAC are an important cause of

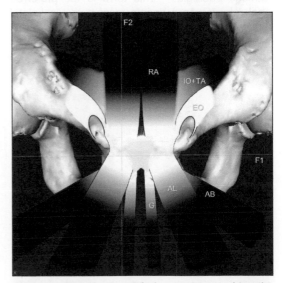

Fig. 3. A coronal view of the anterior pubis. This schema demonstrates the major components of the prepubic aponeurotic complex located over the anterior pubis bilaterally. The dotted lines represent the level of Fig. 1 (F1) and Fig. 2 (F2). RA, rectus abdominis; IO+TA, internal oblique and transversus abdominis; EO, external oblique aponeurosis forming superficial inguinal ring; AL, adductor longus; AB, abductor brevis; G, gracilis.

groin pain. The anatomic relationships suggest that a shear or avulsion injury to the P-PAC could potentially result in chronic microavulsion of the attachment of the inguinal ligament medially, and additionally weaken the common attachment of the transversus abdominis/internal oblique/rectus abdominis at the pubic crest, thus producing symptoms referable to the inguinal region. As this results in pain in the inguinal region (despite the lack of discrete hernia formation), athletes presenting with pain in this region likely represent the clinical entity previously referred to as the "sportsman's hernia."

Of note, as each ligamentous or tendinous component is connected with each other on the same and contralateral side through the P-PAC, injury of one of its components may cause pubic symphysis instability and also difficulty in localizing symptoms, hence causing diagnostic confusion from a clinical perspective. The complex interrelated anatomy of this anatomic area has led to the use of confusing diagnoses and terminology when describing the causes of groin pain, which are almost certain to be linked pathophysiologically.

ETIOLOGY OF GROIN PAIN

A catch-all term for all the causes of groin pain is "athletic pubalgia."[9] This term is the preferred label referring to a spectrum of musculoskeletal injuries that occur in and around the pubic symphysis and that share similar mechanisms of injury and common clinical manifestations.[9] The literature supports that the commonest causes of athletic pubalgia originate from the muscles and tendons of the adductor group and rectus abdominis, pubic symphysis (osteitis pubis), and inguinal wall.[1,9,17]

Groin pain in athletes can be acute (secondary to a single event), chronic (secondary to altered biomechanical load and repetitive microtrauma), or a combination of the two. It can be postulated that an injury to a structure inserting into the P-PAC (typically adductor longus or rectus abdominis) may secondarily affect the remaining structures that rely on the aponeurotic complex for their integrity.

COMMON ADDUCTOR-RECTUS ABDOMINIS INJURY

Although there are many causes of athletic pubalgia described, most investigators conclude that the commonest cause of groin pain in athletes is adductor dysfunction, as this is the strongest muscle group acting on the pubic symphysis.[29,30] Although the exact frequency of injury to specific structures around the pubic symphysis will be sport specific, injury to the adductor longus is consistently the commonest, especially in soccer players.[29] The prevalence of adductor dysfunction ranges from 44% to 60% in published series.[8,31,32] There are several risk factors for adductor injury, including a history of strain and low levels of sport-specific preseason training.[33] The hip adductors include the adductor longus, adductor brevis, adductor magnus, pectineus, and the gracilis (the obturator externus is occasionally included in this group). The pectineus muscle arises from the

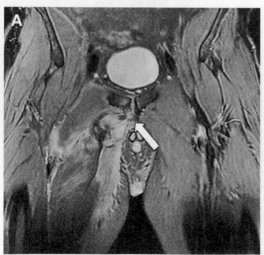 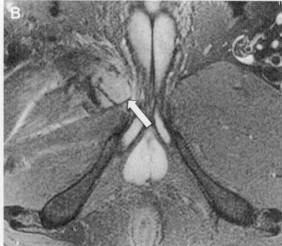

Fig. 4. (*A*) Coronal fat-saturated T2-weighted MR image. Large acute proximal right adductor longus origin tear with hematoma formation, edema, and distal retraction of the tendon (*arrow*). This condition is potentially disruptive for the prepubic aponeurotic complex. (*B*) Axial fat-saturated T2 MR image demonstrating a hematoma and retracted adductor longus tendon (*arrow*).

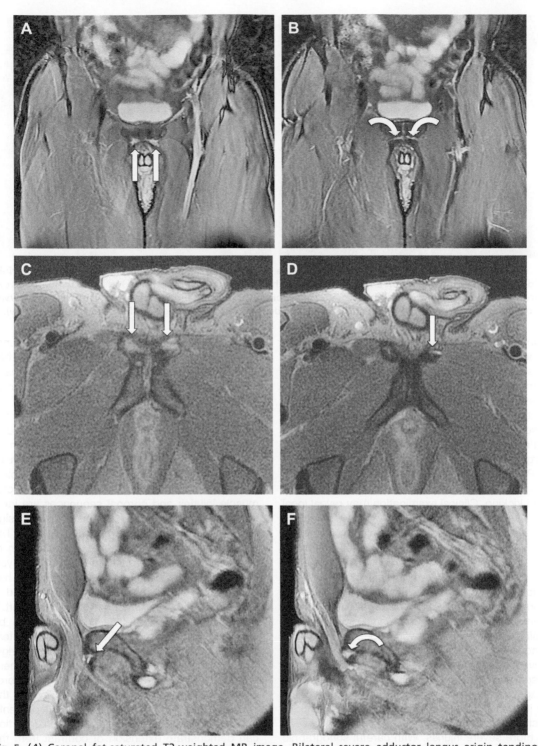

Fig. 5. (A) Coronal fat-saturated T2-weighted MR image. Bilateral severe adductor longus origin tendinosis (arrows). (B) Coronal fat-saturated T2-weighted MR image. Bilateral secondary clefts extending from the pubic symphysis into the adductor attachments, indicating some disruption of the prepubic aponeurotic complex tissue (curved arrows). (C) Axial fat-saturated T2-weighted MR image demonstrating bilateral adductor longus tendinosis (arrows). (D) 3D Axial fat-saturated T2-weighted MR image. Small tear of the left adductor longus tendon (arrow). (E) Sagittal fat-saturated T2-weighted MR image. Small tears of the origin of the left adductor longus tendon (arrow) (F) Sagittal fat-saturated T2-weighted MR image. This image demonstrates more severe adductor longus tendinosis that involves the prepubic aponeurotic complex (curved arrow).

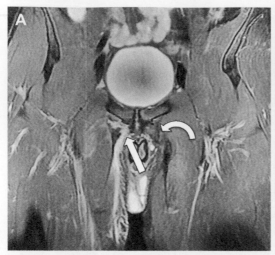 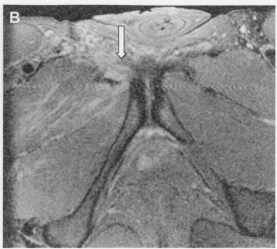

Fig. 6. (A) Coronal fat-saturated T2-weighted MR image. Hyperintense signal abnormality at the origin of the right adductor longus tendon (*straight arrow*) consistent with an acute tear. Chronic tear of left adductor longus as evidenced by thickening and hypointensity with retraction of the tendon and healing with scar formation (*curved arrow*). (B) Axial fat-saturated T2-weighted MR image demonstrating acute right adductor longus tear (*arrow*).

superior pubic ramus just lateral to the pubic tubercle. The adductor magnus arises from the inferior pubic ramus and ischial tuberosity. The remainder (gracilis, adductor longus, and adductor brevis) arise from a small area of the anterior aspect of the pubis (see **Fig. 3**). The adductor muscles insert on the posteromedial aspect of the femur (linea aspera), with the adductor magnus having the largest area of insertion.

Patients with adductor origin injury typically present with groin pain, exacerbated by exercise and kicking. Clinical examination may reveal local muscle tenderness or tenderness over the pubic symphysis, exacerbated by resisted adduction of the thighs. As the adductor longus muscle is the most frequently injured muscle, inflammatory change in the parasymphyseal bone (osteitis pubis) may coexist. Radiographs are generally normal; however, enthesopathy, ill definition of cortical bone at the tendon origin, sometimes is visible. Ongoing healing with repeated injury can lead to a mixed sclerotic-lytic appearance in severe cases (which is separate to osteitis pubis, discussed later). Sonography can also be used to diagnose tendinosis of the adductor longus distal to its origin. Tendinosis manifest as hypoechogenicity to the tendon, with tendon expansion seen in more severe injuries. With careful sonographic examination, a partial-thickness or full-thickness tear can be visualized.[34] A rectus abdominis injury at its origin from the pubic symphysis is also described as a source of pubic pain in athletes, with similar clinical and physical findings seen in adductor origin injury.[30] As Gibbon[31] described in 1999, a common adductor-rectus abdominis

(CA-RA) origin exists as an anatomic and functional unit anterior to the pubis. This unit has been referred to as an aponeurosis by many investigators[9,23,29] and is the main contributor to the P-PAC described.

Magnetic resonance (MR) imaging is the modality of choice in the depiction of adductor tendon, rectus abdominis tendon, and aponeurotic complex injuries (**Fig. 4**). Fat-saturated fluid-sensitive MR sequences in the axial oblique plain will best demonstrate acute or chronic adductor muscle injuries and coronal sequences are ideal for the detection of the "secondary cleft" sign adjacent to the pubic symphysis (**Fig. 5**). The secondary cleft sign is manifest as extension of fluid-bright signal external to the pubic symphysis to one or both sides (the side of extension has been shown to correlate with symptoms) and is continuous with the primary intra-articular cleft.[18] The exact anatomy of this sign has yet to be formally elucidated, but it likely represents a tear or partial avulsion of the adductor longus origin where it gains origin from the P-PAC. The aponeurotic injury likely extends into the underlying fibro-cartilage disc, disrupting the integrity of the anterior aspect of the physiologic cleft (if present). In this circumstance, symphyseal cleft injection can demonstrate extension of contrast from the physiologic cleft into the secondary cleft.[18] Tendinosis manifests as ill-defined increased signal on T2-weighted imaging, with partial thickness tears manifesting as focal areas of T2 hyperintensity similar to fluid signal. Gadolinium enhancement, if used, has been shown to correlate with the symptomatic side.[35] Muscular strains most

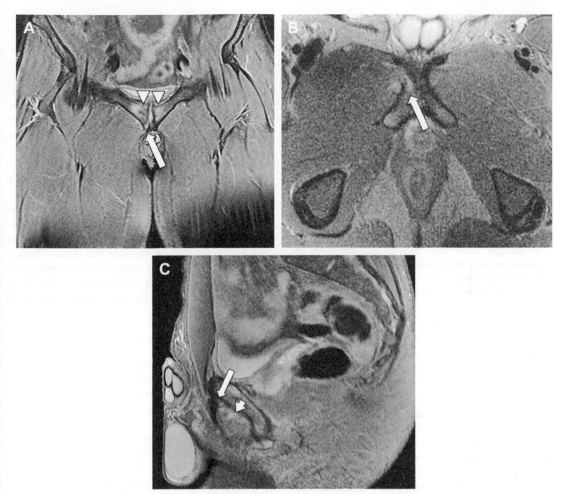

Fig. 7. (*A*) Coronal fat-saturated T2-weighted MR image. Bilateral osteitis pubis, right worse than left, character-ized by bone marrow hyperintensity (*arrowheads*),with microtearing along the medial right obturator externus attachment and disruption of the prepubic aponeurotic complex causing secondary cleft formation (*straight arrow*). (*B*) Axial fat-saturated T2-weighted MR image demonstrating microtearing of the right obturator exter-nus attachment posterior to adductor longus with secondary bony stress reaction (*arrow*). (*C*) Sagittal fat-satu-rated T2-weighted MR image. Edema and microtearing of the origin of the obturator externus (*short arrow*) posterior to adductor longus and brevis, extending posterior to the adductor longus origin from the prepubic aponeurotic complex (*long arrow*).

commonly occur at the musculotendinous junction of the adductor longus, normally anteriorly. In severe injury, a retracted tendon secondary to a full-thickness tear can be visualized on MR imaging (Fig. 6).

As the P-PAC is essentially a common origin for the adductors and the rectus abdominis, signifi-cant injury at the adductor origin, with disruption of the aponeurotic complex, frequently extends to the origin of the rectus abdominis that may be apparent on imaging. The reverse is also possible, with a primary rectus abdominis injury causing disruption of the complex.[30] In addition, it can be seen how injury to the complex can affect adjacent structures causing symptoms to be referred to the inguinal region.

Nonoperative management is the rule in adductor strain, with surgical intervention used in the acute setting for reattachment of full-thickness avulsion injuries. In the context of chronic groin pain, adductor tenotomy can be performed, with surgical excision of granulation tissue.[6,36]

OSTEITIS PUBIS

Osteitis pubis is a painful condition affecting the pubic symphysis that likely represents an inflam-matory response, secondary to altered biome-chanics, and loading at the symphysis. Osteitis pubis is most frequently seen in athletes involved in kicking sports, such as soccer and Australian Rules football. Osteitis pubis can occur in isolation;

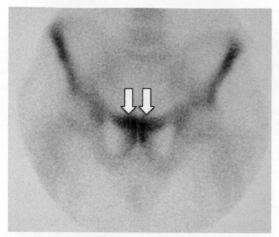

Fig. 8. Isotope bone scan shows concentration of radiotracer activity at the symphysis pubis in a patient with increased marginal osteoblastic activity in a 27-year-old soccer player with osteitis pubis (*arrows*).

however, it is commonly associated with other pathologic entities around the pubic symphysis such as adductor and rectus abdominis injuries (**Fig. 7**).[18,29,30] Patients typically complain of pain localized to the symphysis, radiating to the medial thigh, lower abdomen, and perineum. The pain is exacerbated by exercise, kicking, and running.

Imaging appearances were first described on plain radiography as irregularity of the subchondral bone, erosions, and fragmentation with areas of mixed sclerosis and lysis. If very severe there may be widening of the symphysis. A craniocaudal discrepancy of inferior pubic margins on stress radiography is diagnostic of symphyseal instability. Radioisotope bone scans show increased uptake of radiotracer about the pubic symphysis (**Fig. 8**).[37] Hyperintense signal change on fluid-sensitive sequences in the bone marrow adjacent to the symphysis on MR imaging are presumed to represent bone marrow edema and the earliest manifestation of osteitis pubis. As has been mentioned, the pubic symphysis is intimately connected with the prepubic aponeurotic complex that acts as the origin for many structures around the symphysis. Chronic repetitive injury of a component of the aponeurotic complex may lead to instability at the pubic symphysis and a stress response, with resultant edema in the parasymphyseal subchondral bone. If the bone edema is preferentially unilateral, this likely reflects direct traction effects from a more focal injury. Of note, osteitis pubis with bone marrow edema is usually seen in symptomatic patients and predicts preseason training restriction.[16,29]

MR imaging reveals parasymphyseal hyperintensity on fluid-sensitive sequences, presumably

reflecting edema due to increased stress response and areas of trabecular microtrauma.[38] Histologic sampling of these T2 hyperintense parasymphyseal regions has demonstrated new woven bone formation consistent with a bone stress response.[39] T1-weighted images can show widening of the symphyseal cleft in chronic cases. If stress fractures are also present, these are often manifest as vertically oriented subchondral areas of T1 hypointensity adjacent to the pubic symphysis. Nonsurgical management includes rest, oral anti-inflammatory medications, physical rehabilitation, and image-guided injection of corticosteroid and local anesthetic directly into the joint.[40,41] Surgical management includes curettage, and in the setting of instability arthrodesis may be performed to stabilize the pelvis. Wedge resection of the pubic symphysis is rarely performed in cases that are refractory to nonoperative measures, as this can be eventually complicated by pelvic instability.

SPORTSMAN'S HERNIA

This condition has confusing clinical findings and historically varying terminology. Sportsman's hernia is interchangeably referred to as a sportsman's hernia, prehernia complex, conjoint tendon tear, Gilmore groin, external oblique tear, and inguinal wall deficiency.[1,17,18,30] The symptoms of a sportsman's hernia can generally be described as pain referable to the medial inguinal area without evidence of a typical hernia on physical examination, usually experienced by athletes.[42,43] The P-PAC is possibly a unifying

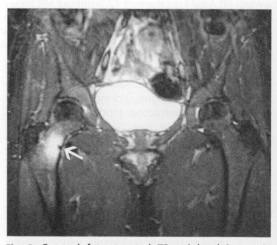

Fig. 9. Coronal fat-saturated T2-weighted image in a 30-year-old female runner shows bone marrow hyperintensity consistent with edema, which surrounds a hypointense line at the inferior aspect of the right femoral neck (*arrow*) compatible with a stress fracture.

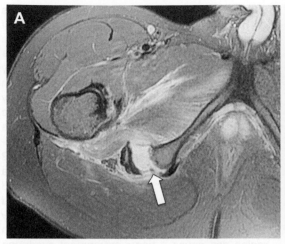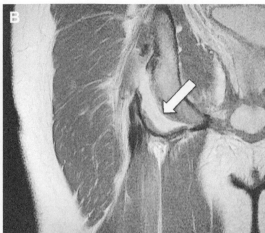

Fig. 10. (A) Axial fat-saturated T2-weighted MR image of a 12-year-old patient shows an avulsion at the attachment of the hamstring to the ischial apophysis on the right (*arrow*). (B) Coronal T1-weighted image of same patient demonstrating the hamstring avulsion injury (*arrow*).

structure to explain many presentations of this condition, as it is a common anchor for the structures of the posteromedial inguinal canal (internal oblique and transversus abdominis via the rectus sheath); for the medial crus of the superficial inguinal ring; for the most medial aspect of the inguinal ligament itself; and for the main stressors around the pubis (adductors and rectus abdominis) (see Fig. 3). An adductor longus or rectus abdominis injury involving the aponeurotic complex may thus affect the structures of the inguinal canal. Depending on the anatomic component and the severity of the injury (from strain to tear), symptoms may range from mild tenderness without palpable protrusion of the inguinal wall, to severe tenderness and palpable protrusion with possible discrete hernia formation.

Gilmore groin is classically described as tenderness over the superficial inguinal ring, with evidence of dilation of the superficial inguinal ring on clinical examination.[44] The pathologic process thus likely relates to the medial attachments of the external abdominis aponeurosis, which is a component of the P-PAC. Whereas the majority of patients cannot localize their symptoms precisely, approximately 40% of patients are found to have concomitant tenderness in the adductor region.[45] Of note, patients can respond to a hernia repair but others experience little or no improvement in their groin pain or develop recurrent symptoms at follow-up.[9,46] Another specific entity in the sportsman's hernia group is posterior inguinal wall deficiency, which has been attributed to an injury of the conjoint tendon. As described earlier, the classic description of the conjoint tendon is not a common finding at cadaveric dissection. The tendon actually merges with the anterolateral aspect of the rectus

abdominis sheath as opposed to inserting onto the pubic crest. This entity of posterior inguinal wall deficiency thus likely relates to an injury at the lateral attachment of the rectus abdominis, possibly secondary to disruption of the P-PAC, which weakens the internal oblique and transversus abdominis components of the inguinal canal. Incompetence of the posterior inguinal canal can be diagnosed with dynamic sonography by demonstrating anterior bulging of the posterior wall on straining.[47]

The sportsman hernia is thus a nonspecific entity that can have variable symptoms and signs. Though this term may be used by clinicians interchangeably with other terms such as athletic pubalgia, it is the authors' opinion that this term not be used as a diagnosis when formulating a radiological report. As MR imaging can reliably identified precisely where an injury has occurred, it is best that the site and extent of injury is

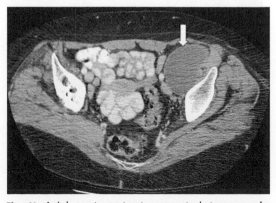

Fig. 11. Axial post contrast computed tomography image shows a distended iliopsoas bursa on the left (*arrow*), anterior to the left hip.

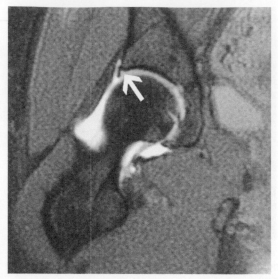

Fig. 12. Direct MRA of the right hip in a 24-year-old gymnast with hip pain. This coronal image shows direct contrast imbibement (*arrow*), into a surgically confirmed hip labral tear.

described, as well as whether any other structures are involved. As groin injuries are commonly secondary to injury of the main muscular attachments at the pubis, these injuries may variably extend to affect the medial inguinal canal components through the P-PAC.

OTHER CAUSES OF GROIN PAIN

As can be seen from **Box 1**, there are several potential causes that may be attributable to an overuse injury to the groin. Stress fractures in athletes mostly occur about the pubic symphysis and proximal femur (**Fig. 9**). Stress fractures are either

fatigue (occurring as a result of abnormal stress on normal bone) or insufficiency (as a result of normal stress on abnormal bone). In general, the term stress fracture is used to describe fatigue fractures rather than insufficiency, and although they occur as a result of chronic stress, they often present as an acute fracture to a site previously weakened over time. There are several pubic region apophyses that can be injured by repetitive muscular contractions in a skeletally immature individual, typically between the ages of 12 and 22 years. Apophysitis may cause athletic pubalgia symptoms (**Fig. 10**).[48] Other conditions that should be considered include muscle contusions and nerve entrapment syndromes. Entrapment of any of the numerous nerves that innervate the groin region can cause a nerve entrapment syndrome (obturator, femoral, genitofemoral, and ilioinguinal nerves). For example, patients with obturator nerve entrapment can present with pain near the adductor origin. Entrapment of the ilioinguinal nerve can cause symptoms similar to athletic pubalgia if it is compressed in the inguinal canal. Findings of muscle denervation-related edema may suggest the diagnosis on MR imaging.[9] Iliopsoas bursitis is an inflammatory condition seen in athletes, secondary to overuse with repetitive hip flexion and extension.[49] The condition causes groin pain in gymnasts, dancers, and runners. On rare occasions patients will present with a groin mass secondary to gross bursal distension (**Fig. 11**). Iliopsoas bursitis can also be seen in association with inflammatory arthropathies, and concomitant exclusion of these conditions may be warranted. MR imaging is the investigation of choice for this condition, as it will more accurately define the size and extent of the distended bursa and also allows

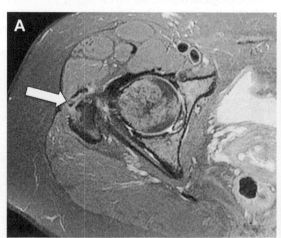
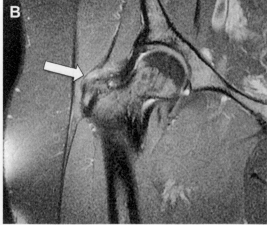

Fig. 13. (*A*) Axial fat-saturated T2-weighted image demonstrating gluteus minimus tendinosis at its insertion on the anterior border of the greater trochanter (*arrow*). (*B*) Coronal fat-saturated T2-weighted image in same patient, demonstrating the abnormal high signal of gluteus minimus tendinosis (*arrow*).

for evaluation of associated hip pathology.[50,51] Fat-saturated fluid sensitive sequences typically show a rounded high signal fluid collection posteromedial to the iliopsoas muscle. Athletic pubalgia also includes pain referred from nearby structures, in particular from hip or spine pathology. An acetabular labral tear in the hip can occur following significant injury, especially after posterior hip subluxation or dislocation. Acute traumatic labral tears are more common in patients who play sports that involve extreme hip rotation and flexion. Patients with preexisting hip dysplasia and with femoroacetabular impingement are more prone to labral tears secondary to altered biomechanics. The pain can be poorly localized, radiating to the groin, where it may be the only area of reported symptoms. Direct magnetic resonance arthrography (MRA) is the gold-standard imaging technique for assessment of the hip labrum (**Fig. 12**).[52] Direct signs of a labral tear on MRA include altered morphology of the labrum and direct contrast imbibition into the labral tear.[53,54] Trochanteric bursitis is also a potential cause of groin and hip pain in the athlete.[55] Trochanteric bursitis typically occurs in athletes who are involved with repeated flexion at the hip joint. It is thought that excess friction between the tensor fascia lata and its underlying bursa gives rise to bursitis. Patients will typically complain of lateral groin and hip pain, exacerbated by adduction and external rotation of the hip. Gluteus minimus tendinosis can cause similar symptoms (**Fig. 13**). Lumbar spondylosis can result in patients presenting with radicular groin pain. In these patients dedicated MR imaging of the lumbar spine may reveal a disc herniation, foraminal stenosis, facet arthropathy, or central canal narrowing. Developmental osseous abnormalities such as transitional anatomy at the lumbosacral junction and spondylolysis may lead to presentation with groin and pelvic pain. Sacroiliitis can also present with groin pain in the athlete. If this is suspected, dedicated MR imaging of the sacroiliac joints should be performed. Full rheumatologic workup of these patients is recommended to evaluate for the potential presence of an underlying inflammatory arthropathy.

REFERENCES

1. Kavanagh EC, Koulouris G, Ford S, et al. MR imaging of groin pain in the athlete. Semin Musculoskelet Radiol 2006;10:197–207.

2. Gilmore J. Groin pain in the soccer athlete: fact, fiction, and treatment. Clin Sports Med 1998;17:787–93, vii.

3. Syme G, Wilson J, Mackenzie K, et al. Groin pain in athletes. Lancet 1999;353:1444.

4. Ekstrand J, Hilding J. The incidence and differential diagnosis of acute groin injuries in male soccer players. Scand J Med Sci Sports 1999;9:98–103.

5. Harris NH, Murray RO. Lesions of the symphysis in athletes. Br Med J 1974;4:211–4.

6. Karlsson J, Sward L, Kalebo P, et al. Chronic groin injuries in athletes. Recommendations for treatment and rehabilitation. Sports Med 1994;17:141–8.

7. Fricker PA. Management of groin pain in athletes. Br J Sports Med 1997;31:97–101.

8. Renstrom P, Peterson L. Groin injuries in athletes. Br J Sports Med 1980;14:30–6.

9. Omar IM, Zoga AC, Kavanagh EC, et al. Athletic pubalgia and "sports hernia": optimal MR imaging technique and findings. Radiographics 2008;28:1415–38.

10. Schilders E, Bismil Q, Robinson P, et al. Adductor-related groin pain in competitive athletes. Role of adductor enthesis, magnetic resonance imaging, and entheseal pubic cleft injections. J Bone Joint Surg Am 2007;89:2173–8.

11. Lynch SA, Renstrom PA. Groin injuries in sport: treatment strategies. Sports Med 1999;28:137–44.

12. Holmich P, Uhrskou P, Ulnits L, et al. Effectiveness of active physical training as treatment for long-standing adductor-related groin pain in athletes: randomised trial. Lancet 1999;353:439–43.

13. Ahumada LA, Ashruf S, Espinosa-de-los-Monteros A, et al. Athletic pubalgia: definition and surgical treatment. Ann Plast Surg 2005;55:393–6.

14. Albers SL, Spritzer CE, Garrett WE Jr., et al. MR findings in athletes with pubalgia. Skeletal Radiol 2001;30:270–7.

15. Morelli V, Weaver V. Groin injuries and groin pain in athletes: part 1. Prim Care 2005;32:163–83.

16. Slavotinek JP, Verrall GM, Fon GT, et al. Groin pain in footballers: the association between preseason clinical and pubic bone magnetic resonance imaging findings and athlete outcome. Am J Sports Med 2005;33:894–9.

17. Koulouris G. Imaging review of groin pain in elite athletes: an anatomic approach to imaging findings. AJR Am J Roentgenol 2008;191:962–72.

18. Brennan D, O'Connell MJ, Ryan M, et al. Secondary cleft sign as a marker of injury in athletes with groin pain: MR image appearance and interpretation. Radiology 2005;235:162–7.

19. Robinson P, Salehi F, Grainger A, et al. Cadaveric and MRI study of the musculotendinous contributions to the capsule of the symphysis pubis. AJR Am J Roentgenol 2007;188:W440–5.

20. Ralphs JR, Benjamin M. The joint capsule: structure, composition, ageing and disease. J Anat 1994;184(Pt 3):503–9.

21. Gamble JG, Simmons SC, Freedman M. The symphysis pubis. Anatomic and pathologic considerations. Clin Orthop Relat Res 1986;203:261–72.

22. Tuite DJ, Finegan PJ, Saliaris AP, et al. Anatomy of the proximal musculotendinous junction of the adductor longus muscle. Knee Surg Sports Traumatol Arthrosc 1998;6:134–7.

23. Gibbon WW, Schilders E. Pelvis, hip and groin. In: Vanhoenacker F, Maas M, Gielen J, editors. Imaging of orthopedic sports injuries. Berlin: Springer; 2007. p. 235–65.

24. Budinoff LC, Tague RG. Anatomical and developmental bases for the ventral arc of the human pubis. Am J Phys Anthropol 1990;82:73–9.

25. Toldt C. The articulations of the lower limb. In: An atlas of human anatomy for students and physicians: osteology. New York: Rebman; 1903. p. 220–1.

26. Ackerman N, Spencer CP. What is your diagnosis? Prepubic tendon injury, with avulsion fracture of the left pubis. J Am Vet Med Assoc 1992;200: 721–2.

27. Condon RE. Reassessment of groin anatomy during the evolution of preperitoneal hernia repair. Am J Surg 1996;172:5–8.

28. Cowan SM, Schache AG, Brukner P, et al. Delayed onset of transversus abdominus in longstanding groin pain. Med Sci Sports Exerc 2004; 36:2040–5.

29. Cunningham PM, Brennan D, O'Connell M, et al. Patterns of bone and soft-tissue injury at the symphysis pubis in soccer players: observations at MRI. AJR Am J Roentgenol 2007;188:W291–6.

30. Zoga AC, Kavanagh EC, Omar IM, et al. Athletic pubalgia and the "sports hernia": MR imaging findings. Radiology 2008;247:797–807.

31. Gibbon WW. Groin pain in athletes. Lancet 1999; 353:1444–5.

32. Walheim GG, Selvik G. Mobility of the pubic symphysis. In vivo measurements with an electromechanic method and a roentgen stereophotogrammetric method. Clin Orthop Relat Res 1984; 191:129–35.

33. Maffey L, Emery C. What are the risk factors for groin strain injury in sport? A systematic review of the literature. Sports Med 2007;37:881–94.

34. Kalebo P, Karlsson J, Sward L, et al. Ultrasonography of chronic tendon injuries in the groin. Am J Sports Med 1992;20:634–9.

35. Robinson P, Barron DA, Parsons W, et al. Adductor-related groin pain in athletes: correlation of MR imaging with clinical findings. Skeletal Radiol 2004; 33:451–7.

36. Van Der Donckt K, Steenbrugge F, Van Den Abbeele K, et al. Bassini's hernial repair and adductor longus tenotomy in the treatment of chronic groin pain in athletes. Acta Orthop Belg 2003;69:35–41.

37. Briggs RC, Kolbjornsen PH, Southall RC. Osteitis pubis, Tc-99m MDP, and professional hockey players. Clin Nucl Med 1992;17:861–3.

38. Gibbon WW, Hession PR. Diseases of the pubis and pubic symphysis: MR imaging appearances. AJR Am J Roentgenol 1997;169:849–53.

39. Verrall GM, Henry L, Fazzalari NL, et al. Bone biopsy of the parasymphyseal pubic bone region in athletes with chronic groin injury demonstrates new woven bone formation consistent with a diagnosis of pubic bone stress injury. Am J Sports Med 2008;36: 2425–31.

40. Holt MA, Keene JS, Graf BK, et al. Treatment of osteitis pubis in athletes. Results of corticosteroid injections. Am J Sports Med 1995;23:601–6.

41. O'Connell MJ, Powell T, McCaffrey NM, et al. Symphyseal cleft injection in the diagnosis and treatment of osteitis pubis in athletes. AJR Am J Roentgenol 2002;179:955–9.

42. Malycha P, Lovell G. Inguinal surgery in athletes with chronic groin pain: the 'sportsman's' hernia. Aust N Z J Surg 1992;62:123–5.

43. Hackney RG. The sports hernia: a cause of chronic groin pain. Br J Sports Med 1993;27:58–62.

44. Holzheimer RG. Inguinal hernia: classification, diagnosis and treatment—classic, traumatic and sportsman's hernia. Eur J Med Res 2005;10:121–34.

45. MacLeod DA, Gibbon WW. The sportsman's groin. Br J Surg 1999;86:849–50.

46. Joesting DR. Diagnosis and treatment of sportsman's hernia. Curr Sports Med Rep 2002;1:121–4.

47. Orchard JW, Read JW, Neophyton J, et al. Groin pain associated with ultrasound finding of inguinal canal posterior wall deficiency in Australian Rules footballers. Br J Sports Med 1998;32:134–9.

48. Long G, Cooper JR, Gibbon WW. Magnetic resonance imaging of injuries in the child athlete. Clin Radiol 1999;54:781–91.

49. Johnston CA, Wiley JP, Lindsay DM, et al. Iliopsoas bursitis and tendinitis. A review. Sports Med 1998; 25:271–83.

50. Kozlov DB, Sonin AH. Iliopsoas bursitis: diagnosis by MRI. J Comput Assist Tomogr 1998;22:625–8.

51. Varma DG, Richli WR, Charnsangavej C, et al. MR appearance of the distended iliopsoas bursa. AJR Am J Roentgenol 1991;156:1025–8.

52. Hong RJ, Hughes TH, Gentili A, et al. Magnetic resonance imaging of the hip. J Magn Reson Imaging 2008;27:435–45.

53. Boutin RD, Newman JS. MR imaging of sports-related hip disorders. Magn Reson Imaging Clin N Am 2003;11:255–81.

54. Kassarjian A, Yoon LS, Belzile E, et al. Triad of MR arthrographic findings in patients with cam-type femoroacetabular impingement. Radiology 2005; 236:588–92.

55. Blankenbaker DG, Ullrick SR, Davis KW, et al. Correlation of MRI findings with clinical findings of trochanteric pain syndrome. Skeletal Radiol 2008; 37:903–9.

MR Imaging of Overuse Injuries of the Hip

Philip A. Hodnett, MD, FFRRCSI, MRCPI, MMedSci[a],*,
Martin J. Shelly, MD, MRCPI[b], Peter J. MacMahon, MD, MRCPI[b],
Eoin C. Kavanagh, MD, MB, FFRRCSI[b],
Stephen J. Eustace, MD, MSc, MB, FFRRCSI[a,c,d,e,f]

KEYWORDS

- MR imaging • Overuse injuries • Hip • Athlete injuries
- Dance injuries • Diagnosis • Treatment

The aim of this article is to emphasize the importance of MR imaging in the evaluation of chronic hip pain and overuse injuries. Image interpretation of the hip can be difficult because of the complex anatomy and the varied pathology that athletes can present with, such as labral and cartilaginous injuries, surrounding soft tissue derangement involving muscles or tendons, and osseous abnormalities. The differential diagnosis in adults is diverse and includes such common entities as stress fracture, avulsive injuries, snapping-hip syndrome, iliopsoas bursitis, femoroacetabular impingement syndrome, tendinosis, and tears of the gluteal musculature.

NORMAL ANATOMY

The hip joint is a ball-and-socket joint allowing motion in a wide range of directions. The femoral head is covered by the spherical acetabular socket except at its inferomedial aspect where the socket is deficient. This deficiency is spanned by the transverse acetabular ligament with stability of the joint in part due to the relationship of the acetabulum to the femur, with the acetabulum directed anterolaterally relative to the pelvis and the femoral neck directed posteriorly. Articular cartilage lines the femoral head except for the fovea capitus, a depression identified on the central surface of the femoral head. The

ligamentum teres arises from this central depression before coursing inferiorly to insert onto the transverse ligament. Horseshoe-shaped articular cartilage, the lunate cartilage, lines the acetabulum except for the central portion of the acetabulum. The acetabular fossa is filled with fibrofatty tissue and lined by synovium.

A fibrocartilaginous labrum, thicker posterosuperiorly than anteroinferiorly, lines the acetabulum, is attached directly to the bony rim, and blends with the transverse ligament at the acetabular notch.[1] The hip capsule inserts onto the acetabular rim directly. Superiorly, the hip joint capsule inserts above the labrum, creating a perilabral recess with a smaller recess between the labrum and joint capsule formed by the capsular insertion along anterior and posterior joint lines.[2,3] The hip is further stabilized by capsular thickenings comprising the iliofemoral, pubofemoral, and ischiofemoral ligaments.

OPTIMAL MR IMAGING PROTOCOL

To optimize MR imaging parameters, consideration must be given to the type of abnormality clinically suspected. Evaluation of the hip may involve one of four standard employed protocols:[4]

Bilateral hip protocol
Unilateral hip protocol

[a] Division of Radiology, Mater Misericordiae University Hospital, Eccles Street, Dublin 7, Ireland
[b] Department of Radiology, Mater Misericordiae University Hospital, Eccles Street, Dublin 7, Ireland
[c] Department of Radiology, Cappagh National Orthopedic Hospital, Finglas, Dublin 11, Ireland
[d] University College Dublin, Belfield, Dublin 4, Ireland
[e] Institute of Radiological Sciences, University College Dublin, Dublin, Ireland
[f] Department of Radiology, Santry Sports Surgery Clinic, Santry Demense, Dublin 9, Ireland
* Corresponding author.
E-mail address: p-hodnett@md.northwestern.edu (P.A. Hodnett).

Magn Reson Imaging Clin N Am 17 (2009) 667–679
doi:10.1016/j.mric.2009.06.005
1064-9689/09/$ – see front matter © 2009 Elsevier Inc. All rights reserved.

Protocol tailored to exclude an occult fracture
Direct magnetic resonance (MR) arthrogram
protocol

When bilateral hip pathology is suspected, routine sequences include T1-weighted and fast inversion recovery sequences in the coronal plane with a torso phased array coil.[5] A fast spin echo sequence is used in the axial plane, often with fat suppression. The addition of a fat-suppressed sequence helps identify areas of bone marrow edema that may be indicative of stress reaction or fracture. The field of view is decreased typically to 17 to 20 cm in patients with suspected unilateral hip pathology with coronal, axial, and sagittal fast spin echo sequences without fat suppression. If the clinical examination or a nonathrographic MR imaging study has suggested a possible labral or intra-articular pathology in the hip, then a direct MR arthrogram is performed.[6] MR arthrography is the preferred examination for evaluation of the joint capsule, labrum, and articular cartilage. Intra-articular needle placement is confirmed under fluoroscopic guidance before 15 mL of 1:200 dilution of gadolinium contrast and normal saline injection. Axial, coronal, sagittal T1-weighted fat-suppressed images are obtained employing a surface coil or torso phased array coil for optimal signal-to-noise ratio.[7] Imaging parameters should include a field of view of 14 to 16 cm, section thickness of 3 to 5 mm for spin echo sequences or 1.5 mm for gradient echo sequences, and a matrix of 192 to 256×256.[8]

STRESS RESPONSE AND FRACTURES

Stress fractures occur when abnormal, repetitive stress is applied to normal bone. The repetitive stresses, none of which is singularly capable of producing fracture, may lead to mechanical failure over time (**Fig. 1**).[9] Running athletes are the most commonly affected with a greater incidence of stress fractures occurring in female athletes because of reduced muscle bulk. Patients typically present with activity-related pain abating with rest, with persisting pain during rest indicating a more advanced stage of injury. Stress fracture of the femoral neck typically occurs at the medial femoral neck in ballet dancers and long-distance runners, with femoral shaft involvement seen in gymnasts (**Fig. 2**). Long-distance runners may also display MR-signal abnormalities, including marrow edema and periostitis of the lesser trochanter, in addition to bone marrow edema in the femoral neck.[10] The absence of a cortical fracture line on MR imaging

allows differentiation of stress response from stress fracture (**Fig. 3**), which represents a spectrum of injury.[11]

The radiographic features of stress fracture vary in accordance with the location and chronicity of injury and may include periosteal reaction, endosteal sclerosis, cortical thickening, and a lucent fracture line.[10] Radiographs are often unrevealing with follow-up films demonstrating abnormalities in only 50%, while bone scintigraphy may result in a false-positive diagnosis in up to 30% of cases.[12,13] Bone scintigraphy has therefore been largely superseded by MR imaging as the imaging modality of choice because of its superior spatial resolution.[14] Edematous marrow has low signal intensity on T1-weighted images and markedly high signal intensity on T2-weighted fat-suppressed or short tau inversion recovery (STIR) images. Edematous marrow, unlike reconversion marrow, is much more intense on STIR images and does not respect boundaries, such as the physis (**Fig. 4**).

MR imaging findings of periosteal and marrow edema are early signs of stress response with low signal intensity most conspicuous on T1-weighted sequences, confirming discrete stress-fracture formation.[15] Stress fractures displaying fragmentation and osteolysis with low signal intensity on T2-weighted sequences are suggestive of more long-standing injury. MR imaging is of greater usefulness in the follow-up imaging of patients with stress fractures. Nondisplaced femoral stress fractures usually show resolution of T2 and STIR high signal intensity within 6 months of the first MR study.[16,17]

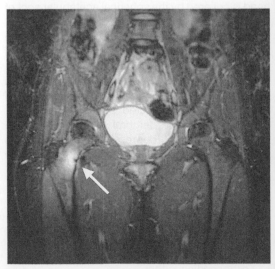

Fig.1. T2 short tau inversion recovery–weighted coronal image showing femoral neck with high signal intensity (*arrow*), consistent with an incomplete stress fracture.

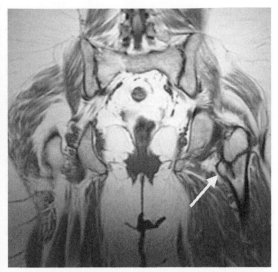

Fig. 2. T1-weighted coronal image demonstrating linear low signal intensity through the femoral neck (*arrow*), consistent with a complete stress fracture.

APOPHYSEAL INJURIES

Apophysitis represents the earliest spectrum of injury to the apophysis with excessive stress the underlying cause. It is most prevalent in the skeletally immature patient, occurring in patients between the ages of 12 and 22 years of age clinically presenting with athletic pubalgia.[13] The clinical term *athletic pubalgia* has been used to encompass patients presenting with symptoms secondary to injuries of pubic symphysis, hip

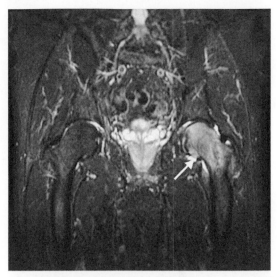

Fig. 4. T2 STIR–weighted coronal image showing florid marrow edema (*arrow*) within the femoral head and neck with incomplete femoral neck stress fracture. Associated joint effusion is also present.

adductor tendon dysfunction, and the pubic attachment of the rectus abdominis.

Apophysitis in the pelvis may involve the anterior superior iliac spine (sartorius and tensor fascia lata muscles) (Fig. 5), the anterior inferior iliac spine (rectus femoris), and the ischial tuberosity (semitendinosus, semimembranosus, long head of biceps, and ischial origin of adductor magnus). Fluid-sensitive sequences reveal marrow edema in the apophysis with associated high signal intensity consistent with edema in the involved muscle and associated peritendinous edema (Fig. 6). Increased signal intensity on fluid-sensitive sequences and mild widening of the physis, often with adjacent bone-marrow edema, are characteristic of apophysitis in adolescent athletes. If these

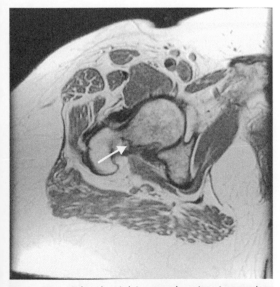

Fig. 3. T1-weighted axial image showing incomplete stress fracture (*arrow*) through the femoral neck. Note the adjacent edematous marrow in the femoral neck mainfesting as low signal intensity.

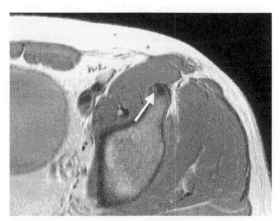

Fig. 5. T1-weighted axial image demonstrating anterior iliac spine apophysitis (*arrow*).

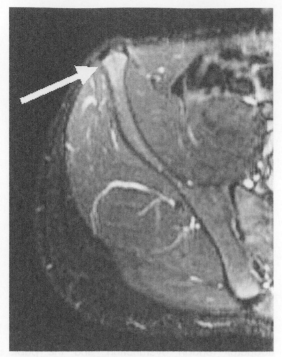

Fig. 6. T2 STIR–weighted axial image of pelvis showing edema (*arrow*) of the anterior superior iliac spine with irregularity typical of apophysitis.

overuse injuries are not recognized, particularly in athletes involved in kicking of sports, avulsive injuries may occur. Initial early diagnosis is crucial to allow conservative management and involves cessation of the offending activity to allow ossification at the zone of transitional cartilage.[13] Avulsive injuries are common amongst participants in organized sports, particularly amongst adolescents. Muscles attach to bone directly or indirectly via tendons, producing movements at joints. In adolescents, tendons and muscles insert directly onto the apophyses, rendering these patients susceptible to this type of injury until their middle 20s when fusion has taken place.[18] Cheerleaders, sprinters, gymnasts, and football, baseball, and track athletes are especially prone to these injuries with multiple avulsions occasionally seen. While acute avulsive injuries result from extreme, unbalanced, often eccentric muscular contractions, chronic injuries are the result of repetitive microtrauma.

When there is no history of a specific traumatic event and plain film findings are confusing, MR imaging can be crucial in avoiding unnecessary imaging and potential biopsy, as well as useful in excluding high-grade tendon injury. Posttraumatic appearance at the site of avulsive injury may simulate osteomyelitis or malignancy.

Avulsion injuries primarily occur at six sites in the pelvis: the iliac crest, the anterior superior the iliac spine, the anterior inferior iliac spine (Fig. 7), the greater trochanter, the lesser trochanter, the body of pubis, and the ischial tuberosity.[19,20] On plain film assessment, acute injuries are associated with avulsed bone fragments, while injuries that are more chronic may have an aggressive appearance of mixed sclerosis and lysis.

Coronal fluid-sensitive images are particularly useful in assessing the pelvis with marrow edema and reactive change in the surrounding soft tissues at the site of repetitive microtrauma. Often, MR images show irregularity and bony protuberance at the avulsive site with the displaced bone fragment visible. Fortunately, the periosteum and surrounding fascia often limit severe displacement (Fig. 8). In nondisplaced avulsions, sharply marginated pieces of bone are seen adjacent to its donor site. Avulsions of both the anterior superior (sartorius) and anterior inferior (rectus femorus) iliac spines tend to be less disabling and symptomatic than avulsions of the ischial tuberosity (Fig. 9) where full athletic potential returns in 5 to 6 weeks.[21,22] Avulsion injuries of the iliac spines are most commonly seen in the sprinting phase of running, in hurdling, and in kicking sports, such as soccer.

Reports of iliac crest avulsion at the abdominal musculature insertion are uncommon, as are lesser trochanter injuries at the iliopsoas insertion.[23,24] Avulsion of the lesser trochanter occurs with vigorous contraction of the iliopsoas tendon during hip flexion. Bertin and colleagues[25] were

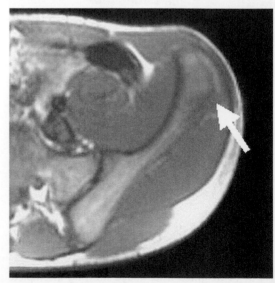

Fig. 7. T1-weighted axial image showing apophysitis of the anterior superior iliac spine and marrow edema (*arrow*) manifest as low signal intensity.

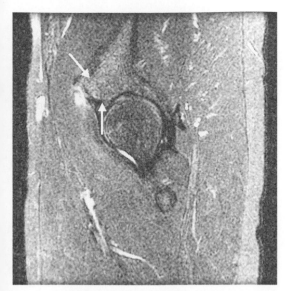

Fig. 8. T2 STIR–weighted sagittal image showing minimally displaced bone fragment (*arrows*) arising from the anterior inferior iliac spine with MR features consistent with acute avulsive injury. Associated reactive changes visible in adjacent soft tissues.

the first to recognize that isolated avulsion fracture of the lesser trochanter in an adult in the absence of trauma is secondary to metastatic disease until proven otherwise. Ischial tuberosity fractures or "hurdlers' fractures" occur during hip flexion with knee extension, causing excessive hamstring muscle tension.[26]

Generally, these injuries are managed conservatively but may result in prolonged symptoms and pain referral to the posterior thigh.[27] Consideration may be given to surgical fixation if the fragment is of sufficient size to contain hardware and the displacement is 2 cm or greater. Reports of late-presentation

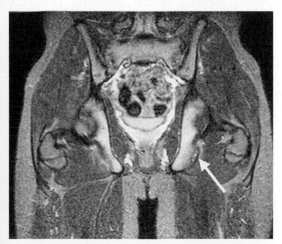

Fig. 9. T2 STIR–weighted coronal image showing acute left ischial tuberosity avulsion (*arrow*).

sciatic nerve palsy that responds to mass excision and neurolysis have been documented.[27–29]

SNAPPING-HIP SYNDROME

Snapping-hip syndrome (coxa saltans, iliopsoas tendonitis, or dancer's hip), a clinical entity referring to an audible snap or click occurring at the hip joint, is commonly seen in such athletes as distance track-and-field runners, ballet dancers, gymnasts, horse riders, and soccer players, where repetitive hip flexion leads to injury (**Fig. 10**). A snapping sensation may be felt when the hip is flexed and extended, which may be accompanied by an audible snapping noise. Less than one third of individuals who experience snapping-hip syndrome have any pain accompanying the snapping-hip sensation. A number of different etiologies, both intra-articular and extra-articular, have been described. Taking into account the localization of the causes for snapping hip, three different syndromes are described.

The lateral (external) extra-articular type of snapping-hip syndrome occurs when movement of the iliotibial band, tensor fascia lata, or gluteus medius is partially obstructed when sliding over the greater trochanter. The medial (internal) extra-articular type involves the iliopsoas tendon as it moves from an anterolateral to a posteromedial position. The iliopsoas tendon comes into contact with an osseous protuberance, most

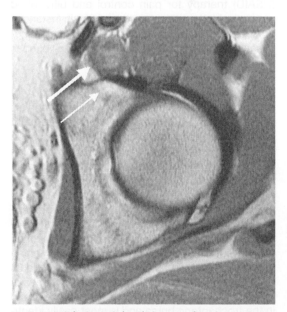

Fig. 10. Axial T1-weighted image showing osseous protuberance anteriorly (*thin arrow*) resulting in intratendinous high signal intensity (tendinosis) within the iliopsoas tendon (*thick arrow*), also referred to as internal snapping-hip syndrome.

commonly the iliopectineal eminence, or a prominent anterior-inferior iliac spinal process during hip extension.[30]

Intra-articular snapping-hip syndrome is often indicative of a torn acetabular labrum, recurrent hip dislocation, ligamentum teres tears, loose bodies, or articular cartilage damage. With chronic repetitive movement, affected patients develop iliopsoas tendon pathology, such as iliopsoas bursitis and tendinosis. Classically, when a snapping iliopsoas tendon was suspected, bursography or tenography procedures were used preoperatively to confirm the diagnosis. Ultrasound, besides detecting bursitis, allows for dynamic visualization of the iliopsoas tendon as it passes over the iliopectineal eminence during dynamic maneuvers.[31] MR imaging allows for more thorough assessment of patients with snapping-hip syndrome than ultrasound does, allowing evaluation of potential intra-articular causes of snapping-hip syndrome. The diagnosis should be considered when thickening of the iliopsoas tendon in association with altered intrasubstance signal intensity is identified next to an osseous spur arising from the iliopectineal eminence. Treatment is generally conservative with physiotherapy that employs passive and active exercises, stretches the hip into extension, and limits excessive knee flexion, thereby maximizing the stretch to the iliopsoas tendon. Treatment also usually involves nonsteroidal anti-inflammatory drug (NSAID) therapy for pain control and ultrasound image–guided corticosteroid injection in instances of bursitis.[13] If nonsurgical treatment is unsuccessful, surgical lengthening of the iliopsoas tendon may be performed.[32]

Lateral (external) snapping-hip syndrome is the most frequent snapping-hip syndrome.[33] It is caused most commonly by the iliotibial band as it slides over the greater trochanter and is frequent in runners, dancers, and basketball players. It can be asymptomatic or accompanied by pain, which may be especially intense in patients who develop trochanteric bursitis. External snapping hip is caused by excessive tightness of the iliotibial band, which can result from leg-length discrepancies. Ultrasound demonstrates the abnormal motion of the iliotibial band or gluteus maximus tendon but is highly user-dependent. MR imaging may demonstrate a number of findings in patients with external snapping-hip syndrome. In cases with iliotibial band involvement, fluid may be found in the trochanteric bursa and is most easily identified on T2-weighted images.[34] In cases with iliopsoas tendon involvement, the tendon may be thicker relative to the contralateral side, which is most obvious on coronal pelvic images. Additional MR imaging findings commonly seen include changes consistent with iliopsoas tendonitis, tendinosis, or both. Tendinosis is demonstrated on spin-echo T1-weighted images as an area of higher signal intensity within the tendon with less marked signal change on T1-weighted images. In cases of tendonitis, increased fluid in the iliopsoas peritendinous tissues is conspicuous on spin-echo T2-weighted images or STIR sequences as a focus of high signal intensity surrounding a normal tendon.[33,34] Nonoperative treatment of external snapping hip consists of rest, avoidance of painful movements, iliotibial band–stretching exercises, strengthening of hip flexors, and NSAID therapy. In refractory cases, ultrasound-guided corticosteroid injection into iliopsoas peritendinous tissues or the iliopsoas bursa may allow return to sporting activity.

GREATER TROCHANTERIC PAIN SYNDROME

Lateral hip pain is often a challenging diagnostic problem with a wide range of diagnostic considerations that may present in a similar fashion.[35] Many pathologic processes, such as trochanteric bursitis, tendinosis and tears of the gluteal medius and minimus muscles, degenerative hip arthropathy, stress fractures, and entrapment syndromes may all present with similar symptoms.

Modern high-field MR imaging has increased our understanding of pathologies affecting the soft tissues of the hip. This encompasses not only trochanteric bursitis but also what have been labeled rotator cuff tears of the hip, which are analogous to rotator cuff tears in the shoulder.[36] The term *rotator cuff tear* refers to a tear in one or more tendons of the hip abductors. Typically, this is a circular or oval defect in the gluteus minimus tendon extending posteriorly into the lateral part of the gluteus medius with signs of trochanteric bursitis and gluteal tendon tears frequently coexisting on MR imaging and surgical correlation. The greater trochanteric pain syndrome, a common regional pain syndrome most often clinically diagnosed as trochanteric bursitis, typically presents with pain along the lateral hip aspect.[35] Patients typically present with chronic pain and tenderness over the lateral aspect of the hip with a peak incidence between the fourth and sixth decades of life and with a female preponderance.[36] Trochanteric bursitis is relatively common and occurs in both sedentary and athletic patients, occurring frequently in marathon runners. Clinical examination reveals localized or diffuse tenderness over the greater trochanter with symptom exacerbation occasionally reproduced in abduction and external rotation.

Symptoms are typically worse when lying in the lateral decubitus position on the affected side.[36]

Historically, patients presenting with a clinical diagnosis of trochanteric bursitis refer to inflammatory change of the subgluteus maximus bursa, which lies beneath the iliotibial band at the insertion of gluteus medius tendon insertion (**Fig. 11**).[37] The trochanteric bursal complex comprises the major bursae, subgluteus maximus and medius bursae, and the solitary minor bursa, subgluteus minimus.[38] Studies examining the trochanteric bursal complex and our understanding of the greater trochanteric bursitis reveal that tendinopathy of the gluteus medius and minimus muscles in these patients forms part of a spectrum of injury, commencing with bursitis secondary to impingement followed by tendinopathy and the formation of tears.[39,40]

Trochanteric bursitis is described if distension of the above bursae is evident on T1- or T2-weighted images. This MR finding is quite commonly absent and likely explains why the term *greater trochanter pain syndrome* rather than *trochanteric bursitis* is increasingly employed. Trochanteric bursitis has been demonstrated to coexist with gluteal tendinosis in up to 40% of patients with bursitis and manifests as homogeneous T2 hyperintensity, which may display enhancement post–contrast administration on MR imaging. Gluteal tears typically appear as a circular or oval defect most commonly in the gluteus minimus tendon extending into the adjacent part of the gluteus medius tendon.[41] A partial tear is diagnosed (**Fig. 12**)

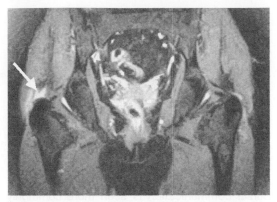

Fig. 12. T2 STIR–weighted coronal image with right gluteus medius (*arrow*) proximal tendon partial tear.

when focal tendon discontinuity is present. A complete tear is diagnosed when a full-thickness abnormality (**Fig. 13**) or tendon retraction is evident. The deepest and most anterior aspects of the gluteal medius tendon are most commonly affected by partial tears with coexistent gluteus minimus tears occurring in 20% to 100% on surgical correlation. The term *bald trochanter* is used when there are full-thickness tears of both gluteus medius and minimus with retraction evident on MR imaging.[42] Partial tears may occur in isolation but often occur on a background of underlying gluteal tendinosis or tendinopathy.[43] Gluteal tendinopathy on MR imaging manifests as thickening of the tendon and T2-weighted signal intermediate to high signal intensity. The abnormality is important to identify as radiologists play an important role in conservative management by performing ultrasound-guided corticosteroid injection into the bursa.

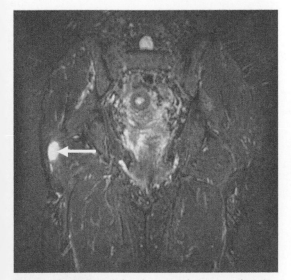

Fig. 11. T2 STIR–weighted coronal image showing signal hyperintensity within a distended trochanteric bursal complex (*arrow*), historically referred to as trochanteric bursitis.

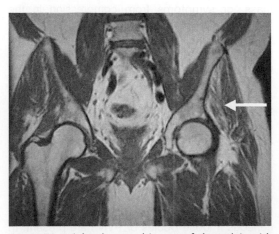

Fig. 13. T1-weighted coronal image of the pelvis with asymmetry (*arrow*) within left gluteal musculature. MR findings compatible with left gluteus medius tendon full-thickness tear and muscle atrophy.

ILIOPSOAS BURSITIS AND TENDINOSIS

The iliopsoas musculotendinous unit is becoming recognized as an important cause of hip pain in the general and athletic population with iliopsoas tendinosis, snapping-hip syndrome, iliopsoas bursitis, and avulsion injuries, which are all recognized entities.[44] The iliopsoas tendon inserts on the lesser trochanter, allowing hip flexion and external rotation of the femur. The iliopsoas bursa is found in 98% of subjects, communicates with the cavity of the hip in about 15% of cases, and is readily demonstrated on hip arthrography. Bursal communication is seen more commonly after hip arthroplasty, possibly because of surgical disruption of the bursal wall or increased intra-articular pressure from excess joint fluid. This communication may be congenital or caused by friction of the iliopsoas tendon on the bursa, resulting in small synovial tears.[45] Patients typically present with insidious onset of anterior hip or groin pain.

The average time from initial onset of symptoms to diagnosis ranges from 32 to 41 months. Pain, first occurring after onset of aggravating activity, may eventually occur during activity and rest.[44] Tenderness on palpation of the lesser trochanter under the gluteal fold may be elicited with the patient in the prone position. If the patient sits with knees extended and the heel on the affected side elevated, pain may be reported. This is known as a positive Ludloff sign.[44]

The normal iliopsoas bursa separates the iliopsoas tendon from the hip joint articular capsule and is collapsed on MR imaging. The iliopsoas muscle is of intermediate signal intensity on routine T1- or T2-weighted images.[46] Iliopsoas bursitis may present with hip pain, a palpable mass, or symptoms from compression in the inguinal and pelvic areas. Inflammation of the iliopsoas bursa may occur secondary to overuse, trauma, osteoarthritis, rheumatoid arthritis, avascular necrosis, gout, pigmented villonodular synovitis (PVNS), and pyogenic infection.[47] The distension present within the iliopsoas bursa on MR imaging is variable and characteristically extends along the iliopsoas muscle. Imaging characteristics of iliopsoas bursitis are a well-defined cystic mass posterior to the iliopsoas tendon (Fig. 14). The signal characteristics of the fluid within the bursa are typically similar to those of water and thus homogeneously hyperintense on fluid-sensitive sequences, but may appear heterogeneous if loose bodies or PVNS are present. In most cases, the bursal wall displays peripheral contrast enhancement.[48] Concurrent hip effusion is often seen in patients with iliopsoas bursitis

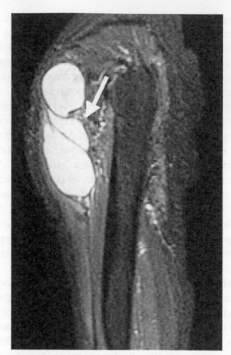

Fig. 14. Coronal T2-weighted sagittal image of the pelvis with well-defined cystic mass (*arrow*) posterior to the iliopsoas tendon, consistent with iliopsoas bursitis.

with bursal distension caused by overproduction of synovial fluid within an arthritic hip decompressing into the bursa (Fig. 15). The identification of iliopsoas bursitis allows subsequent ultrasound

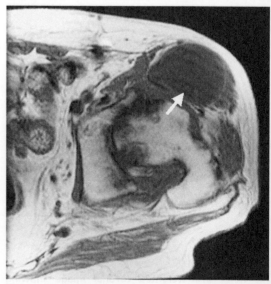

Fig. 15. T1-weighted axial image with features of erosive hip arthropathy with hip joint effusion and associated (*arrow*) iliopsoas bursitis.

image-guided bursal aspiration and corticosteroid injection, which may provide long-term pain relief.[49,50] Ultrasound-guided lidocaine injection through the femoral triangle can be performed with the lidocaine challenge test deemed positive if resolution of symptoms occurs after injection. Other treatments occasionally employed for refractory bursitis include those that address causes for excess joint fluid, such as removal of a loose joint prosthesis, oral NSAID therapy, use of sclerosant agents, and, rarely, surgical bursectomy.[50]

The iliopsoas tendon should appear with uniformly low signal intensity on T1- and T2-weighted images. MR imaging in iliopsoas tendinosis shows focal high signal intensity on the spin-echo T1-weighted imaging within the iliopsoas tendon with less marked abnormality on spin-echo T2-weighted images. The use of MR imaging also allows exclusion of acute musculotendinous injury, which displays conspicuous T2 increased signal intensity associated with inflammation and swelling. However, in instances of more severe injury, both the T1-weighted images and T2-weighted images depict high signal change.[51,52] In instances of iliopsoas tendinosis where MR imaging is unremarkable, the previously described lidocaine challenge test may be performed using ultrasound guidance. Most patients respond to conservative treatment measures with surgical intervention rarely used for iliopsoas tendinosis. In carefully selected patients in whom prolonged nonsurgical management has failed, two surgical techniques have been employed.[51] These involve either complete release of the iliopsoas tendon or, alternatively, partial release by transection of the posteromedial aspect of the iliopsoas tendon with good results in terms of pain relief and return to previous level of athletic involvement.[52]

LABRUM AND HIP JOINT CAPSULE

Radiographs are typically normal in patients with internal derangement as a cause for hip pain. Multiple pathologies, including osteoarthritis, occult fracture, avascular necrosis, synovial osteochondromatosis, and PVNS, may all present with similar symptoms. Labral tears have been reported in patients with a previous history of trauma and developmental dysplasia of the hip and in patients with no previous injury referable to the hip. The increased risk for labral injury in patients with developmental dysplasia is secondary to deficient acetabular coverage of the femoral head increasing the weight-bearing load on the labrum. Labral lesions have a strong

correlation with anterior hip pain, transient locking, and subluxation of the hip, with pain reproduced during internal rotation and flexion of the hip and with an audible click occasionally heard.[8]

MR arthrography has emerged as the gold standard for the preoperative diagnosis of labral tears. In addition to identifying labral lesions, usually visible previously only at arthroscopy, loose bodies and other intra-articular causes for hip pain are demonstrated. Once intra-articular needle placement has been confirmed in the fluoroscopy suite, a dilute solution (0.2 mmol/L) of gadopentetate dimeglumine is injected. The high-signal intra-articular gadopentetate solution is most conspicuous on T1-weighted imaging with fat saturation routinely employed to increase contrast. Images are obtained in the three orthogonal planes given the spherical nature of the hip joint with the normal labrum showing uniformly low signal intensity on T1-weighted images with internal intermediate signal intensity at the junction of the articular cartilage and labrum.[53] Both acetabular and glenoid labral tears share common features on MR arthrography. Labral tears in both instances begin at the junction of labral fibrocartilage and hyaline cartilage and may extend into the labral substance or extend to the bony labral attachment.[54] Detachments occur more frequently than tears and are visible as contrast material interposed at the acetabular-labral junction. Sports-related labral tears occur anterosuperiorly on the acetabular rim (**Fig. 16**), visible as a labral detachment separating the base of the labrum from underlying bone.[8,53] In cases of hip dysplasia, labral tears are identified superior

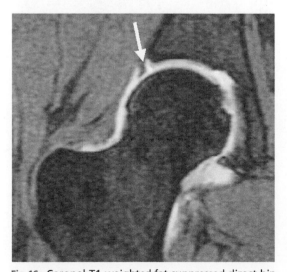

Fig. 16. Coronal T1-weighted fat-suppressed direct hip arthrogram showing an anterosuperior labral tear (*arrow*).

(lateral) on the acetabular rim secondary to repeated femoral head impaction.[54] Paralabral cysts may develop adjacent to labral tears with extrusion of fluid into the periarticular soft tissues and should provoke careful search for a labral tear (**Fig. 17**) with other ancillary findings, including subchondral marrow edema and subchondral cystic change. In most cases, gadolinium injected at arthrography fails to fill these cysts. As a torn labral fragment becomes detached from the acetabular rim, its protection of adjacent articular cartilage decreases and weight-bearing forces become unevenly distributed over the cartilaginous surface. This predisposes to degenerative joint disease and chondral defects, the latter accompanying 30% of labral tears and detachments. For the radiologist, it is these labral tears, loose bodies, and chondral abnormalities that must be identified, as these may be amenable to arthroscopic intervention that may halt or delay potential premature degenerative joint disease.

Femoroacetabular impingent (FAI) occurs when the configuration between the acetabular rim and proximal femur is abnormal. Each FAI is classified as either a cam FAI or a pincer FAI, depending on the presence of either a femoral or an acetabular abnormality respectively. FAI leads to premature osteoarthritis, typically becoming symptomatic in the second and third decades in the athletic population. In cases of cam-type impingement, the nonspherical shape of the femoral head at the femoral head-neck junction and reduced depth of the femoral waist leads to abutment of femoral head-neck junction against the acetabular rim (**Fig. 18**).[8] The abnormal femoral head can be measured by assessment of the α angle at the anterior aspect of the femoral head-neck junction. A cut-off angle of 55° has been described in the diagnosis of FAI, emphasizing the need for radial images around the center line of the femoral neck for visualization of the anterosuperior femoral neck.[53] With cam impingement, articular cartilage injury and labral tears usually occur along the anterior and superolateral acetabular rim.

In pincer-type impingement, overcoverage of the acetabulum as in protrusio acetabuli or localized in patients with acetabular retroversion is the underlying cause. Pincer-type impingement results in more severe cartilage damage at the posterior and posteroinferior acetabulum. In pincer-type FAI, chondral acetabular injury occurs in a narrow band at the anterior and superolateral acetabular labrum where forces are greatest and as a contre-coup injury in the posterior labrum due to the femoral head levering out of the hip socket during hip flexion.

In both types of impingement, labral and bony acetabular changes frequently coincide, with an osseous deformity visible at the femoral head-neck junction (**Fig. 19**).[54] The majority of patients

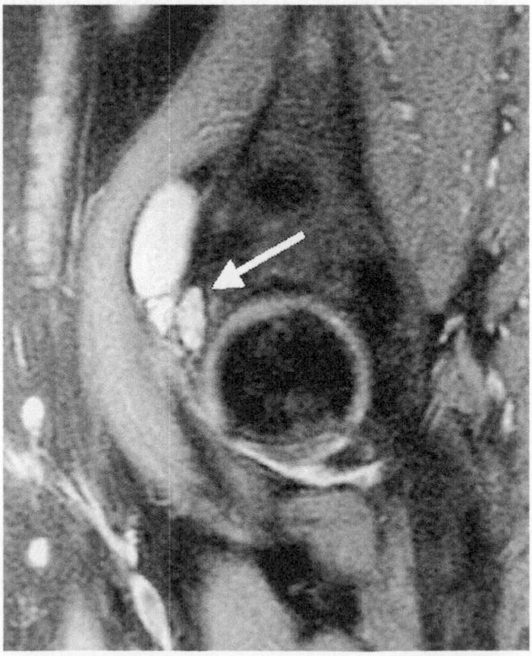

Fig. 17. T1-weighted sagittal fat-suppressed direct arthrogram showing paralabral cyst (*arrow*) formation in patient with arthroscopically proven labral tear.

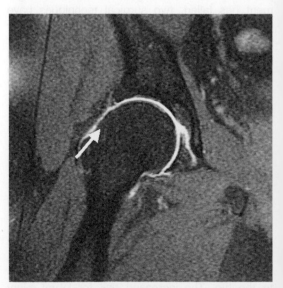

Fig. 18. T1-weighted fat-suppressed coronal direct arthrogram showing the nonspherical shape of the femoral head at the femoral head-neck junction (*arrow*) and reduced depth of the femoral waist. MR image features typical in cam-type FAI.

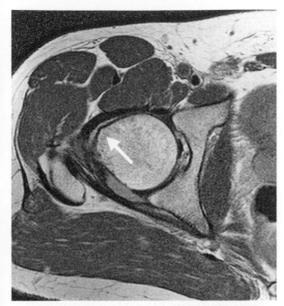

Fig. 19. T1-weighted axial image showing osseous deformity (*arrow*), visible at the femoral head-neck junction, which has a strong association with cam-type FAI.

with proven labral tears have an abnormality on hip radiographs.[55] The irregular ossification and osteophyte formation of the acetabular rim lead to progressive overcoverage of the femoral head and exacerbates the FAI. Frequently, an os acetabuli, which initially develops at 8 years of age before uniting with the os pubis in late adolescence, is identified on MR in patients with FAI and is secondary to abnormal stresses causing fragmentation of the bony fragment.[56–58]

FAI leads to premature osteoarthritis in the hip joint and early detection allows surgical correction and possible delay or halt of end-stage osteoarthritis. In cam-type impingement, surgical correction is achieved by reshaping the nonspherical portion of the femoral head and proximal femur. Surgical intervention in pincer-type FAI includes trimming the acetabular rim to reduce overcoverage of the acetabulum and periacetabular osteotomy to reorient the acetabulum in patients with acetabular retroversion. In patients with advanced cartilage delamination, joint-preserving surgery may no longer be possible and therefore accurate assessment is vital. Unfortunately, the diagnosis of cartilage delamination is difficult even with MR arthrography. Shearing forces strip the acetabular labrum from the subchondral bone. The diagnosis of cartilage delamination is paramount because procedures that can be joint preserving, such as open or arthroscopic osteochondroplasty, can provide improved function, relieve pain, and allow

return to sport participation. The difficulty arises in diagnosis because, in delamination, the cartilage surface may be intact but the cartilage layer moves relative to the underlying bone plate.[59] Overall, the sensitivity of MR arthrography for assessment of the acetabular cartilage in FAI ranges from 65% to 100% with specificity falling to 40% to 80%.[60] Initial reports on delamination described the "inverted Oreo cookie" sign, where the cartilage flap appears as a linear articular low-signal filling defect surrounded by intra-articular contrast material.[61] This is infrequently found, however, with hypointensity of the articular cartilage on intermediate-weighted fat-saturated images and on T1-weighted images a more helpful finding in the diagnosis of cartilage delamination.[61–65]

SUMMARY

Athletes presenting with hip pain can have diverse causes for presentation, including stress fractures, traction injuries of the apophysis, tendon injuries, bursitis, and intra-articular derangement encompassing labral and cartilaginous injuries. Modern high-field MR imaging is an excellent diagnostic modality for the assessment of extra- and intra-articular hip pathology. Labral abnormalities and cartilage damage previously only seen at invasive arthroscopy can now be visualized with direct MR arthrography. MR arthrography of the hip has emerged as a valuable tool for detecting internal derangement of the hip and allowing detection of intraosseous bodies, cartilage, and labral injuries, precursors to the development of premature osteoarthritis. Familiarity with the complex hip anatomy and MR findings encountered typically in overuse injuries of the hip will allow the radiologist to continue to make a significant contribution in the diagnosis and treatment of these athletes.

REFERENCES

1. Czerny C, Hofmann S, Neuhold A, et al. Lesions of the acetabular labrum; accuracy of MR imaging and MR arthrography in detection and staging. Radiology 1996;200:225–30.
2. Keene GS, Villar RN. Arthroscopic anatomy of the hip; an in vivo study. Arthroscopy 1994;10:392–9.
3. Williams PL, Warwick R, editors. Arthrology; the joints of the lower limb-the hip (coaxial) joint. Gray's anatomy. 36th edition. Philadelphia: Saunders; 1980. p. 477–82.
4. Abe I, Harada Y, Oinima K, et al. Acetabular labrum: abnormal findings on MR imaging in asymptomatic hips. Radiology 2000;216(2):576–81.
5. Bogost GA, Lizerbram EK, Crues JV. R imaging in evaluation of suspected hip fracture: frequency of

unsuspected bone and soft tissue injury. Radiology 1995;197:263–7.

6. Conway WF, Totty WG, McErney KW. CT and MR imaging of the hip. Radiology 1996;198:297–307.

7. Teh J. Imaging the hip. Imaging 2007;19(3):234–48.

8. Petersilge CA. Chronic adult hip pain: MR arthrography of the hip. Radiographics 2000;20:S43–52.

9. LeBlanc KE, LeBlanc KA. Groin pain in athletes. Hernia 2003;7:68–71.

10. Nguyen JT, Peterson JS, Biswal S, et al. Stress related injuries around the lesser trochanter in long distance runners. AJR Am J Roentgenol 2008;190:1616–20.

11. Deutsch AL, Coel MN, Mink JH. Imaging of stress injuries to bone: radiography, scintigraphy and MR imaging. Clin Sports Med 1997;16:275–90.

12. Spitz D, Newberg A. Imaging of stress fractures in the athlete. Radiol Clin North Am 2002;40:313–31.

13. Omar IM, Zoga AC, Kavanagh EC, et al. Athletic pubalgia and "sports hernia": optimal MR imaging technique and findings. Radiographics 2008;28:1415–38.

14. Brittenden J, Robinson P. Imaging of pelvic injuries in athletes. Br J Radiol 2005;78:457–68.

15. Gaeta M, Minutoli F, Scribano E, et al. CT and MR imaging findings in athletes with early tibial stress injuries; comparison with bone scintigraphy findings and emphasis on cortical abnormalities. Radiology 2005;235:553–61.

16. Slocum KA, Gorman JD, Puckett ML, et al. Resolution of abnormal MR signal intensity in patients with stress fractures of the femoral neck. AJR Am J Roentgenol 1997;168:1295–9.

17. Lee JK, Yao L. Stress fractures; MR imaging. Radiology 1988;169:217–20.

18. Anderson K, Strickland SM, Warren R. Hip and groin injuries in athletes. Am J Sports Med 2001;29:521–33.

19. Zarins B, Cuillo JV. Acute muscle and tendon injuries in athletes. Clin Sports Med 1983;2:167–82.

20. Wooton JR, Cross MJ, Holt KWG. Avulsion of the ischial apophysis. J Bone Joint Surg Br 1990;72:625–7.

21. Schneider R, Kaye JJ, Ghelman B. Adductor avulsive injuries near the symphysis pubis. Radiology 1976;120:567–9.

22. Tehranzadeh J. The spectrum of avulsion and avulsive like injuries of the musculoskeletal system. Radiographics 1987;7:945–74.

23. Combs JA. Hip and pelvis avulsion fractures in adolescents. Phys Sports Med 1994;22:41–9.

24. Metzmaker JN, Pappas AM. Avulsion of the pelvis. Am J Sports Med 1985;13:349–58.

25. Bertin KC, Horstman J, Coleman SS. Isolated fracture of the lesser trochanter in adults: an initial manifestation of metastatic malignant disease. J Bone Joint Surg Am 1984;66:770–3.

26. Gamble JG, Kao J. Avulsion fracture of the lesser trochanter in a preadolescent athlete. J Pediatr Orthop B 1993;2:188–90.

27. Kujala UM, Orava S, Karpakka J, et al. Ischial tuberosity apophysitis and avulsion among athletes. Int J Sports Med 1997;149–55.

28. Miller A, Stedman GH, Beisaw NE, et al. Sciatica caused by an avulsion fracture of the ischial tuberosity. J Bone Joint Surg Am 1987;69:143–5.

29. Spinner RJ, Atkinson JL, Wenger DE, et al. Tardy sciatic nerve palsy following apophyseal avulsion fracture of the ischial tuberosity. J Neurosurg 1998;89:819–21.

30. Peck DM. Apopyseal injuries in the young athlete. Am Fam Physician 1995;1:1891–5.

31. Cardinal E, Buckwater KA, Capello WN, et al. US of the snapping iliopsoas tendon. Radiology 1998;198:521–2.

32. Blakenbaker DG, Tuite MJ. The painful hip: new concepts. Skeletal Radiol 2006;35(6):352–70.

33. Jacobson M, Allen WC. Surgical correlation of the snapping iliopsoas tendon. Am J Sports Med 1990;18:470–4.

34. Gruen G, Scioscia T, Lowenstein J. The surgical treatment of internal snapping hip. Am J Sports Med 2000;30:607–13.

35. Williams RL, Warwick R. Gray's anatomy. Philadelphia: Saunders; 1980. p. 390–4, 477–82, 600–3.

36. Kagan A II. Rotator cuff tears of the hip. Clin Orthop 1999;36:135–40.

37. Karpinski MRK, Piggot H. Greater trochanteric pain syndrome. J Bone Joint Surg Br 1985;67:762–3.

38. Raman D, Haslock I. Trochanteric bursitis—a frequent cause of hip pain in rheumatoid arthritis. Ann Rheum Dis 1982;41:602–3.

39. Bird PA, Oakley SP, Shnier R, et al. Prospective evaluation of magnetic resonance imaging and physical examination findings in patients with greater trochanteric pain syndrome. Arthritis Rheum 2001;44(9):2138–45.

40. Bywaters EGL. The bursae of the body [editorial]. Ann Rheum Dis 1965;24:215–8.

41. Kingzett-Taylor A, Tirman PFJ, Feller J. Tendinosis and tears of gluteus medius and minimus muscles as a cause for hip pain. AJR Am J Roentgenol 1999;173:1123–6.

42. Chung CB, Robertson JE, Cho GJ, et al. Gluteus medius tendon tears and avulsive injuries in elderly women: imaging findings in six patients. AJR Am J Roentgenol 1999;173(2):351–3.

43. Bunker TD, Esler CN, Leach WJ. Rotator cuff tears of the hip. Clin Orthop 1999;368:135–40.

44. Gordon EJ. Trochanteric bursitis and tendonitis. Clin Orthop 1961;20:193–202.

45. Slawski DP, Howard RF. Surgical management of refractory trochanteric bursitis. Am J Sports Med 1997;25:86–9.

46. Blankenbaker DG, Tuite MJ. Iliopsoas musculotendinous unit. Semin Musculoskelet Radiol 2008;12(1): 13–27.

47. Chandler SB. The iliopsoas bursa in man. Anat Rec 1934;58:235–40.

48. Varma DG, Richli W, Charnsangavej C, et al. MR appearance of the distended iliopsoas bursa. AJR Am J Roentgenol 1991;156:1025–8.

49. Binek R, Levinsohn ME. Enlarged iliopsoas bursa: an unusual cause of thigh mass and hip pain. Clin Orthop 1987;224:158–63.

50. Wunderbaldinger P, Bremer C, Schellenbrger E, et al. Imaging features of iliopsoas bursitis. Eur Radiol 2002;12:409–15.

51. Blankenbaker DG, De Smet AA, Keene JS. Sonography of the iliopsoas tendon and injection of the iliopsoas bursa for diagnosis and management of the painful snapping hip. Skeletal Radiol 2006; 35(8):565–71.

52. Johnston CA, Wiley JP, Lindsay DM, et al. Iliopsoas bursitis and tendonitis. A review. Sports Med 1998; 25(4):271–83.

53. Newman JS, Newberg AH. MRI of the painful hip in athletes. Clin Sports Med 2006;25:613–33.

54. McCarthy JC, Busconi B. The role of hip arthroscopy in the diagnosis and treatment of hip disease. Can J Surg 1995;38(Suppl 1):S13–7.

55. Notzli HP, Wyss TF, Stoecklin CH, et al. The contour of the femoral head-neck junction as a predictor for the risk of anterior impingement. J Bone Joint Surg Br 2002;84:556–60.

56. Ito K, Minka MA II, Leunig M, et al. Femoroacetabular impingement and the cam-effect: a MRI-based quantitative anatomical study of the femoral head-neck offset. J Bone Joint Surg Br 2001;83:171–6.

57. Jager M, Wild A, Westhoff B, et al. Femoroacetabular impingement caused by a femoral osseous head-neck bump deformity: clinical, radiological and experimental results. J Orthop Sci 2004;9: 256–63.

58. Wenger DE, Kendell KR, Miner M, et al. Acetabular labral tears rarely occur in the absence of bony abnormalities. Clinical Orthopaedics & Related Research 2004;426:145–50.

59. Dora C, Zurbach J, Hersche O, et al. Pathomorphologic characteristics of posttraumatic acetabular dysplasia. J Orthop Trauma 2000;14:483–9.

60. Kassarjian A, Yoon LS, Belzile E, et al. Triad of MR arthrographic findings in patients with cam-type femoroacetabular impingement. Radiology 2005; 236:588–92.

61. Klaue K, Durnin CW, Ganz R. The acetabular rim syndrome: a clinical presentation of dysplasia of the hip. J Bone Joint Surg Br 1991;73:423–9.

62. Tannast M, Goricki D, Beck M, et al. Hip damage occurs at the zone of femoroacetabular impingement. Clin Orthop Relat Res 2008;466:273–80.

63. Schmid MR, Notzli HP, Zanetti M, et al. Cartilage lesions in the hip: diagnostic effectiveness of MR arthrography. Radiology 2003;226:382–6.

64. Beaule PE, Zaragoza EJ. Surgical images; musculoskeletal acetabular cartilage delamination demonstrated by magnetic resonance arthrography—inverted "Oreo" cookie sign. Can J Surg 2003;46:463–4.

65. Pfirrman CW, Due SR, Duc SR, et al. MR arthrography of acetabular cartilage delamination in femoroacetabular cam impingement. Radiology 2008;249: 236–41.

Traumatic Injuries of the Hip

Nina Marshall, MBBS, FRANZCR[a],*,
George Koulouris, MBBS, GrCertSpMed, MMed, FRANZCR[b]

KEYWORDS

- Athletes • Traumatic injury • Hip • Sports medicine
- MR imaging • MR arthrogram

Imaging of the hip in the athlete has undergone a recent resurgence of interest and understanding because of the increasing accessibility and use of hip arthroscopy, which expands the treatment options available for intra-articular pathology. MR imaging and MR arthrography are the diagnostic tools best suited to guide the referring clinician in the diagnosis of intra-articular and extra-articular soft tissue, chondral, and osseous pathology.

Traumatic hip injury in the athletic population is not common, accounting for 5% to 8% of athletic injuries in adults[1,2] and 2% to 27%[3,4]% in children. Soccer players, runners, and dancers are particularly susceptible.[2,3] Soft tissue injuries (eg, contusions and sprains) are most frequent, typically self-limiting, and do not warrant further imaging. Although intra-articular lesions are uncommon, they do account for a significant amount of time lost from play, up to 120 days in one 10-year review of National Football League American football players.[5]

THE ROLE OF MR IMAGING

Plain radiography is an essential screening tool in the diagnosis of hip pathology and is often all that is required for fracture imaging. CT adds further information to allow operative intervention. Ultrasound is an invaluable tool not only in allowing dynamic assessments (as in snapping hip) but to guide intervention.

MR imaging has steadily been more frequently used, particularly given that arthroscopy is not without risks, with complication rates of 1.4% to 5% reported, including serious complications,

such as sciatic or femoral nerve palsy and avascular necrosis (AVN).[6,7]

The accuracy of MR imaging when correlated with arthroscopic and surgical findings has increased over the years with improvements in field strength and techniques.[8] Three-Tesla MR imaging has limited published material pertaining to efficacy at this stage but early reports document improved visualization of labral and chondral pathology.[9]

TECHNIQUE

Standard MR imaging of the hip uses a large field of view for the entire pelvis with the use of an array coil. The authors perform coronal T1, spin echo, short tau inversion recovery (STIR), axial T1, proton density, and fast spin echo T2 fat-saturated sequences (Table 1). An oblique axial (also termed "oblique sagittal" in some of the literature) in the plane of the femoral neck is obtained to assess the femoral head neck offset in the assessment for femoroacetabular impingement and also allows for better assessment of the labrum. These standard sequences enable evaluation of the entire pelvis including pelvic viscera for extra-articular and potentially bilateral pathology including AVN, occult fracture, marrow abnormality, and musculotendinous and bursal pathology.

Imaging of the hip can be challenging because of the overlying soft tissues. Unilateral high-resolution imaging of the hip with a surface coil and smaller field of view (16–22 cm) produces better imaging of the labrum and chondral surfaces.

[a] Royal College of Surgeons in Ireland, Beaumont Hospital, Beaumont Road, Dublin 9, Ireland
[b] Melbourne Radiology Clinic, 100 Victoria Parade, East Melbourne, VIC 3002, Australia
* Corresponding author.
E-mail address: ninamarshall@rcsi.ie (N. Marshall).

Magn Reson Imaging Clin N Am 17 (2009) 681–696
doi:10.1016/j.mric.2009.06.009

Table 1
Standard MR imaging hip sequences

	Pelvis				Hip			
	Coronal T1	Coronal STIR	Axial T2 FS	Axial T1	Coronal T2 FS	Sagittal PD FS	Axial PD FS	Axial Oblique T2 FS
TR (ms)	600	—	3000	600	3000	3000	3000	3000
TE (ms)	14	—	90	14	90	30	30	90
IR	—	—	—	—	—	—	—	—
Slice thickness (mm)	5	5	5	5	—	—	—	—
FOV (cm)	36	36	34	34	22	16	16	16
Image matrix size	320 × 256	320 × 256	384 × 224	384 × 224	320 × 256	320 × 224	384 × 224	384 × 224

Abbreviations: FOV, field of view; FS, fat-saturated; PD, proton density; STIR, short tau inversion recovery.

In the absence of a hip joint effusion, diagnostic accuracy for intra-articular structures is significantly improved by MR arthrography. There is a higher sensitivity and accuracy as compared with standard MR imaging (90% and 91% versus 30% and 36%, respectively).[10]

Diagnosis is improved for labral and ligamentum teres tears, intra-articular bodies, osteochondral lesions, and preoperative assessment of developmental hip dysplasia.[11–13] Although MR arthrography is superior to standard MR imaging in detecting chondral loss, it still has a high false-negative rate particularly when advanced.[14–16] For this reason, some authors have suggested a negative MR arthrogram does not obviate the need for arthroscopy.[16] The routine use of intra-articular local anesthesia is suggested to allow a subjective assessment of pathology. Resolution of the pain can confirm an intra-articular location of pathology, with an accuracy of 90%[17] albeit as a nonspecific finding.[18] Conversely, a lack of a response in the face of a positive MR imaging examination implies that any diagnosed intra-articular pathology is likely not to be the cause of a patient's symptoms.[19] A lack of response does not entirely exclude the diagnosis of intra-articular pathology[20] possibly because of the lack of provoking stimulus during the period of action.

Instillation of contrast is performed under fluoroscopic control and using a sterile technique. A 22-gauge needle is placed into the joint and intra-articular position confirmed using a small amount of iodinated contrast. Thereafter, approximately 10 mL of a mixture consisting of 0.1 mL of gadopentetate dimeglumine (Magnevist; Berlex Laboratories, Wayne, New Jersey), 10 mL of normal saline, and 10 mL of 0.25% bupivacaine is then injected. Injection can be performed with a 45-degree anterior angled approach, anteriorly with a perpendicular approach to the skin, or a lateral approach. The authors favor an anterior perpendicular approach to avoid the femoral neurovascular bundle. It is important to avoid the inadvertent injection of air, which may result in magnetic susceptibility artifact, or the appearance of nondependent debris in the joint. Imaging is performed 30 minutes after injection (**Table 2**). Peak contrast-to-noise ratio and joint distention occurs at 30 minutes in the hip with steady decrease after this time.[21]

Use of T1 fat-saturated sequences allows maximum contrast between intra-articular contrast and adjacent soft tissues. STIR or T2 fat-saturated imaging is routine to allow detection of other unsuspected pathology including extra-articular fluid collections and bone marrow lesions.

Table 2
Standard MR imaging arthrogram sequences

	Hip				
	Axial T1 spin echo FS	Sagittal T1 FS	Coronal T1 FS	Coronal T2 Fast Spin echo FS	Axial Oblique PD FS
TR (ms)	600	600	600	3000	3000
TE (ms)	14	14	14	90	30
Slice thickness (mm)	5	5	5	5	5
FOV (mm)	24	24	24	24	24
Image matrix	320 × 224	256 × 224	320 × 224	320 × 224	320 × 224

Abbreviations: FOV, field of view; FS, fat-saturated; PD, proton density.

Indirect MR arthrography is another technique whereby intravenous injection of gadolinium leads to synovial enhancement and then diffusion into the synovial fluid. This does not result in joint distention unless there is a concomitant effusion. Even if an effusion is present indirect arthrography is more successful in joints where the bulk of joint fluid is in close proximity to the synovial membrane and is a less useful technique in the hip.[22] There is less confidence in depicting labral pathology, in particular differentiating between a displaced versus detached tear.

OSSEOUS INJURY

Osseous traumatic injury of the hip forms a minority of the workload of inpatient orthopedic services, recorded as constituting up to 1% of trauma presentations for an adult trauma service[23] and 4% of the presentations to the emergency department in the pediatric setting.[24]

Most pelvic and femoral fractures are adequately diagnosed on plain films. Complex fractures, including those with intra-articular fragments, are better demonstrated with multidetector CT[25] as are subtle undisplaced fractures. CT is accessible and the most appropriate modality in the unstable multitrauma patient, rapidly delineating fracture anatomy while enabling assessment of other injuries.

Bone scan diagnosis is helpful in delayed presentations and in stress injury as a diagnostic tool but provides little in the way of anatomic information and is ultimately nonspecific. Scintigraphy relies on commencement of osteoblastic activity and healing attempts and may not be initially positive for fracture, particularly in elderly patients in the first 24 hours after injury. In the athletic population there is also the potential to miss the early phases of stress injury when the abnormality is limited to the soft tissues or periosteum.[26]

Specificity may be hampered by false-positives because of other processes, such as degeneration, myositis ossificans, calcific capsulitis, and transient osteoporosis of the hip. False-positives occurred at a rate up to 19%[27] in one study in an older population[28] and up to 32% in a small population of endurance athletes.[29]

Osseous injury in the athlete varies depending on activity and age and can be categorized into avulsion injuries, direct trauma, chronic microtrauma, and stress injury. The latter entity is discussed elsewhere in this issue.

Avulsion Injury

These injuries typically occur in the pediatric and adolescent patient and are usually well characterized by plain film. Such patients may present for cross-sectional imaging if the trauma is not recognized, particularly in the subacute and chronic setting. Here the imaging findings can appear aggressive and plain film findings may be confused with osseous neoplasm or infection.

Fractures in children occur at characteristic sites (**Table 3**), with acute fractures usually Salter-Harris type 1 fractures occurring at the physis (**Fig. 1**). Avulsion injuries at ASIS and AIIS tend to have a shorter recovery time than displaced hamstring avulsions.[30] False-positives can occur if a normal unfused apophysis is not recognized. Avulsion fractures seen in the adult are concerning and suggest underlying bony pathology, such as metastasis or less commonly renal osteodystrophy.[30]

In the subacute and chronic presentations, repetitive microtrauma results in apophysitis rather than acute fracture. In these cases the presence of periosteal reaction, callus, and lysis can combine to give a more aggressive appearance on all imaging modalities. MR imaging readily demonstrates soft tissue abnormality, such as hematoma and

Table 3
Common avulsion fracture sites of the pelvis and hip

Fracture	Muscle	Mechanism
Anterior superior iliac spine	Sartorius, tensor fascia lata	Sprinting, kicking
Anterior inferior iliac spine	Rectus femoris	Sprinting, kicking
Inferior pubic ramus	Adductor longus, brevis, gracilis	Soccer players, runners
Ischial tuberosity	Hamstring insertions, adductor magnus	Runners, gymnasts, dancers
Greater trochanter	Gluteal tendon	More common in adults as part of intertrochanteric fracture Associated with femoral head necrosis in the pediatric population
Lesser trochanter	Psoas tendon	More common in adults as part of intertrochanteric fracture

tendon retraction. Small cortical fracture fragments that do not contain bone marrow can be missed. A high index of clinical suspicion is required because occasionally these patients may require operative fixation if there is ongoing symptoms or inability to return to sport. Pain may continue if there is nonunion or malunion secondary to significant fracture fragment displacement or possibly because of irritation of the adjacent sciatic nerve in the case of hamstring avulsions.[31]

Direct Trauma: Dislocation

Dislocation of the hip is a rare athletic injury that can occur in high-velocity, high-impact sports, such as rugby, American football, and skiing and snowboarding.[32] Hip dislocations constitute an orthopedic emergency and may be anterior or posterior. Most sports-related hip dislocations (90%) are posterior, except in alpine skiing where anterior dislocation is more common.[33]

Plain films for associated fractures prereduction and postreduction is routine. Rapid reduction is

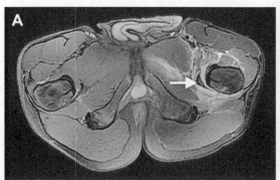
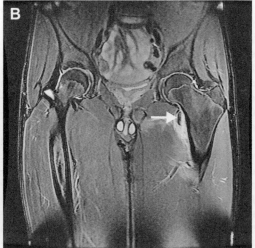

Fig. 1. Axial (A) and coronal (B) T2 fat-saturated (FS) images in a pediatric athlete demonstrating acute avulsion of the lesser trochanter (arrow) involving the insertion of the iliopsoas tendon. Note the surrounding T2 hyperintensity consistent with hemorrhage.

the priority to avoid complicating AVN and imaging should not delay intervention, such as open reduction. CT scan is indicated for failure of reduction to evaluate for loose intra-articular bodies or fracture fragments impeding reduction and for acetabular fracture. Fractures that involve greater than 30% of the weight-bearing surface of the acetabulum are considered for internal fixation.[34] Most athletic injuries have no associated fracture, or a small fracture, and do not often requiring surgical stabilization. MR imaging may be required in the subacute phase to evaluate for associated soft tissue pathology: labral tears, chondral injury, cartilaginous loose bodies, femoral head microfractures, and sciatic nerve injury. This is primarily in the elite athlete where surgical repair is considered for these complications. MR imaging can also document damage to the iliofemoral ligament, which is typically torn before dislocation occurs. There may also be anterior labral injury and chondral shear injuries to the femoral head.[34] Aspiration of a large hemarthrosis can also be performed, primarily for symptomatic relief.

MR imaging can also be used to evaluate for the presence of complicating AVN, best performed at 4 to 6 weeks following injury, before which it may be less accurate.[35] AVN occurs because of disruption of the circumflex vessels in a similar mechanism to that in fracture of the femoral neck. Animal studies have also suggested that a hemarthrosis results in increased intracapsular pressure and reduced flow in the extraosseous vessels, and may be another cause for the development of AVN.[36] Estimates show that AVN in dislocation occurs at a rate of 1% to 17%.[34]

Subluxation and Instability

There is a scarcity of literature on traumatic subluxation of the hip, because it is likely underdiagnosed or misdiagnosed as a hip sprain (Fig. 2). Subluxation can occur with seemingly minimal trauma. This can occur in the setting of a fall forward on flexed knee or impact from behind while on all fours. Traumatic hip subluxation, like dislocation, is most commonly posterior and postulated to occur with a lesser traumatic force than dislocation. It is associated with small posterior acetabular lip fractures and tearing of the iliofemoral ligament. Despite the lesser force, AVN has also been described in this population.[37] There have been recent advances in arthroscopic surgery addressing subluxation, with Philippon[38] reporting an 82% return to preinjury level of athletic competition after labral debridement and thermal capsulorrhaphy.

OSTEOCHONDRAL INJURY

Osteochondral traumatic lesions occur following hip dislocation where the site of injury typically reflects the impaction point (Fig. 2B,C).[39] Osteochondral lesions have also been reported outside of the setting of major trauma in athletes and were seen in 64% of patients in a small series by Weaver and coworkers[40] where the patients recalled no discrete traumatic event. The underlying pathology is suspected to be a chondral laceration and microfracture of the underlying subchondral bone. It has been postulated that these injuries predispose patients to osteoarthritis in later years.

MR imaging is the modality best suited to diagnosis and grading of these lesions and guides management (Table 4). T2-weighted sequences in particular are used to diagnose an unstable fragment as indicated by a high signal intensity line undermining the lesion, representing intervening joint fluid. The presence of T2 hyperintensity in the adjacent subchondral bone is also thought to represent mechanical stress at the fragment-donor interface implying motion and instability. The signal within the fragment requires assessment; necrotic and nonviable fragments are low signal on all sequences, whereas the presence of T1 hyperintensity (normal marrow) indicates viability. Accurate staging can be more difficult in the joint without an effusion, because the distinction between granulation tissue and fluid is problematic and accuracy rates in this context are reported as low as 67% with a sensitivity of 47%.[16] MR arthrography has an improved accuracy of 93% to 99%.[41]

CHONDRAL PATHOLOGY

Chondral evaluation is hampered by the intrinsic anatomy of the hip, a deep ball and socket joint where cartilage surfaces are intimately in contact even with capsular distention. The normal acetabular cartilage is as thin as 1.34 mm and femoral cartilage 1.1 mm; subtle chondral abnormalities remain difficult to detect.[42,43] The increased resolution of 3-T imaging shows promise with one author reporting improved depiction of lesions,[9] but to date there have been no data confirming improved correlation with surgical grading. Unlike the knee, the accuracy of chondral defects reported in the hip is as low as 18% sensitivity on standard MR imaging, with improvement on MR arthrography reported to have 41% to 79% sensitivity and 77% to 100% specificity.[44]

LABRAL INJURY

Similar to glenoid labral tears, labral tears of the hip have long been recognized as secondary to

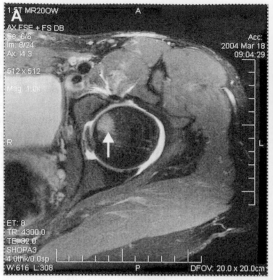
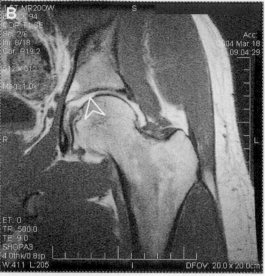
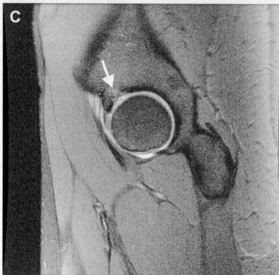

Fig. 2. (A) Axial T2 FS images of the left hip of an athlete following an episode of anterior subluxation. Note an area of subchondral bone marrow edema of the femoral head (*arrow*) consistent with an impaction injury. Hyperintensity is demonstrated in the iliopsoas muscle anteriorly. (B) Coronal proton density image in the same athlete demonstrates a full-thickness osteochondral defect (*arrowhead*). (C) Sagittal T2 FS arthrographic image of the hip demonstrates a full-thickness acetabular chondral defect with associated bone marrow edema (*arrow*).

major trauma, such as dislocation and in the setting of chronic degeneration (Fig. 3).[39] More recently, tears have been recognized after trivial trauma and in hip instability.[45] The role of labral pathology in hip pain has recently generated much literature in the discussion of femoroacetabular impingement.

Trauma can occur from a single event or in a repetitive fashion, such as a golf swing, ballet, and martial arts practitioners.[46] Certain sports may self-select athletes with greater hip rotation (gymnasts) because of mild hip dysplasia;

however, this also implies that such athletes are also more likely to have associated labral pathology. Labral tears are also associated with chondral lesions, which may be caused by secondary degenerative change or as a consequence of the same traumatic event.[2]

Early diagnosis of labral tears allows for early repair and limited resection to allay current pain[47] and potentially slow the onset of osteoarthritis. It has been documented that early detection and intervention results in a more successful outcome in this setting rather than conservatively

Table 4
Grades using arthroscopy and MR imaging

Grade	Description	Treatment
I	Intact articular cartilage, signal change in the subchondral bone	Conservative
II	Partial detachment of the cartilage and subchondral fragment	Surgical: curettage, drilling, allograft
III	Completely detached nondisplaced fragment	Surgical
IV	Detached and displaced fragment away from the donor site	Surgical

monitoring labral degeneration and tearing, with the extent of chondral involvement being the best correlate of symptomatic outcome.[48,49]

Paralabral cysts can be detected on standard MR imaging and the presence of such a cyst is considered a highly specific secondary sign.[50] The distinction between undisplaced tears, detached tears, and anatomic variants of the labrum is made with increased certainty on MR arthrography. MR arthrography is superior in that it provides capsular distention that allows some separation of the capsule from the labrum, which better delineates the morphology of the defect. The shape of the defect helps in distinguishing a tear from the normal labrum and displacement of any tear is helpful in treatment planning. T2-weighted sequences are important to perform in MR arthrography in the detection of cysts because frequently there may be no ongoing communication of the cyst with the joint and no filling with intra-articular gadolinium. Studies directly comparing standard MR imaging with MR arthrography determined that MR arthrography is 15% more sensitive (65% and 80% sensitivity for MR imaging and MR arthrography, respectively) and 23% more accurate (65% and 88%) in depicting labral tears.[51]

The normal labrum on standard MR imaging is of uniform low T1 and T2 signal intensity. The detection of absence of a portion of labrum is to be interpreted with care because absent portions are reported in up to 14% of asymptomatic individuals[52] and may be a normal variant; however, it may also possibly represent the earliest manifestation of the degenerative process. A sublabral sulcus has also been variably described on imaging as being in all quadrants on surgical review[53] most commonly identified posteroinferiorly on MR imaging.[54] This is distinct from the normal perilabral recess, which is seen between

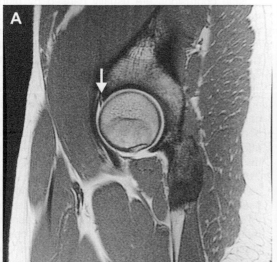 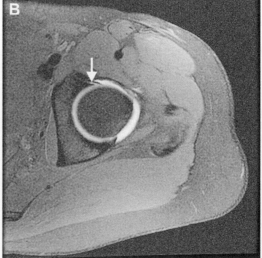

Fig. 3. Axial T1 FS (*A*) and sagittal proton density (*B*) MR arthrographic images demonstrate a characteristic full-thickness anterosuperior labral tear (*arrow*) at the labral-acetabular junction.

the capsule and the labrum, seen most distinctly on coronal images superiorly. A corresponding sublabral abnormality had not been found in preliminary arthroscopic and cadaveric examinations.[52] Labral signal and morphologic abnormalities have previously been attributed to fibrovascular structures or alternatively to degeneration.[55] More recent studies with surgical correlation, however, have been useful in demonstrating sublabral recesses in the anteroinferior portion of the labrum, whereas MR arthrographic abnormalities in the anterosuperior labrum are more likely to represent a tear rather than a recess.[56] In a 2008 study by Studler and colleagues,[56] only 2 of 55 of the cases with MR arthrographic abnormality in the anterosuperior quadrant had a recess on subsequent surgical correlation. They also found that perilabral changes and abnormality extending into the base of the labrum are other useful discriminators in making the diagnosis of a tear over a variant recess. Signal abnormality in the anterosuperior quadrant is believed by many authors to represent a normal variant,[52] possible tears,[30] or definite tear.[57] The presence of these sulci is likely the reason why MR arthrography, although improving the detection rate for a labral tear, has a higher false-positive level than standard MR imaging (20% versus 10% in one study[17]).

Labral tears that located on the posteromedial load zone of the acetabulum have been classified morphologically on arthroscopy as radial flap, radial fibrillated and longitudinal peripheral, and unstable tears.[58] Trauma-related tears are most commonly radial flap tears, similar to a meniscal parrot beak tear, and longitudinal tears.[58] The latter type arises from the labral-acetabular junction and extends along the acetabular rim. As in the knee, these tears are more likely to be unstable in the formation of a bucket handle fragment. Given that arthroscopy and debridement is the uniform approach to these lesions, there is less importance in the typing or classification of the tear than ensuring that it is accurately detected. The postoperative appearance to the labrum may result in truncation; however, if fluid undercuts the labrum or extends into its substance, it is indicative of a residual tear or subsequent reinjury.

MUSCULOTENDINOUS PATHOLOGY

These injuries are the most commonly encountered in clinical practice if not forming a substantial portion of referrals for MR imaging.

Injury mechanism here can be divided into three groups: (1) direct blunt trauma, (2) forceful contraction, and (3) microtrauma caused by overuse or repetitive injury. The subsequent injuries for these mechanisms are muscle contusion, avulsion, and strain, respectively. Fascial involvement is reflected by hematoma, interstitial hemorrhage, and muscle herniation. Finally, the sequelae of injury may include fibrotic scarring or atrophy.

Multiplanar imaging is required to assess the muscle in longitudinal and short axis. A large field of view has the advantage of comparison with the contralateral side and allows measurement from anatomic landmarks useful to the referrer. For this reason coronal and axial planes are usually used for the hip. Use of markers at the patient-reported site of maximal tenderness or mass is also useful.

STIR or T2 fat-saturated sequences are useful to localize pathology and demonstrate edema. Some centers use this as an initial planning sequence with subsequent sequences then planned to optimize assessment of pathology. STIR images tend to be superior to fat-saturated sequences in a larger field of view because of improved homogeneity of fat saturation. T1 images are used to assess fatty atrophic change and the presence of methemoglobin as seen in subacute hemorrhage. Gradient echo T2* sequences also allow detection of hemorrhage depicted as blooming artifact; however, they are rarely used routinely. Gas and metallic foreign bodies also bloom; however, this is uncommonly a diagnostic dilemma. Use of gadolinium has also been suggested to demonstrate subtle abnormality or subacute pathology but is not in routine use.[59,60]

Muscle Contusion

Muscle contusions are usually caused by blunt trauma and are most commonly a feature of sports where there is relatively little protection, such as rugby, soccer, and Australian Rules football. Common sites of trauma include the iliac crest, where there are multiple muscle insertions: internal and external oblique muscles of the anterior abdominal wall, latissimus dorsi, and the paraspinal muscles. Similarly, the quadriceps can be compressed on the femur. The iliopsoas can be affected in contact sports and may be seen in the elderly after a fall.[61]

Although muscular contusions are often clinically diagnosed without difficulty, MR imaging is useful in patients whose symptoms do not resolve as expected. MR imaging can demonstrate persistent or unexpected hematoma or myositis ossificans. Although there are few indications for surgical intervention for muscle injury outside of compartment syndrome, occasionally drainage may be required when the size of the hematoma is such that it limits the range of motion.[4] If there is clinical concern in the acute stages of an arterial injury leading to a rapidly enlarging contusional injury, CT angiography is a more useful investigation. Conversely, muscular injuries can be an occult source of pain and have been reported in patients with pain without fracture on plain film.[62]

The appearance of an intramuscular hematoma varies with age; however, the rate of change is not as predictable as described in the central nervous system. Acute hematoma demonstrates signal that is isointense to muscle on T1- and T2-weighted sequences. Central low signal may be seen indicating deoxyhemoglobin (hyperacute hematoma). In the latter stages, intracellular methemoglobin exhibits high T1 signal leading to a heterogeneous appearance. A peripheral rim or low signal representing fibrosis or hemosiderin may develop, as may fluid-fluid levels, although the latter typically occur in the acute stage. Contusions may have mass effect, enlarging the muscle belly and potentially compressing adjacent nerves. Well-described syndromes include sciatica caused by compression in the buttock and iliopsoas hematoma compressing the femoral nerve in the inguinal canal.[63,64] Similarly, the sciatic neurovascular bundle can be compressed because of avulsion of the ischial tuberosity at the time of injury or because of later callus formation.[65]

Myositis ossificans is the formation of heterotopic bone after traumatic injury (**Fig. 4**). Typically, it occurs in large muscle groups, such as the quadriceps, that have undergone significant contusion, occurring at a rate of 9% of such contusions, with the likelihood increasing to 17% in those with moderate-severe contusions.[66]

Known risk factors include a large hematoma caused by severe or repeated injuries with delays in treatment or use of nonsteroidal anti-inflammatory agents. Early massage, hydrotherapy, or passive forceful stretching and application of heat in the early phases are also postulated as exacerbating factors. The risk is also increased if there is reinjury to the area or if there is too vigorous physical therapy or early return to play.

A process of maturation characterizes the histopathologic changes of myositis ossificans. Trauma to the muscle triggers proliferative repair with activation of perimysial tissue-inducible osteoprogenitor cells.[67] Fibrovascular granulation tissue transforms into new bone. There may occasionally be preceding cartilage formation before the immature bone is replaced by lamellar bone. Repair mechanisms commence at the periphery and progresses centrally. There are three distinct zones histologically: (1) a central undifferentiated zone, (2) surrounding zone of immature osteoid formation, and (3) a peripheral zone of mature bone. These zones are appreciable after 10 days following onset of symptoms. If biopsy is performed before 10 days or if only the central portion is sampled then the appearance can resemble osteosarcoma. When mature the bone is histologically indistinct from normal bone. If biopsy is performed in the acute or subacute phase it can of itself exacerbate the ossification.

On plain film early examination is normal with flocculent calcification evident at 2 to 6 weeks,

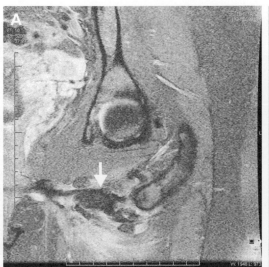
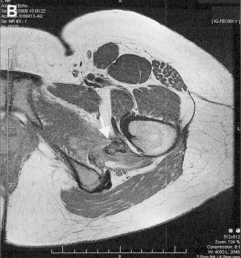

Fig. 4. Coronal short tau inversion recovery (*A*) and axial T2 (*B*) images through the hip of a 25-year-old female athlete demonstrate an area of ill-defined hypointensity (*arrow*) consistent with myositis ossificans. This is surrounded by T2 hyperintensity in keeping with surrounding fibrovascular granulation tissue formation.

becoming more sharply circumscribed at 6 to 8 weeks. Serial radiographs may be required. As the lesion ages it may attach to underlying bone at which point the zonal pattern is less apparent. On MR imaging immature lesions demonstrate heterogeneous T2 signal lesions with surrounding edema and minimal T1 signal abnormality. Mature lesions demonstrate heterogeneous high T1 and high T2 signal. Rim and occasionally central enhancement is also seen, which is in common with soft tissue neoplasm and abscess leading to potential difficulty in diagnosis.[68] This diagnosis is best made on plain film and CT, where the peripheral zone of calcification is demonstrated to best effect. The progression to mature ossification typically occurs in 6 to 12 months after injury, after which time complete or partial resorption can occur.

Strain

Strains occur by indirect trauma from excessive tension and tend to affect the weakest point of the myotendinous unit known as the "musculotendinous junction." The most commonly affected muscle group around the hip is the hamstrings and in particular the proximal myotendinous junction of biceps femoris. The hamstrings are particularly susceptible because they span two joints, undergo eccentric contraction, and are composed of fast-twitch contracting fibers.[69] Biceps femoris may be implicated because it has limited extensibility. Older athletes and those with previous injury are most at risk.[30] Hamstring injury can occur at multiple sites and has been reported with a variable prevalence ranging from 5% to 60%.[69] This divergence may partially reflect the different athletes imaged (Australian Rules football versus track and field athletes). Attempts have been made to prognosticate on recovery time and recurrence risk for hamstring injuries depending on the imaging characteristics, such as which muscle is involved, length of injury, and injury location relative to the musculotendinous junction. These injuries are of particular significance given their slow rehabilitation times and tendency to recurrence. Some authors concluded injuries involving a cross-sectional area of greater than 50% are the most reliably reproducible indicator of a longer rehabilitation time.[69,70] Clinical estimates, however, have also been shown to be accurate in predicting rehabilitation time in one study[71] and other authors have found no MR imaging correlation with outcome.[72] Interestingly, symptomatic relief and return to play tends to occur more quickly than resolution of the imaging

changes and histologic healing, which may explain high injury recurrence rates.[69]

The adductor muscles are also frequently involved, especially in hockey, soccer, and football players, leading to groin pain.[73] Such injuries uncommonly present for imaging in the acute setting. Much of the literature in this area is focused on adductor and rectus abdominis enthesopathy, osteitis pubis, and posterior inguinal wall deficiency (described in further detail elsewhere in this issue).

The quadriceps muscles, in particular the rectus femoris, also frequently undergo strain either at the central musculotendinous junction or peripherally. The rectus femoris is similar to the hamstring muscles in the presence of a long central tendon and aponeurosis, Strains at the central tendon have been associated with a prolonged rehabilitation period (**Fig. 5**).[74]

A combination of rectus strain, adductor strain, and labral tear has been described in American football players, referred to as the "sports hip triad" by Feeley and colleagues.[5] These authors postulate that muscle strains around the hip result in altered and unbalanced mechanics leading to labral injury.

Strain injuries are classified clinically as shown in **Table 5**. An important mimic of grade 1 muscle strain on MR imaging is the normal postexercise hyperintensity seen on T2-weighted sequences. This is caused by increased water content in muscle that is predominately extracellular. This phenomenon can be useful, for example in study of muscle recruitment and diagnosis in chronic exertional compartment syndrome.

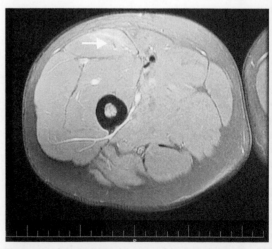

Fig. 5. Axial T2 FS image in an athlete presenting with acute thigh pain. Feathery T2 hyperintensity at the proximal musculotendinous junction (*arrow*) is consistent with a grade 1 strain of the central tendon slip.

Table 5
Grading of muscular strain: radiologic pathological correlation

	Clinical Classification	Underlying Pathology	MR imaging Features
First degree	Stretch injury Heal within 2 wk with conservative management	Minor fiber disruption Fluid leaking through the endomysium, which surrounds each muscle fiber Interstitial edema and hemorrhage at MT junction, which extends into fascicles	Feathery appearance on T2-weighted images
Second degree	Partial tear Mild functional impairment Require at least 4 wk of conservative management	Partial tear without retraction	Hematoma at MT junction Intramuscular and extramuscular fluid collection
Third degree	Complete tear Complete loss of function	Complete rupture	Retraction can be measured

Abbreviation: MT, musculotendinous.

Delayed-onset Muscle Soreness

Delayed-onset muscle soreness occurs after unaccustomed periods of exertion and is not uncommon in professional or recreational athletes. This phenomenon can also occur at submaximal workloads.[75] Symptoms commence 1 to 2 days after exercise and largely resolve by day 7. MR imaging appearances are similar to grade 1 muscle strain with T2 hyperintensity. The distinction between the two entities is clinical because strain symptoms occur at the time of injury and resolve over a 2-week period.

Tendon Tear

Tendon tears are more significant injuries for the athlete than muscle strains because of a prolonged rehabilitation time. A rectus femoris tear, for example, sees a return to play in 6 to 12 weeks,[76] whereas a grade 1 or 2 muscle strain usually results in a return in 9 to 26 days.[74] Any of the muscle groups may be affected; however, these injuries are very uncommonly related to exertion in the athlete. Most complete tendon tears (excepting Achilles tears) occur outside of sport.[77] Similarly, partial tears are more a feature of tendinopathy and most commonly present for imaging in the setting of acute or chronic pain.

Tears can occur because of underlying problems including use of fluoroquinolones, rheumatoid arthritis, hydroxyapatite deposition, and tendinosis. Underlying tendinosis is more likely to result in a partial-thickness tear or interstitial tear.

Tears of the gluteal (abductor) tendons have been termed "rotator cuff tears of the hip" and are most commonly seen in older patients, particularly elderly women.[78] They have been described in the setting of total hip arthroplasty (as have iliopsoas tears[79]). Tears of the rectus femoris origin can occur in the acute setting, as may avulsion fracture and more commonly affecting the indirect head.[80] Adductor origin tears may occur as avulsion fractures or rarely tendon ruptures[81] in the acute setting but much more commonly as microtears in the setting of chronic groin pain.

Ultrasound is comparable with MR imaging in documenting tendon tears in many joints, such as the shoulder[82] and ankle.[83,84] In the hip, however, MR imaging is superior because of the small size of many of the short muscles and also their relative depth as when compared with tendons related to other joints.[78]

Tendinosis is demonstrated by tendon thickening and increased signal on proton density sequences with intermediate signal on T2-weighted sequences. Interstitial tears may not demonstrate tendon contour abnormality. A partial (**Fig. 6**) or full-thickness tear (**Fig. 7**) demonstrates loss of fiber continuity and high T2 signal, particularly conspicuous on fat-saturated sequences. This signal reflects hemorrhage in the acute setting or granulation tissue later in the subacute period. Tendon retraction may occur with full-thickness

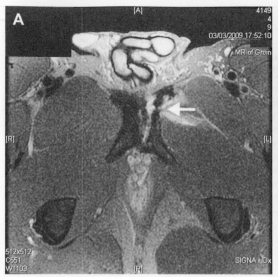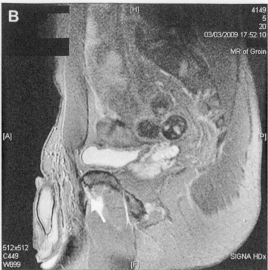

Fig. 6. Axial (A) and sagittal (B) images through the groin of a male athlete demonstrating hyperintensity of the origin of the adductor longus tendon (arrow) consistent with an extensive partial-thickness tear.

tears and may be missed if there is no comparison with the contralateral side (see Fig. 6). The degree of tendon retraction can be measured on MR imaging, which allows surgical planning and prognostication.[85] Fatty atrophy may be seen as a consequence of tendon tear. The process of fatty atrophy is best described in the rotator cuff musculature where the likelihood of atrophy has been found to correlate with the degree of retraction of fibers[86] and tear site within the tendon.[87] This is best appreciated on T1-weighted sequences and is diagnosed when there is a 25% or more loss of muscle volume as compared with the contralateral side.

Depending on the site of injury, most patients improve with conservative treatments including the RICE protocol (rest, ice, compression, elevation) and physical therapy. Steroid injections, although useful in tendinopathy, have historically been believed to constitute a risk of tendon tear and in the setting of a partial tear may cause conversion to a full-thickness tear. The bulk of evidence is, however, related to tears in the Achilles tendon[88] and there is limited literature on the risk in imaging-guided practice. Other therapeutic injections, such as platelet-enriched autologous blood[89] and polidocanol[90] injections, have been trialed for tendinopathy, but there have as yet been no large-scale trials to prove benefit conclusively of one treatment method over the other. Again, most studies are focused on Achilles and patella tendinopathy and lateral epicondylitis.

Surgery is required when there is a need for hematoma evacuation or tendon reattachment. In the minority of hamstring injuries, however, repair

of a complete hamstring avulsion is recommended to improve strength and endurance.[91] Surgery for gluteal tendon tears has been reported in the management of chronic trochanteric pain syndromes[92] including using an endoscopic approach.[93]

Subcutaneous Injury

Posttraumatic hematomas in the subcutaneous fatty tissues are common. A more significant lesion is named after the French surgeon who first described them in 1863, the Morel-Lavallee lesion. These are most common in the trochanteric region

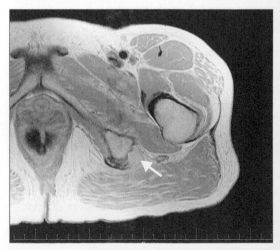

Fig. 7. Axial proton density image demonstrates full-thickness disruption of the hamstring muscle origin with the typical appearances of a "bald" ischial tuberosity (arrow).

and proximal thigh, although they may also occur over the flank or lumbodorsal region.

The initial insult is a closed degloving-type injury where the subcutaneous fat tears away from the fascia or dissects the perifascicular planes adjacent to the fascia lata and iliotibial band. Perforating vessels are torn leading to collections of blood and lymph in the space. The collection can undergo subsequent organization with peripheral granulation tissue. Occasionally, there may be ongoing bleeding and subsequent growth.[94] Such injuries are associated with complex pelvic fractures, classically in motor bike accidents.[95] They can complicate fracture management because of the increased risk of infection and as such these fractures are regarded as compound injuries.

CT,[96,97] ultrasound,[97] and MR imaging can all demonstrate soft tissue hematomas. The appearance of these fluid collections on MR imaging depends on their age and contents, ranging from seroma to infected collection. A capsule may be present in the later organizing lesions. A comprehensive MR imaging classification system has been proposed by Mellando and Bencardino.[94] In the absence of underlying fracture conservative treatment, such as percutaneous drainage, has been advocated by some authors.[98] Surgical excision is often recommended because of the tendency for recurrence and high incidence of infection. Rates of infection have been quoted as up to 46%[99] in one study where cultures were taken from lesions occurring within the setting of trauma with pelvic fracture.

Ligamentous Teres Injury

Injuries to ligamentum teres are not uncommon but are underreported on imaging. One study reported a 13% incidence of tear in a series of hip arthroscopies performed in athletes with groin pain.[100] Preoperative diagnosis is the exception with reported rates being as low as 5%,[101] often only being recognized if there is an associated bony fracture fragment. Injuries to the ligamentum teres can be assumed in the setting of hip dislocation[39] but can also occur with minimal trauma and degeneration.[102] Partial tears in particular have been associated with sports injury.[103] If undiagnosed, there is a risk of ongoing subluxation and instability, premature osteoarthritis, and AVN. Importantly, prompt recognition of this diagnosis allows for arthroscopic debridement, which can result in symptomatic relief.[104] Armfield and colleagues[57] reported the advantage of axial oblique images in detecting pathology of the significant partial volume averaging on standard sagittal and coronal sequences. Armfield's group

defined a tear as abnormal T2 signal and morphology in a ligament of normal thickness. Abnormality of either of these criteria was believed to represent a partial tear. Hypertrophy of the ligament (defined as extending more than 2 mm beyond foveal insertion) has also been described as a sign of chronic instability.[57] MR arthroscopy may add confidence by demonstrating contrast pooling in the acetabular attachment.

The accuracy of MR arthrography is, however, still suboptimal for this pathology with a 9% detection rate in one series of 23 arthroscopic proved ruptures.[101] Arthroscopy remains the most reliable tool for diagnosis.

SUMMARY

Traumatic lesions of the hip in athletes can be clinically challenging because of the overlap in symptomatology with various conditions and the presence of multiple injuries. MR imaging and MR arthrography have a unique role in diagnosis of these pathologies, guiding the surgeon, arthroscopist, and referring clinician in their management of bony and soft tissue injury.

REFERENCES

1. Borowski LA, Yard EE, Fields SK, et al. The epidemiology of US high school basketball injuries, 2005–2007. Am J Sports Med 2008;36:2328–35.
2. Boutin RD, Newman JS. MR imaging of sports-related hip disorders. Magn Reson Imaging Clin N Am 2003;11:255–81.
3. Giza E, Micheli LJ. Soccer injuries. Med Sport Sci 2005;49:140–69.
4. Anderson K, Strickland SM, Warren R. Hip and groin injuries in athletes. Am J Sports Med 2001; 29:521–33.
5. Feeley BT, Powell JW, Muller MS, et al. Hip injuries and labral tears in the National Football League. Am J Sports Med 2008;36:2187–95.
6. Byrd JW, Jones KS. Prospective analysis of hip arthroscopy with 2-year follow-up. Arthroscopy 2000;16:578–87.
7. Clarke MT, Arora A, Villar RN. Hip arthroscopy: complications in 1054 cases. Clin Orthop Relat Res 2003;406:84–8.
8. Ziegert A, Blankenbaker D, De Smet A, et al. Comparison of hip MR arthrography imaging sequences in identification and characterization of arthroscopically-proven labral tears. AJR Am J Roentgenol 2009;192(5):1397–400.
9. Ramnath RR. 3T MR imaging of the musculoskeletal system (part II): clinical applications. Magn Reson Imaging Clin N Am 2006;14:41–62.

10. Czerny C, Hofmann S, Neuhold A, et al. Lesions of the acetabular labrum: accuracy of MR imaging and MR arthrography in detection and staging. Radiology 1996;200:225–30.

11. Toomayan GA, Holman WR, Major NM, et al. Sensitivity of MR arthrography in the evaluation of acetabular labral tears. AJR Am J Roentgenol 2006;186:449–53.

12. Freedman BA, Potter BK, Dinauer PA, et al. Prognostic value of magnetic resonance arthrography for Czerny stage II and III acetabular labral tears. Arthroscopy 2006;22:742–7.

13. Kawaguchi AT, Otsuka NY, Delgado ED, et al. Magnetic resonance arthrography in children with developmental hip dysplasia. Clin Orthop Relat Res 2000;374:235–46.

14. Sekiya JK, Ruch DS, Hunter DM, et al. Hip arthroscopy in staging avascular necrosis of the femoral head. J South Orthop Assoc 2000;9:254–61.

15. Newberg AH, Newman JS. Imaging the painful hip. Clin Orthop Relat Res 2003;406:19–28.

16. Keeney JA, Peelle MW, Jackson J, et al. Magnetic resonance arthrography versus arthroscopy in the evaluation of articular hip pathology. Clin Orthop Relat Res 2004;429:163–9.

17. Byrd JW, Jones KS. Diagnostic accuracy of clinical assessment, magnetic resonance imaging, magnetic resonance arthrography, and intra-articular injection in hip arthroscopy patients. Am J Sports Med 2004;32:1668–74.

18. Illgen RL II, Honkamp NJ, Weisman MH, et al. The diagnostic and predictive value of hip anesthetic arthrograms in selected patients before total hip arthroplasty. J Arthroplasty 2006;21:724–30.

19. Martin RL, Irrgang JJ, Sekiya JK. The diagnostic accuracy of a clinical examination in determining intra-articular hip pain for potential hip arthroscopy candidates. Arthroscopy 2008;24:1013–8.

20. Fitzgerald RH Jr. Acetabular labrum tears: diagnosis and treatment. Clin Orthop Relat Res 1995; 311:60–8.

21. Wagner SC, Schweitzer ME, Weishaupt D. Temporal behavior of intraarticular gadolinium. J Comput Assist Tomogr 2001;25:661–70.

22. Steinbach LS, Palmer WE, Schweitzer ME. Special focus session: MR arthrography. Radiographics 2002;22:1223–46.

23. Schneider S, Seither B, Tonges S, et al. Sports injuries: population based representative data on incidence, diagnosis, sequelae, and high risk groups. Br J Sports Med 2006;40:334–9 [discussion: 339].

24. O'Toole P, Butt A, Orakzai S, et al. Epidemiology of sporting and recreational injuries in a paediatric orthopaedic outpatients department. Ir Med J 2008;101:173–4.

25. Resnik CS, Stackhouse DJ, Shanmuganathan K, et al. Diagnosis of pelvic fractures in patients with acute pelvic trauma: efficacy of plain radiographs. AJR Am J Roentgenol 1992;158:109–12.

26. Gaeta M, Minutoli F, Scribano E, et al. CT and MR imaging findings in athletes with early tibial stress injuries: comparison with bone scintigraphy findings and emphasis on cortical abnormalities. Radiology 2005;235:553–61.

27. Garcia-Morales F, Seo GS, Chengazi V, et al. Collar osteophytes: a cause of false-positive findings in bone scans for hip fractures. AJR Am J Roentgenol 2003;181:191–4.

28. Lewis SL, Rees JI, Thomas GV, et al. Pitfalls of bone scintigraphy in suspected hip fractures. Br J Radiol 1991;64:403–8.

29. Shin AY, Morin WD, Gorman JD, et al. The superiority of magnetic resonance imaging in differentiating the cause of hip pain in endurance athletes. Am J Sports Med 1996;24:168–76.

30. Bencardino JT, Kassarjian A, Palmer WE. Magnetic resonance imaging of the hip: sports-related injuries. Top Magn Reson Imaging 2003;14:145–60.

31. Kujala UM, Orava S. Ischial apophysis injuries in athletes. Sports Med 1993;16:290–4.

32. Pallia CS, Scott RE, Chao DJ. Traumatic hip dislocation in athletes. Curr Sports Med Rep 2002;1: 338–45.

33. Matsumoto K, Sumi H, Sumi Y, et al. An analysis of hip dislocations among snowboarders and skiers: a 10-year prospective study from 1992 to 2002. J Trauma 2003;55:946–8.

34. Shindle MK, Ranawat AS, Kelly BT. Diagnosis and management of traumatic and atraumatic hip instability in the athletic patient. Clin Sports Med 2006; 25:309–26, ix–x.

35. Poggi JJ, Callaghan JJ, Spritzer CE, et al. Changes on magnetic resonance images after traumatic hip dislocation. Clin Orthop Relat Res 1995;319: 249–59.

36. Moorman CT, Warren RF, Hershman EB, et al. Traumatic posterior hip subluxation in American football. J Bone Joint Surg Am 2003;85:1190–6.

37. Cooper DE, Warren RF, Barnes R. Traumatic subluxation of the hip resulting in aseptic necrosis and chondrolysis in a professional football player. Am J Sports Med 1991;19:322–4.

38. Philippon MJ. New frontiers in hip arthroscopy: the role of arthroscopic hip labral repair and capsulorrhaphy in the treatment of hip disorders. Instr Course Lect 2006;55:309–16.

39. Philippon MJ, Kuppersmith DA, Wolff AB, et al. Arthroscopic findings following traumatic hip dislocation in 14 professional athletes. Arthroscopy 2009;25:169–74.

40. Weaver CJ, Major NM, Garrett WE, et al. Femoral head osteochondral lesions in painful hips of athletes: MR imaging findings. AJR Am J Roentgenol 2002;178:973–7.

41. Kramer J, Stiglbauer R, Engel A, et al. MR contrast arthrography (MRA) in osteochondrosis dissecans. J Comput Assist Tomogr 1992;16:254–60.

42. Nishii T, Sugano N, Sato Y, et al. Three-dimensional distribution of acetabular cartilage thickness in patients with hip dysplasia: a fully automated computational analysis of MR imaging. Osteoarthr Cartil 2004;12:650–7.

43. Nakanishi K, Tanaka H, Sugano N, et al. MR-based three-dimensional presentation of cartilage thickness in the femoral head. Eur Radiol 2001;11: 2178–83.

44. Schmid MR, Notzli HP, Zanetti M, et al. Cartilage lesions in the hip: diagnostic effectiveness of MR arthrography. Radiology 2003;226:382–6.

45. Bharam S. Labral tears, extra-articular injuries, and hip arthroscopy in the athlete. Clin Sports Med 2006;25:279–92, ix.

46. Kelly BT, Williams RJ III, Philippon MJ. Hip arthroscopy: current indications, treatment options, and management issues. Am J Sports Med 2003;31: 1020–37.

47. Robertson WJ, Kadrmas WR, Kelly BT. Arthroscopic management of labral tears in the hip: a systematic review of the literature. Clin Orthop Relat Res 2007;455:88–92.

48. McCarthy JC, Lee JA. Arthroscopic intervention in early hip disease. Clin Orthop Relat Res 2004; 1429:57–62.

49. Farjo LA, Glick JM, Sampson TG. Hip arthroscopy for acetabular labral tears. Arthroscopy 1999;15: 132–7.

50. Magee T, Hinson G. Association of paralabral cysts with acetabular disorders. AJR Am J Roentgenol 2000;174:1381–4.

51. Czerny C, Kramer J, Neuhold A, et al. [Magnetic resonance imaging and magnetic resonance arthrography of the acetabular labrum: comparison with surgical findings]. Rofo 2001;173:702–7 [in German].

52. Petersilge C. Imaging of the acetabular labrum. Magn Reson Imaging Clin N Am 2005;13:641–52, vi.

53. Saddik D, Troupis J, Tirman P, et al. Prevalence and location of acetabular sublabral sulci at hip arthroscopy with retrospective MRI review. AJR Am J Roentgenol 2006;187:W507–11.

54. Dinauer PA, Murphy KP, Carroll JF. Sublabral sulcus at the posteroinferior acetabulum: a potential pitfall in MR arthrography diagnosis of acetabular labral tears. AJR Am J Roentgenol 2004;183: 1745–53.

55. Petersilge CA. MR arthrography for evaluation of the acetabular labrum. Skeletal Radiol 2001;30: 423–30.

56. Studler U, Kalberer F, Leunig M, et al. MR arthrography of the hip: differentiation between an anterior sublabral recess as a normal variant and a labral tear. Radiology 2008;249:947–54.

57. Armfield DR, Towers JD, Robertson DD. Radiographic and MR imaging of the athletic hip. Clin Sports Med 2006;25:211–39, viii.

58. Lage LA, Patel JV, Villar RN. The acetabular labral tear: an arthroscopic classification. Arthroscopy 1996;12:269–72.

59. Robinson P, Barron DA, Parsons W, et al. Adductor-related groin pain in athletes: correlation of MR imaging with clinical findings. Skeletal Radiol 2004;33:451–7.

60. el-Noueam KI, Schweitzer ME, Bhatia M, et al. The utility of contrast-enhanced MRI in diagnosis of muscle injuries occult to conventional MRI. J Comput Assist Tomogr 1997;21:965–8.

61. Shabshin N, Rosenberg ZS, Cavalcanti CF. MR imaging of iliopsoas musculotendinous injuries. Magn Reson Imaging Clin N Am 2005;13:705–16.

62. Oka M, Monu JU. Prevalence and patterns of occult hip fractures and mimics revealed by MRI. AJR Am J Roentgenol 2004;182:283–8.

63. Weiss JM, Tolo V. Femoral nerve palsy following iliacus hematoma. Orthopedics 2008;31(2):178.

64. Chakravarthy J, Ramisetty N, Pimpalnerkar A, et al. Surgical repair of complete proximal hamstring tendon ruptures in water skiers and bull riders: a report of four cases and review of the literature. Br J Sports Med 2005;39:569–72.

65. Dosani A, Giannoudis PV, Waseem M, et al. Unusual presentation of sciatica in a 14-year-old girl. Injury 2004;35:1071–2.

66. Ryan JB, Wheeler JH, Hopkinson WJ, et al. Quadriceps contusions: West Point update. Am J Sports Med 1991;19:299–304.

67. Beiner JM, Jokl P. Muscle contusion injury and myositis ossificans traumatica. Clin Orthop Relat Res 2002;(Suppl 403):S110–9.

68. Ledermann HP, Schweitzer ME, Morrison WB. Pelvic heterotopic ossification: MR imaging characteristics. Radiology 2002;222:189–95.

69. Bencardino JT, Mellado JM. Hamstring injuries of the hip. Magn Reson Imaging Clin N Am 2005;13: 677–90, vi.

70. Connell DA, Schneider-Kolsky ME, Hoving JL, et al. Longitudinal study comparing sonographic and MRI assessments of acute and healing hamstring injuries. AJR Am J Roentgenol 2004;183:975–84.

71. Schneider-Kolsky ME, Hoving JL, Warren P, et al. A comparison between clinical assessment and magnetic resonance imaging of acute hamstring injuries. Am J Sports Med 2006;34:1008–15.

72. Askling CM, Tengvar M, Saartok T, et al. Proximal hamstring strains of stretching type in different sports: injury situations, clinical and magnetic resonance imaging characteristics, and return to sport. Am J Sports Med 2008;36:1799–804.

73. Maffey L, Emery C. What are the risk factors for groin strain injury in sport? A systematic review of the literature. Sports Med 2007;37:881–94.

74. Cross TM, Gibbs N, Houang MT, et al. Acute quadriceps muscle strains: magnetic resonance imaging features and prognosis. Am J Sports Med 2004;32:710–9.

75. Evans GF, Haller RG, Wyrick PS, et al. Submaximal delayed-onset muscle soreness: correlations between MR imaging findings and clinical measures. Radiology 1998;208:815–20.

76. Gamradt SC, Brophy RH, Barnes R, et al. Nonoperative treatment for proximal avulsion of the rectus femoris in professional American football. Am J Sports Med 2009;37:1370–4.

77. Kannus P, Natri A. Etiology and pathophysiology of tendon ruptures in sports. Scand J Med Sci Sports 1997;7:107–12.

78. Cvitanic O, Henzie G, Skezas N, et al. MRI diagnosis of tears of the hip abductor tendons (gluteus medius and gluteus minimus). AJR Am J Roentgenol 2004;182:137–43.

79. Bui KL, Ilaslan H, Recht M, et al. Iliopsoas injury: an MRI study of patterns and prevalence correlated with clinical findings. Skeletal Radiol 2008;37:245–9.

80. Ouellette H, Thomas BJ, Nelson E, et al. MR imaging of rectus femoris origin injuries. Skeletal Radiol 2006;35:665–72.

81. Lohrer H, Nauck T. [Proximal adductor longus tendon tear in high level athletes. A report of three cases]. Sportverletz Sportschaden 2007;21:190–4 [in German].

82. Shahabpour M, Kichouh M, Laridon E, et al. The effectiveness of diagnostic imaging methods for the assessment of soft tissue and articular disorders of the shoulder and elbow. Eur J Radiol 2008;65:194–200.

83. Rockett MS, Waitches G, Sudakoff G, et al. Use of ultrasonography versus magnetic resonance imaging for tendon abnormalities around the ankle. Foot Ankle Int 1998;19:604–12.

84. Gerling MC, Pfirrmann CW, Farooki S, et al. Posterior tibialis tendon tears: comparison of the diagnostic efficacy of magnetic resonance imaging and ultrasonography for the detection of surgically created longitudinal tears in cadavers. Invest Radiol 2003;38:51–6.

85. Sallay PI, Ballard G, Hamersly S, et al. Subjective and functional outcomes following surgical repair of complete ruptures of the proximal hamstring complex. Orthopedics 2008;31(11):1092.

86. Nakagaki K, Ozaki J, Tomita Y, et al. Fatty degeneration in the supraspinatus muscle after rotator cuff tear. J Shoulder Elbow Surg 1996;5:194–200.

87. Shimizu T, Itoi E, Minagawa H, et al. Atrophy of the rotator cuff muscles and site of cuff tears. Acta Orthop Scand 2002;73:40–3.

88. Blanco I, Krahenbuhl S, Schlienger RG. Corticosteroid-associated tendinopathies: an analysis of the published literature and spontaneous pharmacovigilance data. Drug Saf 2005;28:633–43.

89. Connell DA, Ali KE, Ahmad M, et al. Ultrasound-guided autologous blood injection for tennis elbow. Skeletal Radiol 2006;35:371–7.

90. Zeisig E, Fahlstrom M, Ohberg L, et al. Pain relief after intratendinous injections in patients with tennis elbow: results of a randomised study. Br J Sports Med 2008;42:267–71.

91. Wood DG, Packham I, Trikha SP, et al. Avulsion of the proximal hamstring origin. J Bone Joint Surg Am 2008;90:2365–74.

92. Kagan A II. Rotator cuff tears of the hip. Clin Orthop Relat Res 1999;135–40.

93. Voos JE, Shindle MK, Pruett A, et al. Endoscopic repair of gluteus medius tendon tears of the hip. Am J Sports Med 2009;37:743–7.

94. Mellado JM, Bencardino JT. Morel-Lavallee lesion: review with emphasis on MR imaging. Magn Reson Imaging Clin N Am 2005;13:775–82.

95. Phillips TJ, Jeffcote B, Collopy D. Bilateral Morel-Lavallee lesions after complex pelvic trauma: a case report. J Trauma 2008;65:708–11.

96. Reddix RN Jr, Carroll E, Webb LX. Early diagnosis of a Morel-Lavallee lesion using three-dimensional computed tomography reconstructions: a case report. J Trauma 2008 [Epub ahead of print].

97. Neal C, Jacobson JA, Brandon C, et al. Sonography of Morel-Lavallee lesions. J Ultrasound Med 2008;27:1077–81.

98. Luria S, Applbaum Y, Weil Y, et al. Talc sclerodhesis of persistent Morel-Lavallee lesions (posttraumatic pseudocysts): case report of 4 patients. J Orthop Trauma 2006;20:435–8.

99. Hak DJ, Olson SA, Matta JM. Diagnosis and management of closed internal degloving injuries associated with pelvic and acetabular fractures: the Morel-Lavallee lesion. J Trauma 1997;42: 1046–51.

100. Bohnsack M, Lekkos K, Borner CE, et al. [Results of hip arthroscopy in sports related groin pain]. Sportverletz Sportschaden 2006;20:86–90 [in German].

101. Byrd JW, Jones KS. Traumatic rupture of the ligamentum teres as a source of hip pain. Arthroscopy 2004;20:385–91.

102. Yamamoto Y, Villar RN, Papavasileiou A. Supermarket hip: an unusual cause of injury to the hip joint. Arthroscopy 2008;24:490–3.

103. Rao J, Zhou YX, Villar RN. Injury to the ligamentum teres: mechanism, findings, and results of treatment. Clin Sports Med 2001;20:791–9, vii.

104. Yamamoto Y, Usui I. Arthroscopic surgery for degenerative rupture of the ligamentum teres femoris. Arthroscopy 2006;22:689, e1–3.

MR Imaging of Knee Instability

W. James Malone, DO[a],*, Franco Verde, MD[a], David Weiss, MD[a],
Gregory C. Fanelli, MD[b]

KEYWORDS

- Posteromedial corner • Medial collateral ligament
- Posterior oblique ligament • Lateral collateral ligament
- Popliteofibular ligament • MR imaging
- Posterolateral corner

The knee is the most commonly imaged joint, with many cases requiring imaging for the evaluation of possible ligamentous injury. The stability of the femorotibial joint is maintained by a number of structures, including the bony anatomy of the femoral condyles and tibial plateau, and the menisci, which increase contact area between the tibia and femur. The static, or ligamentous, stabilizers are the cruciate ligaments, the medial collateral ligament (MCL) and lateral collateral ligament (LCL), and the posteromedial and posterolateral corners. Dynamic stabilizers include the musculature that crosses the knee joint. In addition, there are thin capsular knee ligaments that are aponeurotic extensions of the thigh and leg musculature that terminate on the menisci, which function to activate motion of the joint and impart stability as ligament tension is modulated by the attached musculature.[1]

A thorough clinical examination is necessary to evaluate for instability resulting from injury, especially the multiple ligament–injured knee.[2–4] This may be difficult, however, because of the pain.[5,6] Furthermore, the accuracy of the clinical examination decreases as the number of injuries increases.[7] Given these limitations, MR imaging is vital in evaluating for ligamentous injury and provides critical information in

planning primary repair or reconstruction when needed.

MEDIAL AND POSTEROMEDIAL STRUCTURES

Numerous blended structural layers stabilize the medial knee.[8,9] In daily practice, and in the surgical and radiologic literature, these structures are often collectively called the MCL or tibial collateral ligament. The MCL, or more accurately the medial stabilizers, functions to prevent valgus stress when the knee is flexed to 30 degrees with a secondary function of limiting anterior or posterior translation and rotation of the tibia.[1] Although the MCL has been studied extensively, little consideration has been given to the posteromedial corner structures located in the posterior third of the knee.[10] Hughston and Eilers[9] first suggested a separate function of the posteromedial corner. It is known that the posteromedial corner primarily functions to resist posteromedial tibial translation relative to the femur and secondarily to resist valgus stress at the knee.[1]

Medial structures. Warren and Marshall[8] initially introduced the layered approach in describing the medial knee anatomy. This approach illustrates the anatomy of the middle third of the knee, where three distinct layers can be discerned before they

[a] Department of Radiology, MC 20-07, Geisinger Medical Center, 100 North Academy Avenue, Danville, PA 17822, USA
[b] Department of Orthopedic Surgery, Geisinger Medical Center, 100 North Academy Avenue, Danville, PA 17822, USA
* Corresponding author.
E-mail address: wjmalone@geisinger.edu (W.J. Malone).

Magn Reson Imaging Clin N Am 17 (2009) 697–724
doi:10.1016/j.mric.2009.06.008
1064-9689/09/$ – see front matter © 2009 Published by Elsevier Inc.

blend with one another when moving from the anterior to the posterior thirds of the knee (**Fig. 1**).

Layer I: crural or sartorius fascia. The most superficial layer is the crural fascia. In the posterior knee, it blends with fascia from the sartorius muscle as it overlies the medial gastrocnemius, semitendinosus, and gracilis tendons. Anteriorly, it blends with fascia from the MCL to form the medial patellar retinaculum. The crural fascia is also reinforced anterosuperiorly by fascia from the vastus medialis muscle. Although it is not an important stabilizer, the crural fascia is the first layer encountered at surgery.[8]

Layer II: superficial MCL. The superficial MCL (sMCL) is the largest of the medial ligaments, having one femoral and two tibial attachments. The proximal or femoral attachment is immediately posterior to the medial epicondyle.[8,11] The primary and most distal attachment is the medial tibia, approximately 6 cm below the joint line.[8,11] The pes anserine tendons overly the distal attachment of the sMCL and insert just anteriorly.[11] LaPrade and colleagues[11] describe a second nonosseous attachment on the more proximal tibia, where deep fibers of the sMCL blend with the underlying anterior arm of the semimembranosus.

Layer III: deep MCL or middle third capsular ligament. The deep MCL is a thick condensation of the joint capsule that underlies the sMCL and can be separated into a long thin meniscofemoral (MF) ligament and a short thick meniscotibial (MT) ligament.[8,11] Both adhere to and stabilize the medial meniscus. They are separated from the sMCL by intervening fat and a thin MCL bursa.[12,13] Further posteriorly, the deep MCL blends with the posterior oblique ligament (POL) in the posteromedial corner.[8,9,11] On MR imaging, the MT and MF ligaments are consistently identified; however, they can be difficult to separate from the overlying sMCL in places and often cannot be followed on a single image from their meniscal attachment to their respective bony attachments.

Posteromedial corner. The posteromedial corner is made up of the POL and semimembranosus tendon, and their aponeurotic extensions that make up the posteromedial joint capsule (**Fig. 2A**). The capsular structures of the posteromedial corner are quite thin, and evaluation can be challenging. The coronal oblique plane and intra-articular gadolinium have been shown to improve evaluation,[13] but neither is typically included in standard knee protocols. Despite the challenges, these structures can usually be accurately assessed with knowledge of their anatomy and normal MR imaging appearance.

The primary function of the posteromedial corner structures is to resist posteromedial tibial translation.[1] In addition, the POL functions to

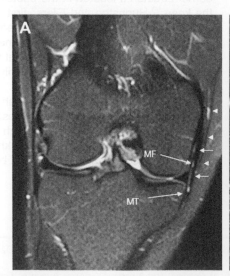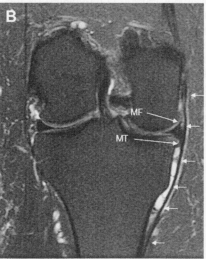

Fig. 1. Layered anatomy of the middle third of the knee. (*A*) The most superficial layer is the crural fascia (*arrowheads*). The middle layer is the tibial collateral ligament (MCL) (*short arrows*). The deep MCL is made up of the meniscofemoral (MF) and meniscotibial (MT) ligaments (*long arrows*). (*B*) The MCL is seen in almost its entirety, which is displaced in this patient with bursitis. The meniscal and tibial attachments of the MT ligament are demonstrated but only the meniscal attachment of the MF ligament is seen.

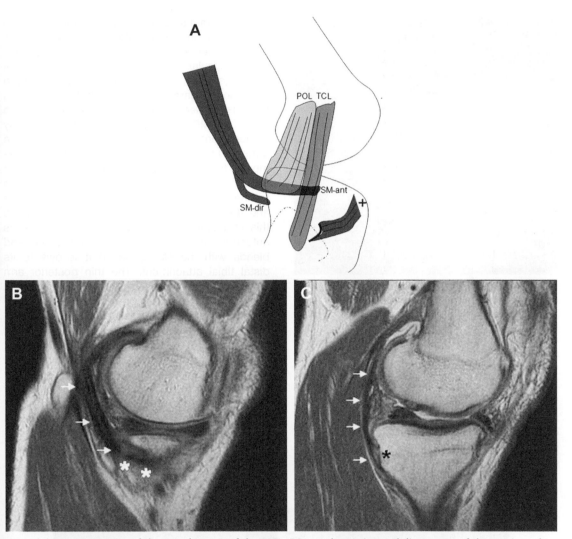

Fig. 2. (*A*) Demonstration of the attachments of the MCL, POL, and anterior and direct arms of the semimembranosus. The anteriorly reflected pes anserinus tendon attachments (sartorius, gracilis, and semitendinosus) are denoted by the (+). SM-ant, anterior semimembranosus; SM-dir, direct semimembranosus; TCL, tibial collateral ligament. (*B*) Demonstration of the anterior arm of the semimembranosus (*arrows*), with its tibial attachment located just superior to the asterisks. (*C*) Note the direct arm of the semimembranosus (*arrows*), with its tibial attachment just posterior to the asterisk.

bridge the meniscus and the semimembranosus tendon. This coupling provides motor function to the meniscus by its capsular attachments resulting in meniscal retraction during knee flexion, preventing meniscal impingement.[10,14]

Semimembranosus. The semimembranosus tendon fans out and attaches to the tibia posteromedially in helping to form and reinforce the capsule. There are two major arms of the semimembranosus. The anterior arm attaches just distal to the joint line along the medial aspect of the tibia, deep to the sMCL and distal to the MT ligament.[11] Fibers from the anterior arm blend largely with the POL in forming the capsule posteromedially. The direct arm attaches to the posteromedial tibia just below the joint line. Thin fibers from the direct arm blend primarily with the popliteal oblique ligament in forming the posterior capsule (**Fig. 2**B, C).[8,9,11]

POL. The POL is approximately 5 cm long and courses 25 degrees relative to the long axis of the tibia (see **Fig. 2**A).[13] The common femoral

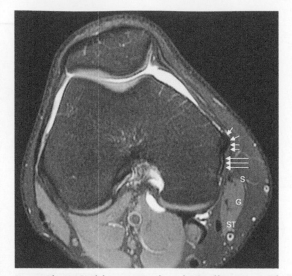

Fig. 3. The MCL (*short arrows*) and POL (*long arrows*) can be separated from one another on axial images. The thickness differential that distinguishes these ligaments is best appreciated near their femoral attachments and becomes less apparent as the ligaments travel distally below the joint line. Note the overlying sartorius (S), gracilis (G), and semitendinosus (ST).

attachment of the POL is separate from the adjacent attachment of the sMCL, which is located just proximal and posterior.[9,11] The POL is comprised of three anatomically distinct ligaments (arms) that blend together and are inseparable on MR imaging. These arms were originally termed the "superficial," "central," and "capsular" arms.[9] Despite consisting of three ligaments, the POL can be conceptualized as a single ligament that contributes in forming the posteromedial capsule, which like the deep MCL has MF and MT components. The aptly named central arm (the thickest of the three arms) is reinforced by the true MT and MF ligaments from the middle third of the knee.[11] Similar to the MF and MT ligaments, it attaches to the posterior horn of the medial meniscus and the posteromedial tibia, helping to stabilize this structure. The thin superficial arm extends anteriorly from the central arm. It parallels and blends with the sMCL, which it follows to its distal tibial attachment. The thin posterior arm blends with the popliteal oblique ligament and fibers of the semimembranosus in helping to form the posterior capsule.[9,11]

The POL and sMCL are separate structures that blend with one another, as seen on MR images. The POL and sMCL can be differentiated by noting their differing thickness, their location with respect to one another (posterior versus anterior), and their tibial attachments (proximal versus distal) (**Figs. 3** and **4**). The coupling of the semimembranosus and the medial meniscus by the POL can be appreciated by correlating the axial with the coronal images of the posterior knee (**Fig. 5**).

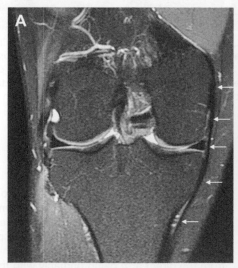
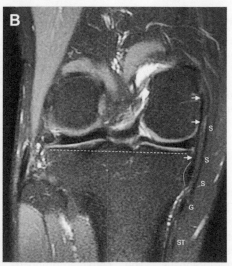

Fig. 4. Illustration of how the MCL and POL can be separated from one another on coronal images by noting their differing locations and tibial attachments. (*A*) The arrows denote the MCL, whose tibial attachment is well below the joint line. (*B*) Same patient at the level of the posterior third of the knee (three cuts posterior to *A*). The arrows are denoting the POL, which attaches to the proximal tibia (relative to MCL). The appearance is that of thickened meniscotibial and meniscofemoral ligaments. Also note the blending of POL with the anterior arm of semimembranosis (*bracket*). The overlying sartorius (S), gracilis (G), and semitendinosus (ST) are present.

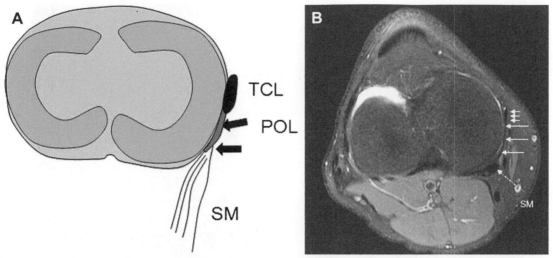

Fig. 5. (A) The coupling of the posteromedial capsule and the medial meniscus. Injury at the periphery of the meniscus where the POL attaches, injury to the POL itself, or injury to the semimembranosus can decouple these structures.[10] (B) Axial image one slice below the femorotibial joint (at level of dashed line in Fig. 4B). This demonstrates the anterior arm of the semimembranosus (SM) tendon as it blends with fibers of the POL (*long arrows*). The POL also is seen to blend with the MCL (*short arrows*).

MEDIAL AND POSTEROMEDIAL STRUCTURES: INJURY AND PITFALLS

Clinical grading of injury to the medial stabilizers is similar to that of other ligaments.[15,16] Grade 1 injuries are mild without instability. Grade 2 injuries are partial tears with some instability. Grade 3 injuries are complete tears with gross instability. Clinical grading becomes more difficult as the number of injuries increases and is also prone to overlap and interobserver variation.[17]

Correlating clinical MCL grade with imaging has been difficult. In respect to the posteromedial corner, there are no studies that have directly graded these injuries. It is reasonable, however, to use the same schema that is in place to define injury to the tibial collateral and other ligaments (Fig. 6–9).[18,19] Typically, grade 1 injuries demonstrate periligamentous edema or hemorrhage without internal morphologic changes or detachment. Grade 2 injuries demonstrate periligamentous or intrasubstance signal changes with areas of partial discontinuity. Grade 3 tears demonstrate complete discontinuity and often a lax or wavy ligament. At the authors' institution, they typically describe the injury using the previously mentioned terminology in the body of the report and classify them as mild, moderate, or severe in the conclusion. For injuries that fall in between, they are described as mild-moderate or moderate-severe; however, this is a more subjective assessment.

It is important to be aware of imaging pitfalls in diagnosing injuries to the medial stabilizers. First, periligamentous edema is not specific for MCL sprain because it is also seen to accompany meniscal tears, osteoarthritis,[20,21] or edema tracking from ruptured Baker cyst. The authors have noted periligamentous to be more commonly seen with the previously mentioned entities than with ligamentous injury. Another common pitfall is misdiagnosing MCL sprain in the case of patella dislocation. Although injuries can occur to all the patellofemoral, medial, and posteromedial stabilizers simultaneously, the authors have noted that more commonly the soft tissue edema accompanying injury to the patellofemoral stabilizers tracks posteriorly along the middle and posterior thirds of the knee (MCL and posteromedial stabilizers), simulating injury to these structures (Fig. 10).

LATERAL LIGAMENTS AND POSTEROLATERAL CORNER

The primary function of the lateral stabilizers is to prevent varus stresses when the knee is flexed to 30 degrees. A secondary function is to limit anterior or posterior translation and rotation of the tibia. The posterolateral corner (PLC) resists

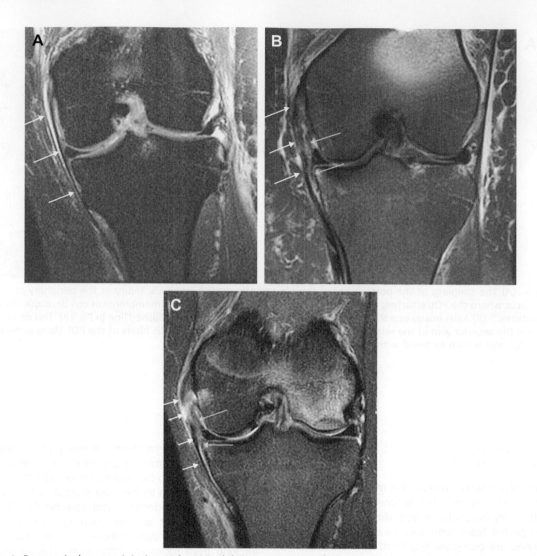

Fig. 6. Progressively worse injuries to the MCL. (*A*) Demonstration of a low-grade (grade I) injury as demonstrated by per-ligamentous edema superficial and deep to the MCL (*arrows*). (*B*) Moderate (grade 2) MCL injury with per-ligamentous edema, thickening, and intrasubstance edema (*white arrows*). Note edema surrounding the menis-cofemoral and meniscotibial ligaments (*light grey arrows*). (*C*) Moderate-high (grade 2–3) MCL injury (*white arrows*) with focal discontinuity proximally. The meniscofemoral and meniscotibial ligaments (*light grey arrows*) demonstrate intrasubstance and per-ligamentous edema.

posterolateral tibial rotation and secondarily limits posterior tibial translation relative to the femur.[1] Like their medial counterparts, clinical evaluation of the PLC can be difficult, especially in the acutely injured and painful knee.[22] Missed PLC injuries can cause secondary osteoarthritis[23,24] and graft failure following cruciate ligament reconstruction.[22,25,26]

In general, the large lateral and posterolateral stabilizers, such as the iliotibial band, biceps fem-oris tendon, LCL (fibular collateral ligament), and popliteus tendon, are well assessed on MR imaging. The smaller ligaments, however, vary in their configuration anatomically, are inconsistently present, and are obliquely oriented, all of which may make MR imaging evaluation a challenge.

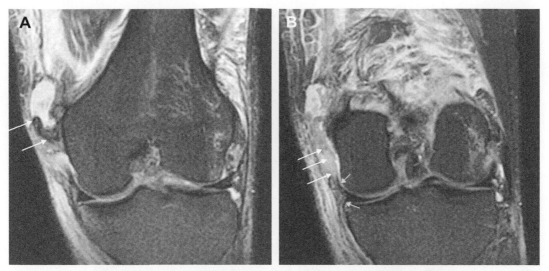

Fig. 7. Patient with high-grade medial injury. (*A*) Coronal image through the middle third of the knee showing complete proximal disruption with retracted and balled up MCL (*arrows*). (*B*) Image through the posterior knee showing nonvisualization of the femoral attachment of the POL caused by high-grade injury (*white arrows*). Note intact MF and MT portions of the POL and their attachments to the meniscus (*light grey arrows*). Compare findings with **Fig. 4**B.

The lateral stabilizers have similarities to the medial structures. First, like the medial structures, the PLC structures are closely situated and some blend with one another. Because of this, when injury occurs it is uncommonly isolated. There is also varying terminology for identical structures in the literature, with numerous names used historically for the popliteofibular ligament.[27,28] Because

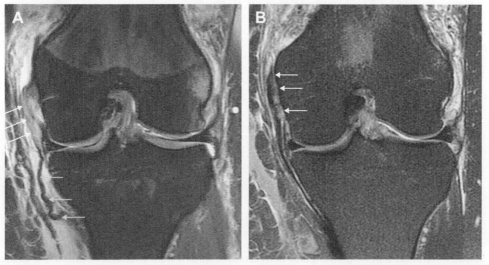

Fig. 8. Two patients with high-grade injuries. (*A*) Marked thickening and intrasubstance edema at the femoral attachment of the MCL (*white arrows*) and avulsion of the distal tibial attachment with retraction (*light grey arrow*). (*B*) Fluid gap between the MCL and its femoral attachment (*arrows*). At surgery the femoral attachment was peeled off the bone along with the medial patellofemoral ligament (not shown). The tibial attachment is intact.

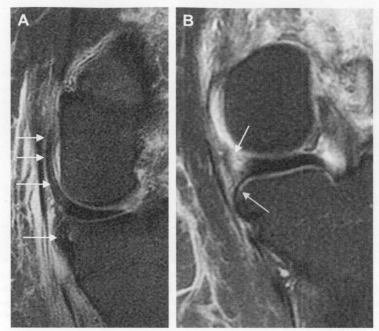

Fig. 9. Two patients with posteromedial corner injuries. (A) Note the markedly thickened MF and MT portions of the POL (*arrows*) with surrounding edema. (B) Note the thin intact meniscotibial portion of the POL (*light grey arrow*). There is disruption of the meniscofemoral attachment of the POL (*white arrow*).

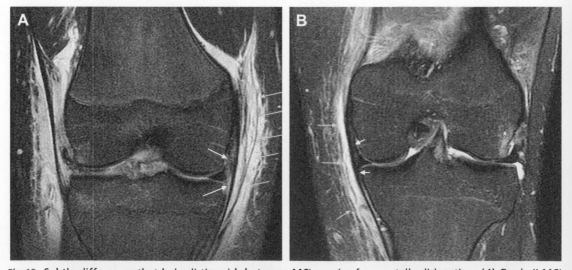

Fig. 10. Subtle differences that help distinguish between MCL sprains from patella dislocation. (A) Grade II MCL sprain. The edema is superficial and deep to MCL (*light grey arrows*) with poor delineation of the injured MT and MF ligaments (*white arrows*). (B) Patella dislocation. The edema is superficial to (*light grey arrows*) but not deep to the MCL and there is no involvement of the MF and MT ligaments (*white arrows*). The characteristic bone contusion pattern seen with patellofemoral dislocation,[95] edema in the anterolateral femoral condyle (*), and medial facet of the patella (not shown) confirms the diagnosis of patella dislocation.

of this, it is important to ensure that the terminology used in reporting is at all times consistent and understood by referring clinicians. Despite these difficulties, evaluation of the PLC can be accomplished with a thorough understanding of the anatomy and an awareness of the patterns of injury.

ANATOMY AND INJURY
Iliotibial Band

The iliotibial band is the terminal extension of the tensor fascia lata. It has five interdigitating layers that insert onto Gerty's tubercle of the lateral tibia.[29] These layers are not consistently separate on MR imaging with standard imaging. The normal and injured iliotibial band is best visualized in the coronal plane (**Fig. 11**).

LCL and Biceps Femoris

The proximal or femoral attachment of the LCL is located approximately 2 cm above the joint line, just anterior to the lateral gastrocnemius origin on the lateral femoral epicondyle (**Figs. 12** and **13**).

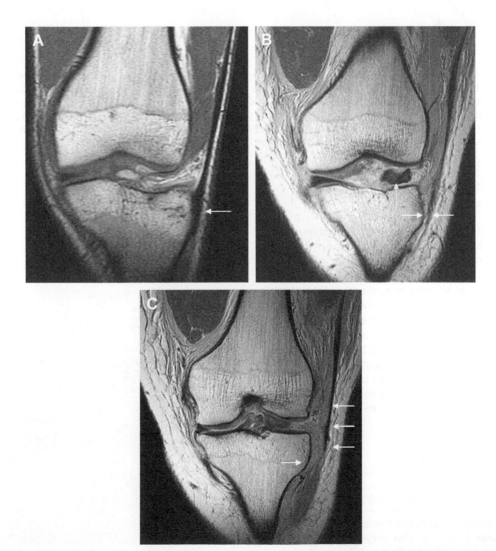

Fig. 11. (*A*) Normal attachment of the iliotibial band (ITB) onto Gerty's tubercle. (*B, C*) Selected coronal images showing fluid gap where the ITB was peeled off the tibia (*white arrows*). Note also the flipped meniscal fragment in *B* (*light grey arrow*).

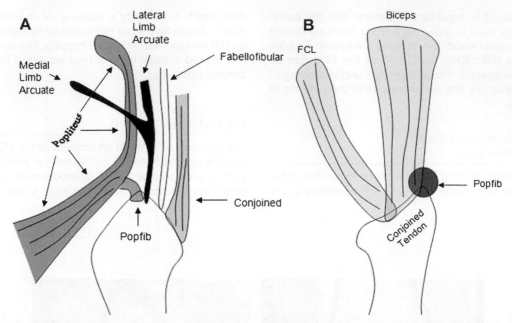

Fig. 12. Insertional geometry of lateral structures onto the fibula head in anteroposterior and lateral views, respectively.[39] (*A*) the popliteofibular ligament attaches medially to the fibula styloid, the conjoined tendon of the biceps and LCL attach far laterally, and when present the fabellofibular and Y-shaped arcuate ligament between them. (*B*) Attachment of the conjoined tendon spans most of the fibular head from anterior to posterior with the exception of the far anterior aspect. The popliteofibular ligament is seen to attach at the apex of the fibula head (styloid). The arcuate and fabellofibular ligaments are not shown in B. FCL, fibular collateral ligament.

The distal LCL shares a conjoined attachment with the biceps femoris tendon on the head of the fibula far laterally.[30,31] The biceps femoris muscle has a short head and a long head, each head possessing two arms: an anterior arm and a direct arm.[30] Both arms of the long head and the direct arm of the short head insert onto the fibular head. The anterior arm of the short head inserts onto the tibia.[30] The obliquely oriented biceps femoris and LCL are most accurately evaluated on successive coronal images, but can also be seen in the axial plane and can sometimes be seen on the far lateral sagittal image. Varying degrees of injury to the LCL may occur (**Fig. 14**).

Popliteus Complex: Popliteus Tendon, Popliteofibular Ligament, and Popliteal Meniscal (Popliteomeniscal) Fascicles

The popliteus complex is made up of a number of structures (**Fig. 15**). The origin of the popliteus tendon is intra-articular from a sulcus on the lateral femoral condyle, inferior and anterior to the proximal attachment of the LCL.[30,31] Injuries of

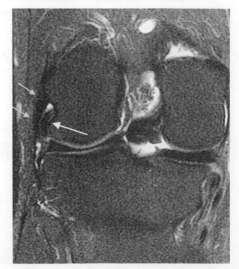

Fig. 13. Normal proximal attachment of the LCL (*light grey arrows*). Also seen is the normal popliteus tendon origin (*white arrow*) just inferiorly.

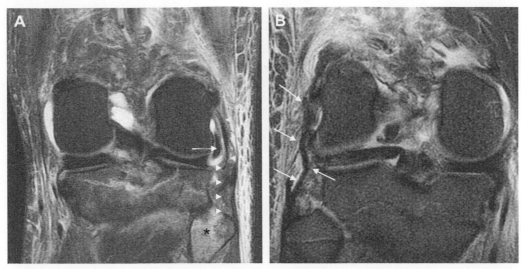

Fig. 14. (A) High-grade conjoined tendon injury (*white arrowheads*). Note the marked edema in the fibula head (*). White arrow shows intact popliteus tendon just proximal to its origin. LCL origin demonstrates per-ligamentous edema but is intact (*light grey arrowheads*). (B) The LCL (*arrows*) is wavy and is thickened with intrasubstance signal alteration proximally, consistent with a moderate high-grade injury.

popliteus may occur at its origin (**Fig. 16**) or more commonly at its myotendinous junction.

The intra-articular portion of the tendon extends distally as it wraps posteromedially, deep to the fabellofibular and arcuate ligaments.[30,31] As the popliteus tendon passes the posterior horn of the lateral meniscus it gives off a thin anteroinferior popliteomeniscal fascicle and a thicker posterosuperior popliteomeniscal fascicle. Both are best seen in the sagittal plane but can sometimes be seen in the coronal plane (**Fig. 17**). These are the two most consistently seen of a number of meniscal fascicles about the posterior joint, along with a third but inconsistent posteroinferior fascicle.[32] The popliteomeniscal fascicles are thought to be important in tethering the lateral meniscus in place, preventing impingement and tear.[33–35] Tear at the periphery of the meniscus where these fascicles attach, or tear of the fascicles themselves, may allow the meniscus to displace into the joint, causing locking (**Fig. 18**). Absence of these fascicles has been associated with tears of the lateral meniscus.[36] The anteroinferior and posterosuperior fascicles reinforce the joint capsule as they parallel and essentially envelope the popliteus tendon as it wraps posteromedially, eventually forming the floor and roof of the popliteus hiatus, respectively.[31,32,37,38] This hiatus is the boundary between the intra- and extra-articular components of the popliteus tendon, with its intra-articular portion being extrasynovial like the cruciate ligaments.[39]

As the popliteus tendon exits the hiatus (**Fig. 19**) it becomes extra-articular and shortly afterward it gives off its fibular attachment, known as the "popliteofibular ligament" (**Fig. 20**). The popliteofibular ligament arises laterally from the popliteus at its myotendinous junction. It inserts medial to

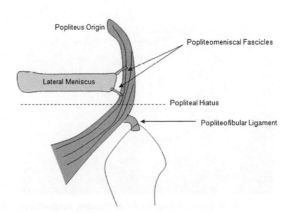

Fig. 15. Anatomy of the popliteus complex.

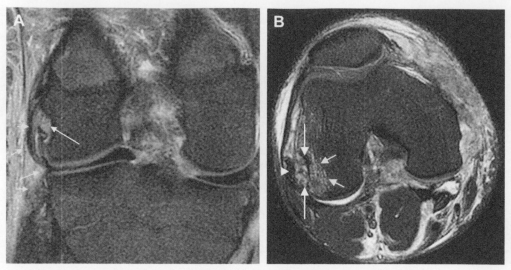

Fig. 16. (*A*) Coronal image showing proximal avulsion of popliteus (*white arrow*) and a wavy LCL secondary to distal avulsion (*light grey arrows*). (*B*) Corresponding axial image in same patient shows an empty popliteus sulcus (*between white arrows*) with adjacent marrow edema (*light grey arrows*). *Arrowhead* is on LCL.

the attachments of the fabellofibular ligament and arcuate ligament, far posteriorly on the fibula styloid.[30,31,40] The popliteofibular ligament is quite variable in morphology. The most common configuration is a single band, but double bands arising from the popliteus (**Fig. 21**) and an inverted Y

variant have been described.[30,31,38,41] The thick but short and obliquely oriented popliteofibular ligament is difficult to image[30,42] despite being nearly always present on anatomic dissection.[43] On average it courses 37 degrees oblique to the horizontal plane.[44] Visualization is improved but

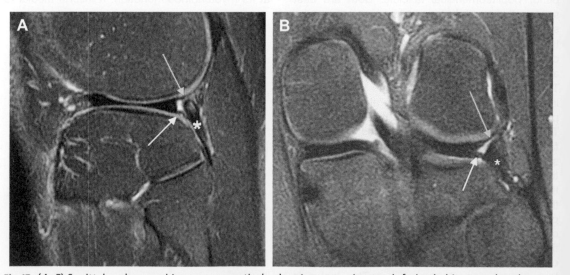

Fig. 17. (*A, B*) Sagittal and coronal images, respectively, showing normal anteroinferior (*white arrow*) and posterosuperior (*light grey arrow*) popliteomeniscal fascicles. Popliteus (*).

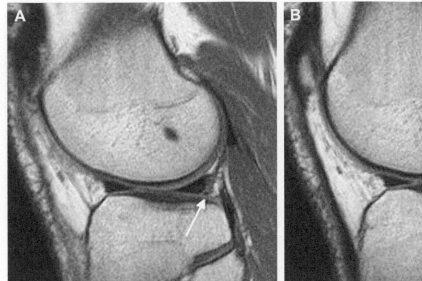

Fig. 18. (A, B) Successive sagittal images in a patient with history of knee locking. There is a subtle discontinuity at the meniscal attachment of the posteroinferior popliteomeniscal fascicle (*arrow*). At surgery the meniscus was displaceable into the joint.

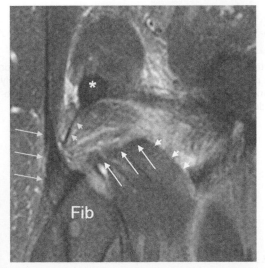

Fig. 19. Short white arrows show the normal appearing and nonedematous popliteus myotendinous junction. The overlying posterior knee capsule is edematous from injury, which nicely demarcates where the popliteus goes from being intra-articular to extra-articular at the popliteus hiatus (*long white arrows*). Note also the normal attachment of the conjoined tendon (*long light grey arrows*) and a variant of the fabellofibular ligament (*short light grey arrows*) that was seen to attach more laterally than normal. Fabella (*).

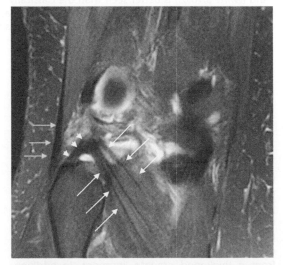

Fig. 20. Classic single band of the popliteofibular ligament (*short white arrows*) coming off the popliteus (*between long white arrows*). Also seen is the biceps contribution to the conjoined tendon insertion (*light grey arrows*).

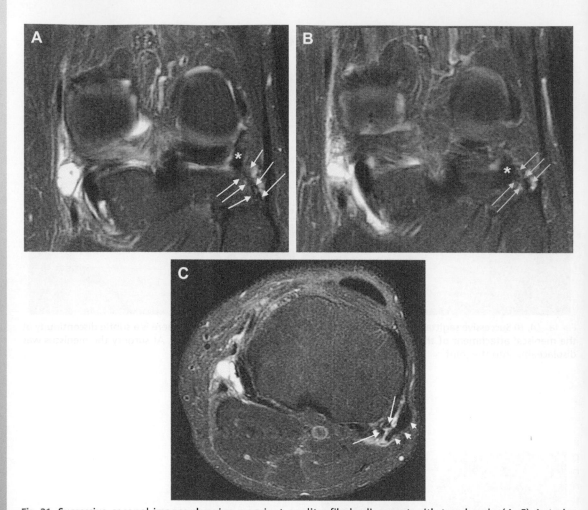

Fig. 21. Successive coronal images showing a variant popliteofibular ligament with two bands. (*A, B*) Anterior band (*white arrows*) is better seen than the classically seen posterior band (*light grey arrows*), which is partially imaged in *B*. Popliteus (*) (*C*) Correlation with the axial plane shows the two separate bands of the popliteofibular ligament (*long arrows*) arising from the popliteus tendon. Short arrows show the conjoined tendon.

remains difficult with the coronal oblique imaging plane.[45] Nevertheless, imaging in the coronal plane frequently depicts popliteofibular ligament injuries (**Figs. 22** and **23**). Correlation with the axial plane is often helpful distinguishing double-band or single-band variation and also distinguishing it from a thickened arcuate ligament. In addition, noting marrow edema in the fibular head at the expected attachment suggests injury.[39] In the presence of fibular head edema, the PLC should be carefully scrutinized.

Lateral Gastrocnemius, Fabellofibular Ligament, and Arcuate Ligament

The lateral gastrocnemius tendon arises from or adjacent to the supracondylar process of the femur. It often contains an osseous or cartilaginous body known as the "fabella."[31] When present, the fabellofibular ligament arises from the fabella and inserts distally onto the lateral base of the fibular head, just anterolateral to the popliteofibular ligament.[30] The fabellofibular

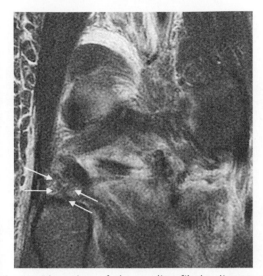

Fig. 22. Disruption of the popliteofibular ligament. Note the disorganization of fibers in the expected location of popliteofibular ligament (*arrows*), which was completely disrupted at surgery. There was a high-grade injury to the popliteus (not shown).

and arcuate ligaments are not consistently present in dissection and can be present alone or in combination.[27,31,43,46,47] The arcuate ligament has both medial and lateral limbs. These two limbs ascend as a single ligament from their fibular attachment just anterior to the fabellofibular ligament (when present together).[30,31] They separate in the form of a Y with the thicker lateral limb coursing straight proximally and attaching to the lateral femoral condyle in reinforcing the lateral joint capsule.[31] The medial limb courses medial and superficial to the popliteal tendon, and then blends with fibers of the popliteal oblique ligament in helping to reinforce the posterior joint capsule.[31]

When present, the thin fabellofibular (**Fig. 24**) may be seen with MR imaging. The medial limb of the arcuate ligament is best seen as the thin hypointense structure immediately posterior to the popliteus tendon on sagittal imaging. When either or both are identified, correlation with the remaining imaging planes is suggested for confirmation given the anatomic variability in this area. For example, the double band of the popliteofibular ligament may be confused with either ligament. The soft tissue edema that often accompanies PLC injury can be helpful in delineating these inconsistently seen structures (**Fig. 25**).

In addition to the injuries shown, typical radiographic signs exist that suggest PLC injury. The anterior oblique band is a thin aponeurotic extension that arises from the anterior LCL at the level of the joint line.[48] The anterior oblique band blends with thin fibers extending posteriorly from the iliotibial band. The blending of these fibers from the LCL and iliotibial band form and reinforce the joint capsule as it attaches to the lateral tibial rim, which is the characteristic location of the Segond fracture (**Fig. 26**).[28] The Segond fracture is highly suggestive of cruciate tear and lateral ligamentous injury, which should be assumed present until proved otherwise.[23,49] Another classic sign of PLC injury is an avulsion fracture of the fibular head termed the "arcuate sign."[50] Huang and colleagues[51] demonstrated in some instances the fracture involves a small piece of bone from the fibular attachment of the arcuate complex (popliteofibular, arcuate, and fabellofibular ligaments) at the posterosuperior apex of the styloid process. In certain cases, a larger bone fragment may be avulsed that also includes the conjoined tendon (**Fig. 27**).[52] Like the Segond fracture, the arcuate sign is highly associated with cruciate tears.[51,52] Cruciate injuries necessitate careful scrutiny of the PLC structures and vice versa.

CENTRAL STABILIZERS
Anterior Cruciate Ligament

The anterior cruciate ligament (ACL) functions to prevent anterior translation of the tibia relative to the femur, limit rotation of the tibia when the knee is in extension, and limit varus and valgus stress when the LCL or MCL are injured.[53,54] The ACL attaches from the posteromedial aspect of the lateral femoral condyle to the anteromedial tibial plateau.[55] The long axis of the ACL is 26 ± 6 degrees tilted from the horizontal.[56,57] It is narrowest in the midsection and is approximately 3.5 times broader at its attachments.[58] The tibial attachment fans out rather broadly and is called the "foot region."[59] The ACL contains two functional bundles named by their relative attachments to the tibia: the anteromedial bundle and the posterolateral bundle. There is, however, no histologic separation between the bundles.[60,61] The anteromedial bundle has a slightly more vertical orientation and the posterolateral bundle a slightly more horizontal course.[56,57] Functionally, both bundles are thought to have reciprocal roles with both restricting anterior tibial translation, the anteromedial bundle during flexion and the posterolateral bundle during extension.[62]

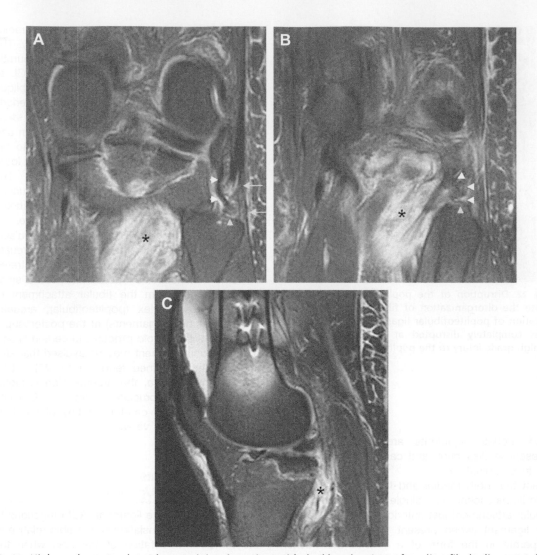

Fig. 23. High-grade posterolateral corner injury in patient with dual band variant of popliteofibular ligament. (A) High-grade injury to the conjoined tendon (*light grey arrows*). The anterior band of popliteofibular ligament is wavy (*white arrowheads*) with fluid gap at site of fibula avulsion (*light grey arrowhead*). (B) Posterior band of the popliteofibular ligament (*white arrowheads*) is seen to be avulsed off the fibula styloid (*light grey arrowhead*). (C) All three images demonstrate the high-grade popliteus myotendinous junction injury (*).

The ACL is evaluated on T2 sequences where it is predominantly hypointense with some linear striations of variable intensity (**Fig. 28**A). Sagittal images often well depict the ACL in its entirety, which parallels the roof of the intercondylar notch following Blumensaat's line.[63] The femoral attachment of the ACL and both the anteromedial bundle and posterolateral bundle are typically well seen in the axial plane (**Fig. 28**B–D). An abnormal appearance (eg, discontinuity, nonvisualization, or abnormal tilt) suggests a tear.[64] These findings are often well seen in the sagittal plane because tears most commonly occur in the midsubstance (**Figs. 29** and **30**). A tear can occur throughout the course of the ligament,[63] however, and uncommonly may avulse with bone. Accordingly,

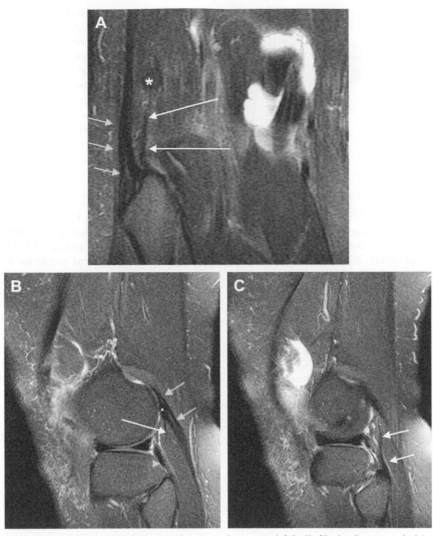

Fig. 24. Coronal and successive sagittal images showing the normal fabellofibular ligament (*white arrows*). (*A*) Note the normal striated appearance of conjoined tendon insertion laterally (*light grey arrows*) and fabella (***). (*B*) Fabella (***) embedded in the lateral gastrocnemius tendon (*light grey arrows*) and the adjacent popliteus tendon (*arrowhead*). The proximal aspect of the fabellofibular ligament is seen (*white arrow*). (*C*) Fibular attachment of the fabellofibular ligament (*arrows*).

it is important to evaluate for an ACL tear in all three imaging planes and not just the sagittal plane. Documentation of the femoral attachment of the ACL in axial plane eliminates the possibility of missing femoral avulsions. This is especially important on open or low-field systems where femoral avulsions are often less obvious (**Fig. 31**).

The pivot shift bone contusion pattern associated with ACL injury is a characteristic clue to the radiologist that an ACL tear has occurred (see **Fig. 29**A). This is identified as a contusion pattern that involves the posterior lateral tibial plateau and sulcus terminalis of the lateral femoral condyle,[65] but can vary depending on

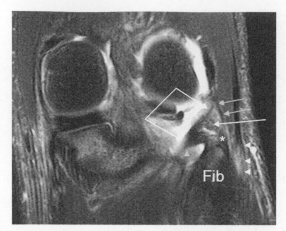

Fig. 25. Soft tissue edema highlights smaller PLC structures as they attach to the fibula (Fib). There is a moderate high-grade injury to the conjoined tendon insertion (*white arrowheads*). Note the popliteus tendon (*connected white arrows*) and take-off of the popliteofibular ligament (*light grey arrowheads*) before attaching on the fibula. The fibular attachment of the Y-shaped arcuate ligament (*) is seen just lateral to the popliteofibular ligament. The thickened medial limb of the arcuate ligament (*long white arrow*) was confirmed on successive sagittal images (versus a dual band variant of the popliteofibular ligament). Light grey arrows show the lateral limb of arcuate ligament. A fabellofibular ligament was not present in this patient.

the degree of flexion when the injury occurred.[63] Associated contre-coup bone bruising is often seen in the posteromedial tibial plateau.[66] Isolated ACL injuries are less common, which should prompt further evaluation of meniscal tears, articular cartilage damage, collateral ligament injury, or bony contusion.[67] Care must be taken not to mistake mucoid degeneration of the ACL for tear, a common pitfall on MR imaging of a patient who does not present with instability (**Fig. 32**).[68]

Posterior Cruciate Ligament

The posterior cruciate ligament (PCL) is located near the center of rotation of the knee.[1] It functions as the primary static stabilizer of the knee and the primary restraint against posterior translation of the tibia. The PCL arises from a broad posterolateral attachment on the medial femoral condyle and attaches to a midline depression 10 to 15 mm below the medial and lateral tibial plateau. Like the ACL it is intra-articular and lies in its own synovial sheath.[69,70] The PCL is larger and stronger than the ACL and like its counterpart it has two functional bundles, the posteromedial bundle and anterolateral bundle, based on their femoral attachments.[71]

On T2 sequences the PCL is seen as a broad homogeneously low signal curved structure

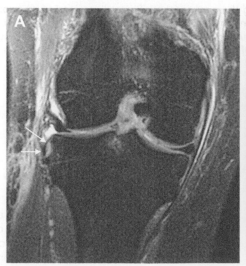

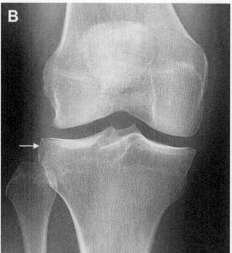

Fig. 26. (*A*) Coronal MR image shows curvilinear hypointense cortical bone fragment (*arrows*) with underlying marrow edema that is seen with a Segond fracture. (*B*) Corresponding radiograph showing a minimally displaced Segond fracture (*arrow*).

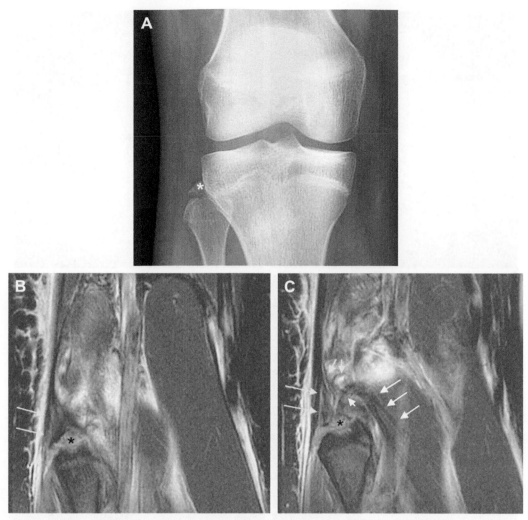

Fig. 27. (*A*) Asterisk denotes the classic "arcuate sign" on radiographs. (*B*) Corresponding MR image shows the large avulsed bone fragment (*) that includes the conjoined tendon (*arrows*). (*C*) More posterior coronal image showing the popliteus (*white arrows*). The popliteofibular ligament take-off (*white arrowhead*) is seen along with its attachment to the avulsed bone fragment. Long light grey arrows are on the conjoined tendon insertion to the bone fragment. Between the popliteofibular ligament and conjoined tendon are some fibers of the medial and lateral limbs of the Y-shaped arcuate ligament (*short light grey arrows*).

extending from the intercondylar notch to the posterior tibial plateau (**Fig. 33**). Unlike the ACL, the PCL bundles are uncommonly if ever differentiated with standard imaging. Criteria for a PCL tear are similar for any ligamentous injury: abnormal curvature, morphology, and the presence of abnormal intrasubstance signal.[64] These findings can occur throughout the ligament and may include bony avulsion (**Figs. 34** and **35**). Dashboard injuries (ie, pretibial impaction in

flexion) account for 50% of all injuries, whereas a fall onto a flexed knee, hyperextension, and flexion account for the remainder.[72,73] Like the ACL, isolated PCL tears are also uncommon.[64,74]

ADDITIONAL INJURIES

In the popliteal fossa, the popliteal artery and vein are separated from the posterior capsule by a layer of fat. The artery is tethered proximally by the

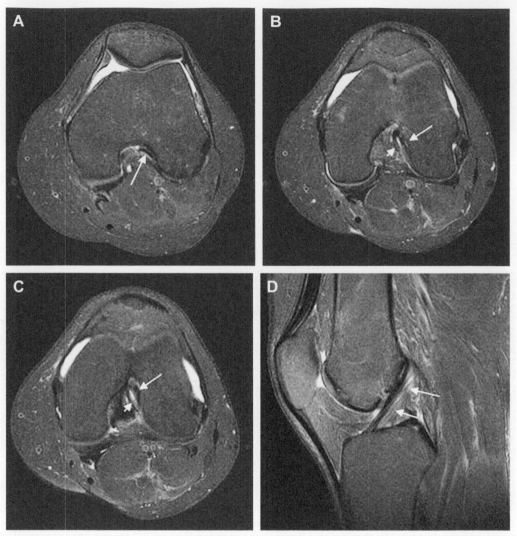

Fig. 28. Successive axial images. (*A*) Normal femoral attachment of the ACL (*arrow*). (*B, C*) Anteromedial (*short arrows*) and posterolateral (*long arrows*) bundles of the ACL. (*D*) Sagittal image demonstrating the normal ACL (*arrows*).

adductor hiatus. The close proximity of the popliteal artery to the joint and its immobility makes it susceptible to damage with high-force injuries, such as dislocation. Recent literature confirms a significant incidence of arterial injury,[75–78] affirming the need for evaluation with CT angiography, MR angiography, or conventional angiography when injury is suspected. Nerve injury is also quite common with dislocation, most commonly

involving the peroneal nerve, which lies posterior to the biceps tendon.[79] These structures are well depicted on MR imaging and must be scrutinized (**Fig. 36**).

SURGICAL PERSPECTIVE

MR imaging in the acute setting is critically important for preoperative planning purposes; however,

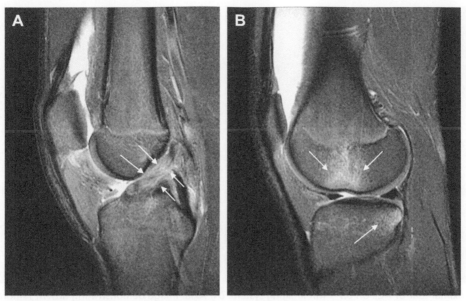

Fig. 29. (*A*) Sagittal image midline demonstrating mid-substance tear of the ACL (*arrows*). (*B*) Lateral image noting the classic pivot shift bruising (*arrows*).

MR imaging is much less helpful in the chronically injured knee. Vascular imaging studies are also essential in any bicruciate injured knee. When the ACL and PCL are disrupted in the adult population it is usually in the midsubstance of the ligament and reconstruction is performed. PLC injuries can be repaired primarily, but require augmentation with autograft or allograft tissue for an optimal result. Some low-grade medial side injuries may heal with bracing; however, higher-grade injuries

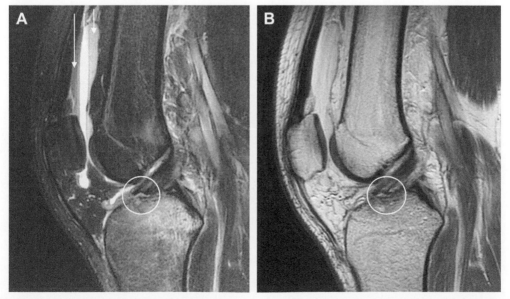

Fig. 30. (*A, B*) Sagittal T2 and proton density images, respectively, showing osseous avulsion of the ACL at the tibial attachment. On the T2 image note the lipohemarthrosis, as denoted by fat, fluid, and hemorrhage layering in the joint (progressively larger *arrows*, respectively) from this intra-articular fracture.

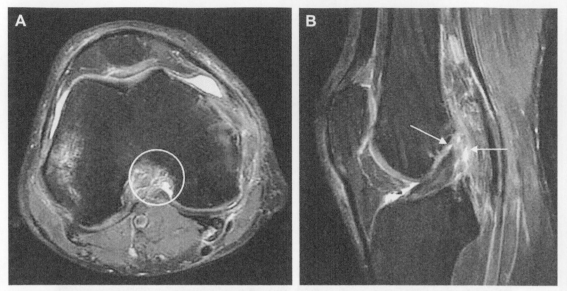

Fig. 31. Proximal tear of ACL on 0.7-T MR imaging system. (*A*) Axial image demonstrating absent femoral attachment (compare with Fig. 28B). (*B*) Sagittal image demonstrating poor delineation of femoral attachment (*arrows*) and abnormal slope.

also require either augmented repair or reconstruction.[80]

Repair of ACL injury was once dominated by single anteromedial bundle reconstruction; however, reconstructing the posterolateral bundle is being investigated clinically.[81] Single bundle reconstructions have up to 95% clinical success rate; however, up to 23% of patients still complain of pain and instability.[82–87] In vitro simulation predicts double bundle reconstruction to improve rotary torque.[88] An extensive literature review and analysis performed by Crawford and

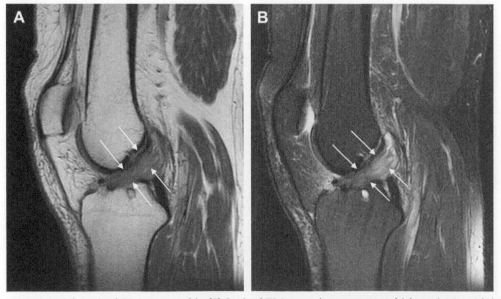

Fig. 32. Arrows in (*A*) Sagittal PD image and in (*B*) Sagittal T2 image demonstrate a thickened ACL with heterogeneous intrasubstance signal alteration in this case of mucoid degeneration. Femoral attachment was normal on the axial sequence (not shown).

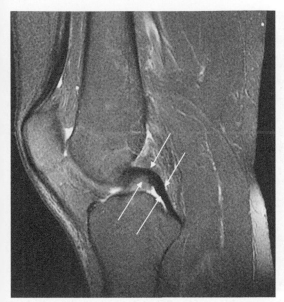

Fig. 33. Sagittal T2 image demonstrating nonstriated homogenously low signal appearance of a normal PCL (*arrows*).

reconstruction; however, further long-term follow-up and larger trials are warranted.

Because the PCL is thicker and stronger, rupture is less common. Partial tearing may be treated conservatively with immobilization.[64] Tibial avulsion is usually internally repaired.[90] If conservative therapy fails, reconstruction using similar ACL single- or double-bundle technique is then performed.[91] Multiple studies have reported favorable outcomes with improved objective stability and return to prior activities.[73,80,92-94]

With high-force injuries and especially with dislocations, patients can present with not only ACL and PCL tears, but with varying combinations of ligamentous involvement. All four major knee ligaments and the posteromedial corners and PLCs can be compromised. These structures frequently require operative attention. Operative treatment of these complex injuries is dependent on many factors, including surgical preference, severity of injury, and patient comorbidity. In general, recent literature supports surgical reconstruction of the multiligament injured knee.[76]

At the authors' institution ACL-PCL tears with low-grade medial-sided injuries (medial or posteromedial stabilizers) may be managed with brace treatment of the medial stabilizers to allow for healing, followed by arthroscopic combined ACL-PCL reconstruction in 4 to 6 weeks. Other more severe injuries to the medial and posteromedial stabilizers require open primary repair or

colleagues[81] show a number of double-bundle reconstruction techniques but few clinical trials to support these newer techniques. Recent trials by Yagi and colleagues[88] and Aglietti and colleagues[89] lend more support to double-bundle

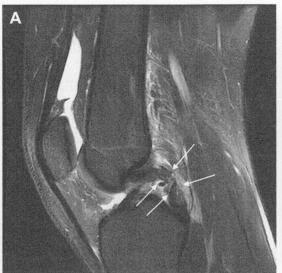
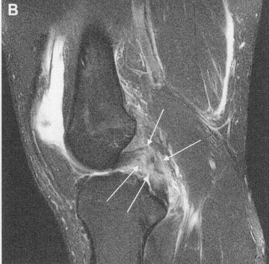

Fig. 34. Two patients with PCL injuries. (*A*) Note thickened PCL with mild intrasubstance signal alteration (*arrows*), consistent with low moderate-grade injury. (*B*) High-grade injury or complete PCL tear (*arrows*).

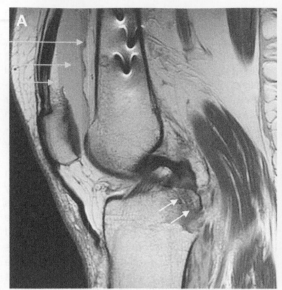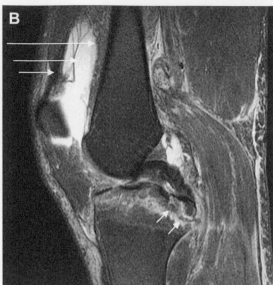

Fig. 35. (*A, B*) Two different patients with mildly displaced bony avulsions of the PCL at its tibial attachment (*short arrows*). Both images also show lipohemarthrosis (*progressively longer arrows*).

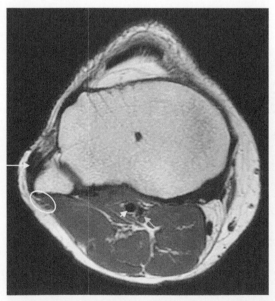

Fig. 36. *Large white arrow* is on conjoined tendon of biceps and LCL. Circle is around peroneal nerve. White arrowhead and *light grey arrow* demonstrate the popliteal artery and vein, respectively.

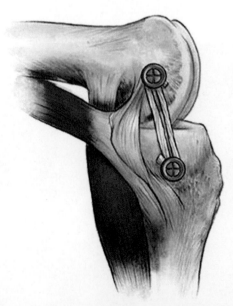

Fig. 37. When MCL reconstruction is indicated, this is performed using allograft or autograft tissue at its anatomic attachments.

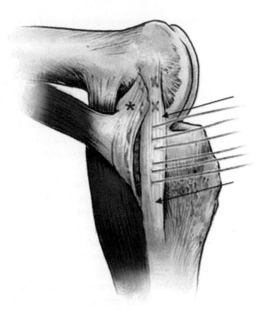

Fig. 38. Posteromedial corner repair. The posteromedial capsule (namely reinforced by the POL and semimembranosus fascial extensions) is repaired and is shifted anterosuperiorly (*). The meniscus attachments of the deep MCL and POL (meniscofemoral and meniscotibial components) are repaired to the new capsular position and finally the shifted capsule is sewn into the MCL (*arrows*).

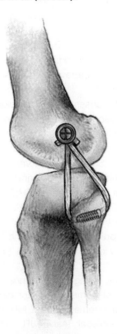

Fig. 39. Posterolateral corner reconstruction. This repair mimics the function of the LCL and popliteofibular ligaments. This is combined with posterolateral capsular shift when needed to tighten the posterolateral capsule. This is similar to posteromedial capsular shift, but with the capsule being reinforced by the arcuate ligament or fabellofibular ligament.

allograft reconstruction (**Figs. 37** and **38**). Combined ACL-PCL and PLC reconstructions are performed between 2 and 3 weeks postinjury to allow for healing of capsular tissues to permit an arthroscopic approach. Staged procedures are used in more severe PLC injuries that require open repair (**Fig. 39**).[1–4,73,80]

SUMMARY

This article demonstrates the anatomic blending of structure and overlapping function that ultimately provides femorotibial stability. An unfortunate corollary is that this interdependence not uncommonly leads to multiligamentous injuries. The different ligaments and other structures have been compartmentalized to help understand the complex anatomy of the knee, but injury patterns often do not obey these boundaries. Particularly in high-grade injuries, such as dislocations, there is no substitute for a thorough understanding of the knee anatomy. This knowledge combined with a meticulous search pattern is the key to identifying the endless combinations of injuries not just to the large stabilizers, but also to the so-called "minor stabilizers." Despite some limitations, a practical description of injuries to even the smallest of these stabilizers provides important information for orthopedic colleagues regarding the need for, type of (repair versus reconstruction), and timing of surgery.

REFERENCES

1. Fanelli GC. Surgical treatment of ACL-PCL-medial side-lateral-side injuries of the knee. Operative Techniques in Sports Medicine 2003;11(4):263–74.
2. Fanelli GC, Gianotti BF, Edson CJ. Arthroscopically assisted combined anterior and posterior cruciate ligament reconstruction. Arthroscopy 1996;12(1):5–14.
3. Fanelli GC, Gianotti BF, Edson CJ. Arthroscopically assisted combined posterior cruciate ligament/posterior lateral complex reconstruction. Arthroscopy 1996;12(5):521–30.
4. Fanelli GC, Gianotti BF, Edson CJ. The posterior cruciate ligament arthroscopic evaluation and treatment. Arthroscopy 1994;10(6):673–88.
5. Jakob RP, Staubli HV, Deland JT. Grading the pivot shift: objective tests with implications for treatment. J Bone Joint Surg Br 1987;69:294–9.
6. Jack EA. Experimental rupture of the medial collateral ligament of the knee. J Bone Joint Surg Br 1950;32:396–402.
7. Oberlander MA, Shalvoy RM, Hughston JC. The accuracy of the clinical knee examination

documented by arthroscopy: a prospective study. Am J Sports Med 1993;21:773–8.

8. Warren LF, Marshall JL. The supporting structures and layers on the medial side of the knee: an anatomical analysis. J Bone Joint Surg Am 1979; 61:56–62.

9. Hughston JC, Eilers AF. The role of the posterior oblique ligament in repairs of acute medial (collateral) ligament tears of the knee. J Bone Joint Surg Am 1973;55:923–40.

10. Sims WF, Jacobson KE. The posteromedial corner of the knee: medial-sided injury patterns revisited. Am J Sports Med 2004;32:337–45.

11. LaPrade RF, Engebretsen AH, Ly TV, et al. The anatomy of the medial part of the knee. J Bone Joint Surg Am 2007;89:2000–10.

12. De Maeseneer M, Van Roy F, Lenchik L, et al. Three layers of the medial capsular and supporting structures of the knee: MR imaging-anatomic correlation. Radiographics 2000;20:S83–9.

13. Loredo R, Hodler J, Pedowitz R, et al. Posteromedial corner of the knee: MR imaging with gross anatomic correlation. Skeletal Radiol 1999;28:305–11.

14. Hughston JC. Knee ligaments: injury and repair. St. Louis (MO): Mosby Year-Book; 1993.

15. Cham DM, Hsu CYC. Cartilage and ligament injuries in sports injuries. In: Renstrum PA, editor. London: Oxford University Press; 1993. p. 54–70.

16. Cheryne S. Disorders of the knee. In: Dee R, Mango M, Hurst LC, editors. Principles of orthopaedic practice, vol. 2. New York: McGraw-Hill; 1989. p. 1283.

17. Reid DC. Sports injury assessment and rehabilitation. New York: Churchill Livingstone; 1992. p. 502–507.

18. Schweitzer ME, Tran D, Deely DM, et al. Medial collateral ligament injuries: evaluation of multiple signs, prevalence and location of associated bone bruises, and assessment with MRI. Radiology 1995;194:825–9.

19. Stoller DW. 3rd Edition. In: Magnetic resonance imaging in orthopaedics and sports medicine, vol. 1. Baltimore (MD): Lippincott Williams & Wilkins; 2007. p. 553–4.

20. Bergin D, Keogh C, O'Connell M, et al. Atraumatic MCL edema in medial compartment osteoarthritis. Skeletal Radiol 2002;31:14–8.

21. Bergin D, Hochberg H, Zoga AC, et al. Indirect soft-tissue and osseous signs on knee MRI of surgically proven meniscal tears. AJR Am J Roentgenol 2008; 191(1):86–92.

22. Hughston JC, Jacobson KE. Chronic posterolateral rotatory instability of the knee. J Bone Joint Surg Am 1985;67:351–9.

23. Hughston JC, Andrews JR, Cross MJ, et al. Classification of knee ligament injuries. Part II. The lateral compartment. J Bone Joint Surg Am 1976; 58:173–9.

24. Kanus P. Nonoperative treatment of grade II and III sprains of the lateral ligament compartment of the knee. Am J Sports Med 1989;17(1):83–8.

25. O'Brien SJ, Warren RF, Paulov H, et al. Reconstruction of the chronically insufficient anterior cruciate ligament with the central third of the patella ligament. J Bone Joint Surg Am 1991;73:278–86.

26. Fleming RE, Blatz DJ, McCarroll JR. Posterior problems in the knee: posterior cruciate insufficiency and posterolateral rotatory insufficiency. Am J Sports Med 1981;9:107–13.

27. Seebacher JR, Ingliez A, Marshall JL, et al. The structure of the posterolateral aspect of the knee. J Bone Joint Surg Am 1982;64:536–41.

28. Campos JC, Chung CB, Lektrakul N, et al. Pathogenesis of the Segond fracture: anatomic and MR imaging evidence of an iliotibial tract or anterior oblique band avulsion. Radiology 2001;219:381–6.

29. Terry GC, Hughston JC, Norwood LA. The anatomy of the iliopatellar band and iliotibial tract. Am J Sports Med 1986;14:39–45.

30. Munshi M, Pretterklieber ML, Kwak S, et al. MR imaging, MR arthrography, and specimen correlation of the posterolateral corner of the knee: an anatomic study. AJR Am J Roentgenol 2003;180: 1095–101.

31. Diamantopoulos A, Tokis A, Tzurbakis M, et al. The posterolateral corner of the knee: evaluation under microsurgical dissection. Arthroscopy 2005;21(7): 826–33.

32. Peduto AJ, Nguyen A, Trudell DJ, et al. Popliteomeniscal fascicles: anatomic considerations using MR arthrography in cadavers. AJR Am J Roentgenol 2008;190:442–8.

33. Simonian PT, Sussmann PS, Wickiewicz TL, et al. Popliteomeniscal fasciculi and the unstable lateral meniscus: clinical correlation and magnetic resonance diagnosis. Arthroscopy 1997;13:590–6.

34. Simonian PT, Sussmann PS, van Trommel M, et al. Popliteomeniscal fasciculi and lateral meniscal stability. Am J Sports Med 1997;25:849–53.

35. LaPrade RF, Konowalchuk BK. Popliteomeniscal fascicle tears causing symptomatic lateral compartment knee pain: diagnosis by the figure-4 test and treatment by open repair. Am J Sports Med 2005; 33:1231–6.

36. De Smet AA, Asinger DA, Johnson RL. Abnormal superior popliteomeniscal fascicle and posterior pericapsular edema: indirect MR imaging signs of a lateral meniscal tear. AJR Am J Roentgenol 2001;176:63–6.

37. Cohn AK, Mains DB. Popliteal hiatus of the lateral meniscus: anatomy and measurements at dissection of 10 specimens. Am J Sports Med 1979;7: 221–6.

38. Stäubli HU, Birrer S. The popliteus tendon and its fascicles at the popliteal hiatus: gross anatomy

and functional arthroscopic evaluation with and without anterior cruciate ligament deficiency. Arthroscopy 1990;6:209–20.

39. Lee J, Papakonstantinou O, Brookenthal KR, et al. Arcuate sign of posterolateral knee injuries: anatomic, radiographic, and MRI data related to patterns of injury. Skeletal Radiol 2003;32:619–27.

40. Brinkman JM, Schwering PJ, Blankevoort L, et al. The insertion geometry of the posterolateral corner of the knee. J Bone Joint Surg Br 2005;87(10): 1364–8.

41. Ullrich K, Krudwig WK, Witzel U. Posterolateral aspect and stability of the knee joint. Part 1. Anatomy and function of the popliteus muscle–tendon unit: an anatomical and biomechanical study. Knee Surg Sports Traumatol Arthrosc 2002; 10:86–90.

42. DeMaeseneer M, Shahabpour M, Vanderdood K, et al. Posterolateral supporting structures of the knee: findings on anatomic dissection, anatomic slices and MR images. Eur Radiol 2001;11: 2170–7.

43. Watanabe Y, Moriya H, Takahashi K, et al. Functional anatomy of the posterolateral structures of the knee. Arthroscopy 1993;9(1):57–62.

44. LaPrade RF, Ly TV, Wentorf FA, et al. The posterolateral attachments of the knee: a qualitative and quantitative morphologic analysis of the fibular collateral ligament, popliteus tendon, popliteofibular ligament, and lateral gastrocnemius tendon. Am J Sports Med 2003;31(6):854–60.

45. Yu JS, Salomen DC, Hodler J, et al. Posterolateral aspect of the knee: improved imaging with a coronal oblique technique. Radiology 1996;198: 199–204.

46. Maynard MJ, Deng X, Wickiewicz TL, et al. The popliteofibular ligament: rediscovery of a key element in posterolateral stability. Am J Sports Med 1996;24(3): 311–6.

47. Sudasna S, Harnsiriwattanagit K. The ligamentous structures of the posterolateral aspect of the knee. Bull Hosp Jt Dis Orthop Inst 1990;50:35–40.

48. Irvine GB, Dias JJ, Finlay. Segond fractures of the lateral tibial condyle: brief report. J Bone Joint Surg Br 1987;69:613–4.

49. Woods GW, Stanley RF, Tullos HS. Lateral capsular sign: x-ray clue to a significant knee instability. Am J Sports Med 1979;7:27–33.

50. Shindell R, Walsh WM, Connolly JF. Avulsion fracture of the fibula: the arcuate sign of posterolateral knee instability. Nebr Med J 1984;69:369–71.

51. Huang GS, Yu JS, Munshi M, et al. Avulsion fracture of the head of the fibula (the arcuate sign): MR imaging findings predictive of injuries to the posterolateral ligaments and posterior cruciate ligament. AJR Am J Roentgenol 2003;180:381–7.

52. Juhng SK, Lee JK, Choi SS, et al. MR evaluation of the arcuate sign of posterolateral knee instability. AJR Am J Roentgenol 2002;178:583–8.

53. Butler DL, Noyes FR, Good ES. Ligamentous restraints to anterior-posterior drawer in the human knee: a biomechanical study. J Bone Joint Surg Am 1980;62:259–70.

54. Wilson SA, Vigorita VJ, Scott WN. Anatomy. In: Scott WN, editor. The knee. St. Louis (MO): Mosby Books; 1994.

55. Giron F, Cuomo P, Aglietii P, et al. Femoral attachment of the anterior cruciate ligament. Knee Surg Traumatol Arthrosc 2006;14(3):250–6.

56. Petersen W, Tillmann B. Anatomy and function of the anterior cruciate ligament. Orthopade 2002;31: 710–8.

57. Zantop T, Petersen W, Fu F. Anatomy of the anterior cruciate ligament. Operat Tech Orthop 2005;15: 20–8.

58. Harner CD, Baek GH, Vogrin TM, et al. Quantitative analysis of human cruciate ligament insertions. Arthroscopy 1999;15:741–9.

59. Arnoczky SP. Anatomy of the anterior cruciate ligament. Clin Orthop Relat Res 1983;172:19–25.

60. Duthon VB, Barea C, Abrassart S, et al. Anatomy of the anterior cruciate ligament. Knee Surg Sports Traumatol Arthrosc 2006;14(3):204–13.

61. Colombet P, Robinson J, Christel P, et al. Morphology of anterior cruciate ligament attachments for anatomic reconstruction: a cadaveric dissection and radiographic study. Arthroscopy 2006;22(9):984–92.

62. Petersen W, Zantop T. Anatomy of the anterior cruciate ligament with regard to its two bundles. Clin Orthop Relat Res 2006;454:35–47.

63. Sanders TG, Medynski MA, Feller JF, et al. Bone contusion patterns of the knee at MR imaging: footprint of the mechanism of injury. Radiographics 2000;20:S135–51.

64. Roberts CC, Towers JD, Spangehl MJ, et al. Advanced MR imaging of the cruciate ligaments. Magn Reson Imaging Clin N Am 2007;1(5):73–86.

65. Murphy BJ, Smith RL, Uribe JW, et al. Bone signal abnormalities in the posterolateral tibia and lateral femoral condyle in complete tears of the anterior cruciate ligament: a specific sign? Radiology 1992; 182:221–4.

66. Kaplan PA, Gehl RH, Dussault RG, et al. Bone contusion of the posterior lip of the medial tibial plateau (contrecoup injury) and associated internal derangements of the knee at MR imaging. Radiology 1999;211:747–53.

67. Piasecki DP, Spindler KP, Warren TA, et al. Intraarticular injuries associated with anterior cruciate ligament tear: findings at ligament reconstruction in high school and recreational athletes: an analysis

of sex-based differences. Am J Sports Med 2003; 31:601–5.

68. Bergin D, Morrison WB, Carrino JA, et al. Anterior cruciate ligament ganglia and mucoid degeneration: coexistence and clinical correlation. AJR Am J Roentgenol 2004;182:1283–7.

69. Gollehon DL, Torzilli PA, Warren RF. The role of the posterolateral and cruciate ligaments in the stability of the human knee: a biomechanical study. J Bone Joint Surg Am 1987;69(2):233–42.

70. Malone AA, Dowd GS, Saifuddin A. Injuries of the posterior cruciate ligament and posterolateral corner of the knee. Injury 2006;37(6):485–501.

71. Amis AA, Gupte CM, Bull AM, et al. Anatomy of the posterior cruciate ligament and the meniscofemoral ligaments. Knee Surg Sports Traumatol Arthrosc 2006;14(3):257–63.

72. Daniel DM, Stone ML, Barnett P, et al. Use of the quadriceps active test to diagnose posterior cruciate-ligament disruption and measure posterior laxity of the knee. J Bone Joint Surg Am 1988;70(3):386–91.

73. Fanelli GC, Edson CJ. Combined posterior cruciate ligament-posterolateral reconstructions with Achilles tendon allograft and biceps femoris tendon tenodesis: 2- to 10-year follow-up. Arthroscopy 2004;20(4): 339–45.

74. Sonin AH, Fitzgerald SW, Hoff FL, et al. MR imaging of the posterior cruciate ligament: normal, abnormal, and associated injury patterns. Radiographics 1995; 15(3):551–61.

75. Almekinders LC, Logan TC. Results following treatment of traumatic dislocation of the knee. Clin Orthop Relat Res 1991;284:203–7.

76. Frassica FJ, Sim FH, Staeheli JW, et al. Dislocation of the knee. Clin Orthop Relat Res 1991;263: 200–5.

77. Shapiro MS, Freedman EL. Allograft reconstruction of the anterior and posterior cruciate ligaments after traumatic knee dislocation. Am J Sports Med 1995; 23(5):580–7.

78. Sisto DJ, Warren RF. Complete knee dislocation: a follow-up study of operative treatment. Clin Orthop Relat Res 1985;198:94–101.

79. Kaplan EB. The iliotibial tract: clinical and morphological significance. J Bone Joint Surg Am 1958; 40:817–32.

80. Fanelli GC, Edson CJ. Arthroscopically assisted combined anterior and posterior cruciate ligament reconstruction: 2- to 10-year follow-up. Arthroscopy 2002;18(7):703–14.

81. Crawford C, Nyland J, Landes S, et al. Anatomic double bundle ACL reconstruction: a literature review. Knee Surg Sports Traumatol Arthrosc 2007; 15:946–64.

82. Bach BR Jr, Tradonsky S, Bojchuk J, et al. Arthroscopy assisted anterior cruciate ligament reconstruction using patellar tendon autograft: five- to nine-year followup evaluation. Am J Sports Med 1998;26:20–9.

83. Beynnon BD, Johnson RJ, Fleming BC, et al. Anterior cruciate ligament replacement: comparison of bone-patellar tendon-bone grafts with two-strand hamstring grafts: a prospective, randomized study. J Bone Joint Surg Am 2002;84:1503–13.

84. Freedman KB, D'Amato MJ, Nedeff DD, et al. Arthroscopic anterior cruciate ligament reconstruction: a metaanalysis comparing patellar tendon and hamstring tendon autografts. Am J Sports Med 2003;31:2–11.

85. Jansson KA, Linko E, Sandelin J, et al. A prospective randomized study of patellar versus hamstring tendon autografts for anterior cruciate ligament reconstruction. Am J Sports Med 2003;31:12–8.

86. Marder RA, Raskind JR, Carroll M. Prospective evaluation of arthroscopically assisted anterior cruciate ligament reconstruction: patellar tendon versus semitendinosus and gracilis tendons. Am J Sports Med 1991;19:478–84.

87. Yunes M, Richmond JC, Engels EA, et al. Patellar versus hamstring tendons in anterior cruciate ligament reconstruction: a metaanalysis. Arthroscopy 2001;17:248–57.

88. Yagi M, Wong EK, Kanamori A, et al. Biomechanical analysis of an anatomic anterior cruciate ligament reconstruction. Am J Sports Med 2002;30:660–6.

89. Aglietti P, Giron F, Cuomo P, et al. Single- and double-incision double-bundle ACL reconstruction. Clin Orthop Relat Res 2007;454:108–13.

90. Torg JS, Barton TM, Pavlov H, et al. Natural history of the posterior cruciate ligament deficient knee. Clin Orthop 1989;246:208–16.

91. Makino A, Aponte Tinao L, Ayerza MA, et al. Anatomic double-bundle posterior cruciate ligament reconstruction using double-double tunnel with tibial anterior and posterior fresh-frozen allograft. Arthroscopy 2006;22(6):684, e1–5.

92. Committee on the Medical Aspects of Sport. Standard nomenclature of athletic injuries. Chicago: American Medical Association; 1976. p. 157.

93. Felsenreich. Klinik der kreuzbandverletzungen. Arch Klin Chir 1934;179:347–408 [in German].

94. Girgis FG, Marshall JL, Monajem A. The cruciate ligaments of the knee joint: anatomical, functional and experimental analysis. Clin Orthop Relat Res 1975;106:216–31.

95. Kirsch MD, Fitzgerald SW, Friedman H, et al. Transient lateral patellar dislocation: diagnosis with MR imaging. AJR Am J Roentgenol 1993; 161:109–13.

Overuse Injuries of the Knee

Sylvia A. O'Keeffe, MB, FFRRCSI[a],*, Brian A. Hogan, MB, FFRRCSI[b],
Stephen J. Eustace, MD, MSc, MB, FFRRCSI[a,b,c,d,e],
Eoin C. Kavanagh, MD, MB, FFRRCSI[a]

KEYWORDS
- Overuse injuries • Knee • Patellofemoral pain
- Bursitis • Tendinitis • Athletic injuries

OVERUSE INJURIES OF THE KNEE

Overuse injuries are a common cause of morbidity in athletes. They occur after repetitive microtrauma, abnormal joint alignment, and poor training technique without appropriate time to heal, with the rate of injury exceeding the rate of adaptation of the soft tissues. Overuse injuries are frequent in the knee joint because of the numerous attachment sites for lower limb musculature and tendons surrounding the joint. MR imaging is the noninvasive imaging modality of choice for the detection of internal derangements of the knee. This article describes the characteristic MR imaging findings of common overuse injuries of the knee.

PATELLAR TENDINOPATHY/JUMPER'S KNEE

Although often referred to as "patellar tendonitis," a more accurate description of "jumper's knee" is that of patellar tendinosis (or tendinopathy), because histopathologic studies have consistently shown that the pathologic changes underlying the disease are degenerative (tendinosis) rather than inflammatory (tendinitis).[1] This is the most common tendinopathy in skeletally mature athletes and the most common athletic injury of the knee joint, with a prevalence of 14% in elite athletes, causing significant functional disability.[2,3] Athletes who participate in activities that demand repetitive, violent contraction of the quadriceps musculature are at risk, with basket ball players, volleyball players, cyclists, and runners being most frequently affected.

Patellar tendinopathy occurs after repetitive microtrauma caused by tendon overload without adequate repair. The diagnosis of patellar tendinopathy is based primarily on clinical examination.[4] It typically affects the deep posterior portion of the patellar tendon adjacent to the lower pole of the patella, although involvement of the tibial insertion of the patellar tendon can occur.[5,6]

Imaging Findings

The patellar tendon originates from the inferior pole of the patella and inserts proximally on the anterior lip of the tibia and distally on the tibial tubercle. The cross-sectional anatomy of the patellar tendon is semilunar in shape with a convex anterior surface. On MR imaging, the normal patellar tendon typically demonstrates homogeneous low signal intensity, with no internal striations on T1, T2, and proton density–weighted images.[7] Occasionally, a thin band of higher signal intensity posterior to the proximal portion of the tendon or a triangular-shaped focus of increased signal intensity near the tibial insertion may be present.[6] Typically, the thickness of the patellar tendon increases from its proximal to its distal extent but does not exceed 7 mm in thickness,

No funding support has been received.
[a] Department of Radiology, Mater Misericordiae University Hospital, Eccles Street, Dublin 8, Ireland
[b] Department of Radiology, Santry Sports Surgery Clinic, Santry Demense, Co. Dublin, Ireland
[c] Institute of Radiological Sciences, University College Dublin, Dublin, Ireland
[d] Department of Radiology, Cappagh National Orthopaedic Hospital, Finglas, Dublin 11, Ireland
[e] University College Dublin, Belfield, Dublin 4, Ireland
* Corresponding author.
E-mail address: sylviaokeeffe@yahoo.co.uk (S.A. O'Keeffe).

and the distinctness of the tendon margin should be preserved throughout its course.[6,8]

The characteristic imaging findings of patellar tendinopathy on MR imaging are best appreciated on sagittal images,[1] which are focal increase in signal on T2-weighted sequences in the deep posterior portion of the tendon adjacent to the lower pole of the patella,[2] alteration in the tendon size, which primarily affects the proximal posterior and medial fibers,[3] indistinct margins of the tendon, especially posterior to the thickened segment, and patellar marrow changes (Figs. 1 and 2).[4] Quadriceps muscle atrophy frequently accompanies chronic symptoms.[9] Although MR imaging is useful in imaging patellar tendinopathy, it is not specific. Positive images for patellar tendinopathy have been shown in asymptomatic tendons, and similarly, symptomatic tendons can appear normal on imaging.[5] Recent studies demonstrated the sensitivity and specificity of MR imaging for the diagnosis to be as high as 78% and 86%, respectively.[5]

The diagnosis of tendinosis is based on a subjective increase in signal intensity, which, coupled with variation of signal intensity of tendons between scanners, may account for false-negative diagnoses. Pitfalls in evaluation include the magic angle phenomenon, which falsely increases the signal intensity in the tendon on T1-weighted and proton density sequences.[10] In studies in which the patellar tendons were placed perpendicular to the main magnetic field to avoid this phenomenon, however, hyperintense signal was still identified in normal asymptomatic tendons.[11] This finding is particularly apparent on modern 3 Tesla (T) scanners and may relate to a slightly different histologic structure of this part of the tendon.[12] The degree of hyperintense signal within the tendon is more extensive in symptomatic patients than in asymptomatic patients and in the appropriate clinical setting enables the diagnosis of patellar tendinopathy to be made.[12]

El-Khoury and colleagues suggested an anteroposterior diameter cutoff point of 7 mm between symptomatic and asymptomatic tendons; however, other authors have shown considerable overlap and variation in tendon thickness.[11,13] Pathologic thickening that is diagnostic of patellar tendinosis characteristically involves the proximal one third of the tendon, and the area of thickening is frequently limited to the medial portion of the proximal tendon. One potential explanation for the asymmetric involvement is that repetitive contraction of the extensor mechanism musculature is unequal because of the lower insertion and larger cross-sectional mass of the vastus medialis muscle compared with the vastus lateralis muscle, which results in the medial portion of the patellar tendon sustaining more tension than its lateral portion.[14]

Loss of definition of the posterior border of the patellar tendon frequently has been reported in

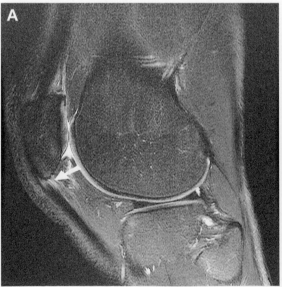
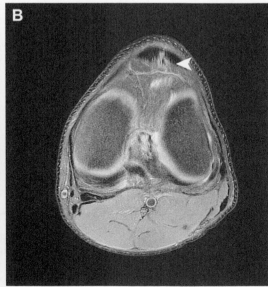

Fig. 1. Moderate patellar tendinopathy. (A) Sagittal T2 fat-saturated image demonstrates focal increased signal in the deep posterior portion of the proximal patellar tendon (arrow) and indistinct posterior margins of the tendon at this point. (B) Axial proton density fat-saturated image of the same patient demonstrates focal high signal in the tendon extending into the retropatellar fat (arrowhead).

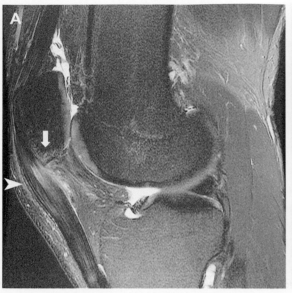
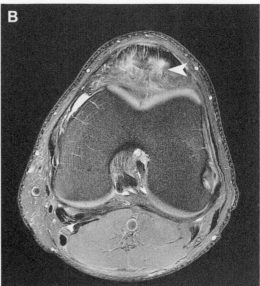

Fig. 2. Severe patellar tendinopathy. (*A*) Sagittal T2 fat-saturated image demonstrates severe hyperintensity of the patellar tendon with increase in tendon size (increased AP diameter at the level of the arrowhead) and patellar marrow changes (*arrow*). (*B*) Axial proton density fat-saturated image of the same patient demonstrates extensive areas of high signal within the patellar tendon (*arrowhead*).

patellar tendinopathy, whereas subcortical bone marrow edema of the patella and Hoffa's fat pad edema may coexist with patellar tendinopathy or cause similar symptoms. Loss of definition of the posterior border of the patellar tendon and increased signal in the infrapatellar fat pad have a high correlation with positive clinical findings.[4]

PATELLOFEMORAL PAIN SYNDROME

Patellofemoral pain syndrome has been suggested as a diagnosis of exclusion reserved for patients with anterior knee pain without an underlying diagnosis. It is believed that the most common causes of patellofemoral pain are overuse, anatomic variations resulting in patellofemoral malalignment, and trauma.[15] Underlying causative factors include developmental patellofemoral joint incongruity (eg, hypoplasia of the femoral trochlea), muscle imbalance and weakness, and extrinsic factors such as excessive training and poor training technique. With overuse, instability of the patella can result in chondromalacia and synovitis (**Fig. 3**). Anatomic factors in women predispose them to this condition, including increased pelvic width with resulting excessive lateral tension on the patella.

Maltracking

There is increasing interest in the role of chronic patellar maltracking and malalignment as causes

of patellofemoral pain, and it is generally recognized that many cases are undiagnosed. Conditions that lead to malalignment and influence patellofemoral stability can be measured with MR imaging. The most common indices described in the literature are the lateral patellofemoral angle (tilt), the congruence angle, the Q angle, the trochlear-tubercle distance, and lateral patellar displacement.[16,17] A static study that acquires axial images at a fixed degree of flexion—usually less than 20°—can be used to obtain accurate indices such as lateral patellar tilt, lateral patellar displacement, sulcus angle, and congruence angle.[18] Advances in fast imaging technology have allowed kinematic studies that acquire images while the knee moves from flexion to extension.[19] Loaded kinematic MR studies, during which the patient performs quadriceps contraction against resistance supplied by weights, have demonstrated improved ability to identify alignment abnormalities compared with unloaded active kinematic examinations.[20,21]

Cartilage Abnormalities

Repetitive, high-frequency overload delivered to a malaligned extensor mechanism may result in persistent and debilitating pain in athletes. Once the patellofemoral joint becomes overloaded, cartilage damage, subchondral bone degeneration, and persistent aggravation of the peripatellar synovium may occur. The resulting cartilage injury

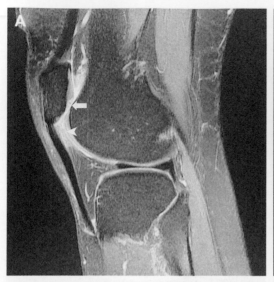
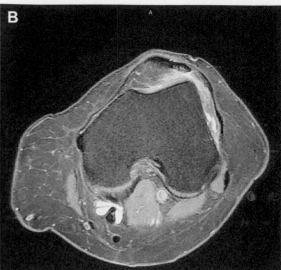

Fig. 3. Patellar maltracking. (A) Sagittal T2 fat-saturated image in a patient with patella alta. High signal intensity in the superolateral fat pad consistent with edema (*arrowhead*) and grade III patellar chondromalacia (*arrow*) are demonstrated. The findings are consistent with a lateral patellar maltracking abnormality, likely secondary to the developmental patellofemoral joint incongruity caused by patella alta. (B) Axial T2 fat-saturated image demonstrates high signal intensity in the superolateral Hoffa's fat pad, consistent with edema (*arrowhead*).

is also known as chondromalacia patella. Abnormalities of cartilage are described using a four-point grading system called the Modified Outerbridge Classification, originally described for the surgical grading of patellar lesions.[22]

> *Grade 1* (low-grade chondromalacia): irregularity of the articular cartilage with swelling and abnormal signal or mild thinning that is less than 50% of the articular cartilage thickness (**Fig. 4**)

> *Grade 2* (intermediate-grade chondromalacia): thinning of the articular cartilage of more than 50% but not all the way to the underlying osseous cortex

> *Grade 3* (high-grade chondromalacia): full-thickness cartilage loss but no underlying marrow signal change

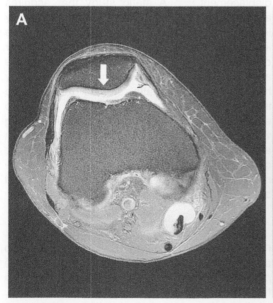
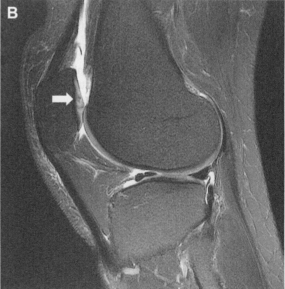

Fig. 4. Grade 1 chondromalacia. (A) Axial proton density fat-saturated image demonstrates fissuring of the superficial patellar cartilage involving less than 50% of the articular cartilage thickness (*arrow*). (B) Sagittal T2 fat-saturated image in the same patient demonstrates the same abnormality (*arrow*).

Grade 4 (high-grade chondromalacia): full-thickness cartilage loss with underlying marrow signal abnormalities (**Fig. 5**).[7]

MR imaging sensitivity and specificity is more than 85% for grade II lesions and higher.[23]

Cartilage appears intermediate in signal intensity on T2-weighted or proton density images with fat saturation. It is clearly distinguishable from the dark signal of the adjacent subchondral plate and the bright signal of joint fluid. Cartilaginous defects of the patella are best demonstrated on the axial images. Alteration of the cartilage surface and areas of fissuring are detected as areas of increased signal intensity on T2-weighted sequences corresponding to the synovial fluid extending down into the cartilage (see **Fig. 4**). Elevated T2-weighted signal in the subchondral bone marrow, which is frequently associated with overlying cartilage injury, also can be detected (see **Fig. 5**).[24] MR imaging findings of cartilaginous delamination consist of linear T2-hyperintensity at the bone cartilage interface (**Fig. 6**).[25]

On three-dimensional, fat-suppressed, T1-weighted, spoiled gradient echo sequences, direct visualization of the cartilage, which has high signal intensity relative to the subchondral bone, facilitates assessment of cartilage thickness and identification of altered signal intensity foci within the cartilage.[26] Although the technique produces reliable high-contrast images of cartilage and subchondral bone, contrast at the articular surface can vary, depending on the amount of protein content or blood degradation products in the synovial fluid. This can lower the sensitivity for the detection of superficial fibrillation or fissures that occur with cartilage injury.[27]

With advances in MR imaging, several cartilage-specific sequences have been developed that are sensitive to changes in cartilage composition that occur in early cartilage lesions before loss of tissue.[28] New techniques based on the steady-state, free-precession, gradient-echo sequences and multi-echo T2*-weighted sequences have been proposed for cartilage imaging.[29–33] These techniques provide high-resolution images of cartilage, with image contrast similar to that obtained with fast spin echo techniques. Although clinical experience with 3.0 T in cartilage imaging is limited, preliminary results suggest that the higher field strength provides greater diagnostic accuracy in detection of focal defects in the knee.[34] The relative insensitivity of conventional MR imaging in detecting early changes of cartilage injury is improved with the use of MR arthrography, using spoiled gradient recalled acquisition.[21] Although invasive, this has demonstrated high sensitivity for detecting early-stage cartilage damage in multiple studies.[35]

Osteochondral Injuries

The knee is the most common joint affected by osteochondritis dessicans. Chronic repetitive microtrauma may produce focal microfracture, necrosis, and healing response of the subchondral bone,

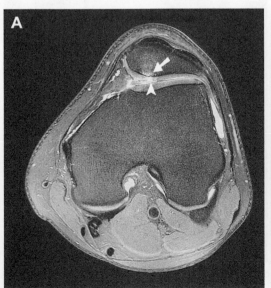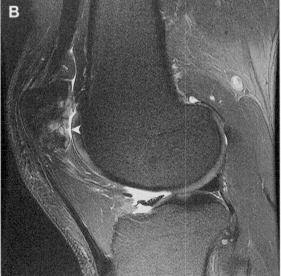

Fig. 5. Grade 4 chondromalacia. (*A*) Axial proton density fat-saturated image demonstrates a full-thickness defect in the patellar cartilage (*arrowhead*) with underlying high signal in the patella consistent with edema (*arrow*). (*B*) Sagittal T2 fat-saturated image in the same patient demonstrates the cartilage defect (*arrowhead*).

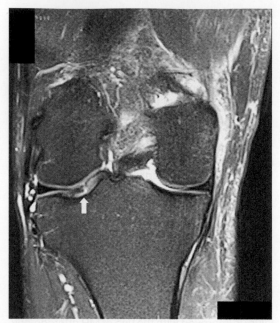

Fig. 6. Cartilage delamination. Coronal T2 fat-saturated image demonstrates linear T2 hyperintensity at the bone cartilage interface on the lateral tibial plateau (*arrow*).

with localized degenerative changes in the overlying cartilage resulting in osteochondritis dessicans. The lateral margin of the medial femoral condyle is the most common site of involvement

(85%) (**Fig. 7**) followed by the inferocentral portion of the lateral femoral condyle (13%) and the anterior lateral femoral condyle (2%).[24] Less frequently, osteochondritis dessicans can involve the patellofemoral joint and can be a source of persistent anterior knee pain in the young athlete (**Fig. 8**).[36] When it involves the femoral trochlea, the lesion is most frequently observed on the anterior lateral femoral condyle close to midline and is typically seen in adolescent athletes who undergo repetitive flexion and extension related to running or jumping activities.[24]

ILIOTIBIAL BAND FRICTION SYNDROME

Iliotibial band friction syndrome is a common cause of lateral knee pain that is often related to intense physical activity, as occurs in long-distance runners, cyclists, and American football players. The iliotibial band functions as a lateral stabilizer of the knee and is formed proximally by the fascia of the tensor fascia lata and gluteus maximus and medius. It distally attaches to the supracondylar tubercle of the lateral femoral condyle and extends below the joint to insert onto the lateral tibial condyle (Gerdy's tubercle). Its distal segment moves freely over the lateral femoral condyle. With the knee extended, the iliotibial band lies anterior to the lateral femoral condyle; with the knee in flexion of 30°, it lies behind the condyle. Repetitive flexion and

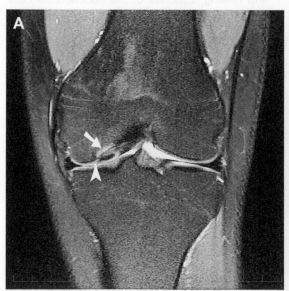
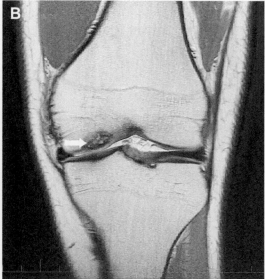

Fig. 7. Osteochondritis dessicans of the medial femoral condyle. (*A*) Coronal T2 fat-saturated image demonstrates a classic osteochondral lesion on the lateral aspect of the medial femoral condyle. High signal intensity surrounding the lesion (*arrow*) indicates instability, and overlying cartilage signal heterogeneity and hypertrophy are evident (*arrowhead*). (*B*) Coronal T1 image demonstrates low signal intensity change in the affected subchondral bone (*arrow*).

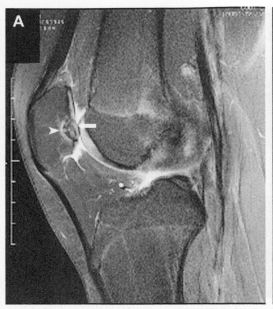 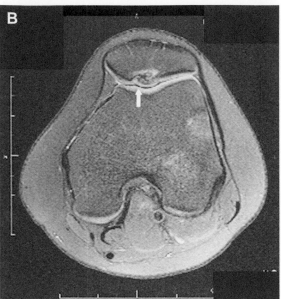

Fig. 8. Osteochondritis dessicans of the patella. (A) Sagittal T2 fat-saturated image demonstrates an osteochondral lesion of the patella with overlying cartilage hypertrophy (*arrow*) and fluid signal intensity tracking deep to the lesion (*arrowhead*), which indicates instability (see Fig. 7). (B) Axial intermediate weighted imaging demonstrating cartilage hypertrophy and signal heterogeneity overlying the osteochondral lesion (*arrow*).

extension of the knee results in excessive friction of the iliotibial band against the lateral femoral condyle and subsequent inflammatory change within the iliotibial band. The patient experiences pain at the lateral aspect of the knee that may radiate inferiorly along the iliotibial band insertion. The diagnosis is based on physical examination; however, it is not uncommon for this syndrome to be misdiagnosed clinically, and imaging modalities, particularly MR imaging, are often requested.

Imaging Findings

The iliotibial band is seen on MR images as a thin band of low signal intensity, parallel to the femur, with an anterolateral insertion. With iliotibial band friction syndrome, T2-weighted or short-tau inversion recovery coronal images show poorly defined hyperintense signal in the fatty tissue deep to the iliotibial band, predominantly beneath the posterior fibers of the iliotibial band (Fig. 9).[37] This is thought to occur because the posterior fibers of the iliotibial band are tighter against the lateral femoral epicondyle than the anterior fibers. This forms the basis of the surgical rationale for release of the more posterior fibers of the iliiotibial band to alleviate the patient of symptoms. The high signal intensity tissue represents an inflammatory reaction with granulation tissue and fibrinous exudates in severe cases.[38] Circumscribed fluid collections can occur but are less common and are thought

to result from chronic inflammation leading to the formation of a secondary (adventitial) bursa rather than from inflammation of a primary bursa.[39] In most patients, the width of the iliotibial band remains comparable to the width in asymptomatic patients; in patients who have chronic disease, however, thickening may occur.[40,41]

BREASTSTROKER'S KNEE

Overuse injuries of the knee rank second to shoulder injuries as a common complaint in competitive swimmers. The particular kicking mechanics used in the breaststroke kick result in high valgus loads on the knee as it is rapidly extended, in association with external rotation of the tibia. High tension stress occurs on the medial side of the knee, as does compressive stress on the lateral compartment, which ultimately results in stretching of the medial collateral ligament secondary to repeated medial collateral ligament sprain.[42] Patellofemoral pain syndrome and cartilage degeneration involving the medial patellar facet are also common in all swimmers.[43]

OSGOOD-SCHLATTER DISEASE

Osgood-Schlatter disease (OSD) is a traction apophysitis of the tibial tubercle that develops during the adolescent growth spurt. It presents with pain localized to the tibial tubercle and can be

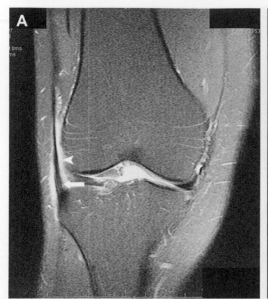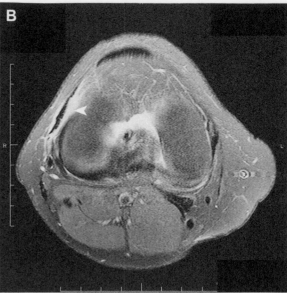

Fig. 9. Iliotibial band friction syndrome. (*A*) Coronal T2 fat-saturated image demonstrates high signal intensity in the fatty tissue deep to the iliotibial band (*arrowhead*) with loss of definition of the normally low signal intensity band (*arrow*). (*B*) Axial T2 fat-saturated image demonstrates high signal intensity in the fatty tissue deep to the iliotibial band consistent with replacement by inflammatory tissue (*arrowhead*).

bilateral in up to 50% of patients.[44] The cause is thought to be skeletal growth that is faster than the elongation of the muscle tendon units, which leads to relative tightness of the soft tissues. This difference creates increased tensile forces at the tendon insertion, causing avulsive fractures of the osseous part of the apophysis of the tibial tubercle.

MR imaging findings depend on the stage on the disease. In early stages of OSD, T1-weighted images show low signal intensity at the secondary ossification center and the adjacent tibia, with T2-weighted images showing high signal intensity within the secondary ossification center (**Fig. 10**). In more advanced stages of OSD, imaging demonstrates cartilaginous damage of the tibial tuberosity and partial avulsion of the anterior part of the secondary ossification center. This damage is also associated with soft tissue swelling anterior to the tibial tuberosity, loss of the sharp inferior angle of the infrapatellar fat pad and surrounding soft tissues, thickening and edema of the infrapatellar tendon, and infrapatellar bursitis.[38] As the disease progresses, MR imaging demonstrates complete detachment and superior retraction of the ossicles. In advanced stages of the disease, TI-weighted images show low signal intensity of the ossicles, indicative of avascular necrosis/fibrosis, and T2-weighted images show low signal intensity of the ossicles accompanied by surrounding high signal intensity. Associated

thickening of the patellar tendon at its insertion site can occur. As healing occurs, the ossicles can fuse to the tibial tubercle or remain detached. High-signal intensity and thickening of the patellar tendon may persist.[45]

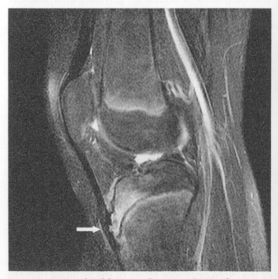

Fig. 10. Osgood-Schlatter disease. Sagittal proton density image in an adolescent demonstrates high signal intensity within the secondary ossification center of the tibial tubercle with mild hyperintensity of the anterior soft tissues (*arrow*) and superficial fibers of the distal patellar tendon.

SINDING-LARSEN-JOHANSSON DISEASE

This disease involves traction apophysitis of the inferior pole of the patella (in rare cases it also affects the superior pole) and is similar to Osgood-Schlatter disease. It primarily affects athletically active adolescents between 10 and 14 years of age and shows a prevalence in boys. MR findings closely match those of OSD.[16]

FAT PAD SYNDROME (HOFFA DISEASE)

The infrapatellar fat pad is bordered by the inferior pole of the patella superiorly, the joint capsule and patellar tendon anteriorly, the proximal tibia and deep infrapatellar bursa inferiorly, and the synovium-lined joint cavity posteriorly.[46] Hoffa disease (also known as a syndrome of infrapatellar fat pad impingement) is a condition first described by Albert Hoffa in 1904, in which acute trauma or repetitive microtrauma to the fat pad causes hemorrhage and inflammation.[47] The resultant changes of enlargement place the fat pad at risk of impingement between the femur and tibia during activities that require constant repetition of maximal extension of the knee.[38] Longstanding inflammatory change results in fibrosis, which rarely may undergo ossification.[16,48]

This cause of anterior knee pain is a diagnosis of exclusion that is characterized by contact tenderness of the fat pad and tenderness during palpation along the edge of the patellar tendon. In the acute setting, there is high T2 signal and mass effect within the fat pad.[47] Bowing of the patellar tendon from mass effect is seen frequently, and a small joint effusion may be present (Fig. 11).[46] Chronically, fibrosis and hemosiderin deposition may occur, which appear dark on T1- and T2-weighted images.[47] Ossification of the fibrous tissue also has low signal intensity on MR imaging. Differentiation of fibrosis from ossification requires correlation with plain radiographs.[48] Hoffa impingement and infrapatellar plica syndrome may be difficult to differentiate on clinical and imaging criteria. If edema or fibrotic thickening within the fat pad follows the course of the infrapatellar plica through Hoffa's fat pad, then infrapatellar plica syndrome may be the preferred diagnosis over Hoffa impingement (Fig. 12). More diffuse and widespread abnormalities involving the posterior aspect of the fat pad would favor the diagnosis of Hoffa impingement. A similar abnormality was described recently in the quadriceps/suprapatellar fat pad, with signal characteristics on MR imaging mimicking those of Hoffa disease and may represent an equivalent disease process (Fig. 13).[49]

Patellar tendon-lateral femoral condyle friction syndrome has been described as a separate

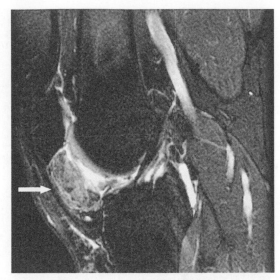

Fig. 11. Hoffa disease. Sagittal T2 fat-saturated image demonstrates high signal and mass effect in the infrapatellar fat pad, which results in anterior displacement of the tendon (*arrow*). Note a small joint effusion.

type of impingement syndrome that results in inflammatory changes of the fat pad interposed between the patellar tendon and the lateral femoral condyle, postulated to occur secondary to patellar maltracking. Although increasingly recognized, it is more common but less reported than the classic variant described by Hoffa and is frequently overlooked.[47] The typical case is associated with patellar alignment abnormalities, including patella alta. MR imaging demonstrates low signal intensity on T1-weighted images and high signal intensity on fat-suppressed T2-weighted or proton density images surrounding the inferolateral aspect of the patellofemoral joint and superolateral aspect of the fat pad. The edema can extend into the central superior aspect of the fat pad. As the edematous fat blends with high signal from the adjacent femoral condyle, the normal three bands of tissue (from anterior to posterior: patellar tendon, Hoffa's fat, femoral condylar cartilage) become two (patellar tendon and edematous fat blending with high-signal cartilage). Associated imaging findings include a focal multilobulated mass with signal intensity characteristics, which suggests simple fluid or cystic change in the lateral soft tissues of the knee between the lateral femoral condyle and the lateral retinaculum. Focal contrast enhancement of the infrapatellar fat pad, patellar tendon abnormalities (including partial tears), and cartilage abnormalities in the lateral facet of the patella also can occur.[16,50]

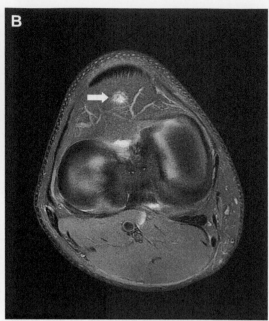

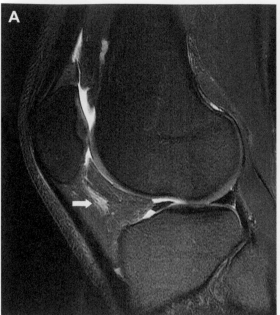

Fig. 12. Infrapatellar plica syndrome. (A) Sagittal T2 fat-saturated image demonstrates linear increased signal intensity in Hoffa's fat pad, which follows the course of the infrapatellar plica (*arrow*). (B) Axial proton density image demonstrating the focal area of increased signal intensity in the region of the infrapatellar plica (*arrow*).

MEDIAL PLICA SYNDROME

Plicae are normal intra-articular structures of the knee and are remnants of the mesenchymal tissue that occupies the space between the distal femoral and proximal tibial epiphyses in the 8-week-old embryo. Incomplete resorption of this mesenchyme results in the formation of residual

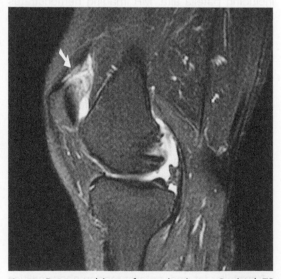

Fig. 13. Retroquadriceps fat pad edema. Sagittal T2 fat-saturated image demonstrates a similar abnormality to Hoffa's disease in the suprapatellar/retroquadriceps fat pad (*arrow*).

synovial pleats known as plicae. The medial plica is present at autopsies in 1 in every 3 to 4 knees.[51] Chronic inflammation secondary to direct trauma, repetitive sports activities, or other pathologic knee conditions affects the pliability of the synovial folds and can become symptomatic. The medial patellar plica is most often symptomatic when it becomes thickened, fibrotic, or bowstrung.[52] It extends from the medial joint wall to the synovium covering Hoffa's fat pad. The thickened plica strikes the medial facet of the patella on flexion and the anteromedial femoral condyle on extension, which leads to chondromalacia at the contact points.[16] Athletes who require repetitive flexion-extension motion (eg, rowing, swimming, and cycling) are affected, particularly adolescents. A palpable, snapping, painful cord medial to the patella is almost pathognomonic for this pathologic condition.[51]

Plicae manifest on MR imaging as linear low signal intensity structures delineated by joint fluid when an effusion is present (**Fig. 14**). Gradient-echo T2-weighted, fat-suppressed T2-weighted and proton density–weighted images are the most valuable for the evaluation of plicae. MR arthrography, performed with fat-suppressed T1-weighting, is a useful technique when no effusion is present and a clinically significant plica is suspected.[52] The size and morphologic features of a given plica seen on MR imaging do not in themselves indicate whether the plica is clinically

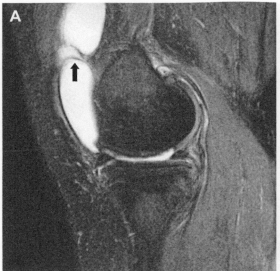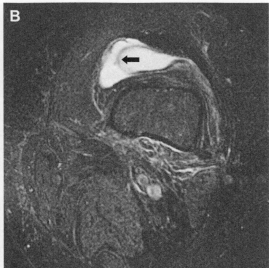

Fig. 14. Medial plica syndrome. (*A*) Sagittal T2 fat-saturated image demonstrates a linear low signal intensity structure representing the medial plica (*arrow*) delineated by a joint effusion. (*B*) Axial T2 fat-saturated image in the same patient demonstrating the medial plica (*arrow*). The diagnosis of medial plica syndrome was confirmed at surgery.

significant. Symptomatic plicae, however, usually appear thickened, and the presence of synovitis and chondromalacic changes in the cartilage overlying the medial femoral condyle and patellar cartilage can support the diagnosis.

OTHER TENDINOPATHIES

Tendinopathies that involve tendons other than the patellar tendon also occur frequently but are less well recognized than patellar tendinopathy. MR imaging demonstrates abnormal signal in the tendon and can be associated with secondary marrow signal alterations at the site of bony insertion. Pes anserinus tendonitis and popliteal tendonitis are rarer forms of tendinopathy; the latter is thought to be caused by excessive or extended pronation of the foot during running.[38,53] Quadriceps tendinopathy manifests as thickening and increased T2 signal within the tendon (Fig. 15). A complete tear of the quadriceps tendon rarely occurs and appears as complete discontinuity of the tendon with retraction of the proximal fibers (Fig. 16).[54]

BURSITIS

Bursae around the knee function to reduce friction between adjacent moving structures and are not normally visible on MR images because they contain only scant amounts of fluid. Inflammation, hemorrhage, or infection can produce accumulation of fluid within the bursa, allowing visualization on MR images.[55]

Anserine Bursitis

The anserine bursa separates the pes anserinus, which is formed by the distal parts of the tendons of the sartorius, gracilis, and semitendinosus muscles, from the subjacent distal portion of the tibial collateral ligament and the bony surface of the medial tibial condyle. Anserine bursitis results from overuse, especially in runners, and manifests clinically with medial knee pain and swelling that

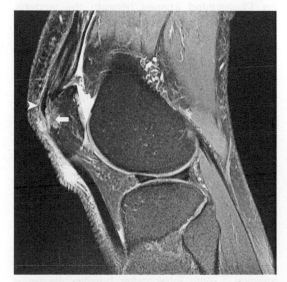

Fig. 15. Quadriceps tendinopathy. Sagittal T2 fat-saturated image demonstrates increased signal intensity and thickening of the distal quadriceps tendon (*arrowhead*) associated with edema at its patellar insertion (*arrow*) and a small joint effusion.

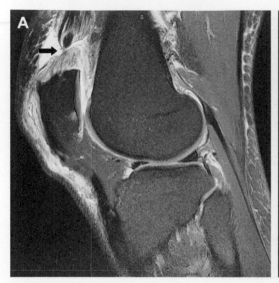
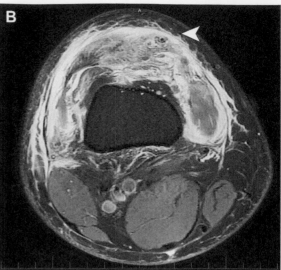

Fig.16. Complete quadriceps rupture. (A) Sagittal T2 fat-saturated image demonstrates complete discontinuity of the quadriceps tendon (*arrow*) with associated fluid signal intensity in the suprapatellar and prepatellar fat. (B) Axial T2 fat-saturated image in the same patient demonstrates extensive increased signal intensity surrounding the distal anterior femoral shaft consistent with hemorrhage and subsequent inflammatory reaction. Note the complete absence of the normal quadriceps tendon anteriorly (*arrowhead*).

may mimic a medial meniscal tear or injury of the medial collateral ligament. Predisposing factors for this syndrome include incorrect training techniques, excessive tightness of the hamstring muscles, valgus alignment of the knee, and excessive rotation of the lower leg in the outward direction.[38] Pes anserinus bursitis has a characteristic MR appearance of a low intensity fluid collection on T1-weighted images beneath the tendons, which shows relatively high homogeneous signal on T2-weighted images and is without communication with the knee joint (**Fig. 17**).[16,56] Prevalence of fluid in the bursa without clinical symptoms has been shown to be as high as 5%, however.[57] Occasionally a Baker's cyst tracking deep to the pes anserinus can mimic anserinus bursitis (**Fig. 18**).

Infrapatellar Bursitis

Bursitis in the deep infrapatellar bursa located directly posterior to the distal third of the patellar tendon and the anterior tibia is often seen in association with patellar tendinopathy and can clinically mimic this condition. A small amount of fluid can be seen in this bursa normally on MR imaging.[56] With infrapatellar bursitis, excessive amounts of fluid accumulate within the bursa, which on MR imaging manifests as T2-weighted hyperintensity with or without inflammatory changes in the adjacent soft tissues and bone.[55]

Medial Collateral Ligament Bursitis

The medial collateral ligament bursa is located between the superficial and deep layers of the medial collateral ligament. MR images show a well-defined fluid collection between the deep and superficial portions of the medial collateral ligament. It is important first to exclude an

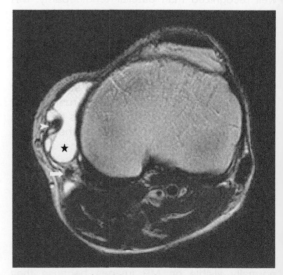

Fig.17. Anserine bursitis. Axial proton density image. A homogenous high signal intensity fluid collection (*asterisk*) is seen deep to the tendons of the pes anserinus. The tendons of sartorius (*arrowhead*) and semitendinosus (*arrow*) are visualized.

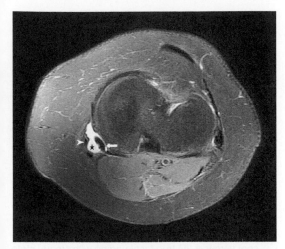

Fig. 18. Baker's cyst mimicking anserinus bursitis. Axial intermediate weighted image of the knee demonstrates a high signal intensity fluid collection (*asterisk*) insinuating deep to the pes anserinus. This communicated with the knee joint on further images consistent with a Baker's cyst. The tendons of sartorius (*arrowhead*) and semitendinosus (*arrow*) are visualized.

underlying medial meniscal tear with parameniscal cyst formation or meniscocapsular separation before making the diagnosis of medial collateral ligament bursitis.[55]

STRESS FRACTURES

Stress fractures about the knee are common and may account for up to 75% of exertional leg pain. They predominantly involve the proximal tibia; however, involvement of the fibula, distal femur, patella, or fabella can occur.[58] The patella is an unusual location for a stress fracture and has been reported in young athletes, football players, high jumpers, and runners. The fracture line may be either transverse or longitudinal.[38] A transverse stress fracture is the consequence of muscular traction stresses, whereas a longitudinal stress fracture results from forces that compress the patella against the femoral condyle. MR imaging is the technique of choice for evaluating stress injuries because periosteal and marrow edema can be detected early on fat-suppressed T2 or short-tau inversion recovery–weighted imaging. One study found the sensitivity, specificity, accuracy, and positive and negative predictive values of MR imaging in detecting stress fractures in the tibia to be 88%, 100%, 90%, 100%, and 62%, respectively. MR imaging is superior at detecting early stress injuries compared with CT and bone scintigraphy (sensitivities 88%, 42%, and 74%, respectively).[58]

SUMMARY

MR imaging provides excellent characterization of overuse injuries in the knee, particularly when a definitive diagnosis cannot be determined by clinical examination alone. As described in this article, many overuse injuries occur in the knee, and MR imaging is an indispensable tool in the evaluation of these lesions in athletes.

REFERENCES

1. Khan KM, Bonar F, Desmond PM, et al. Patellar tendinosis (jumper's knee): findings at histopathologic examination, US, and MR imaging. Victorian Institute of Sport Tendon Study Group. Radiology 1996; 200(3):821–7.
2. Kujala UM, Kvist M, Osterman K. Knee injuries in athletes: review of exertion injuries and retrospective study of outpatient sports clinic material. Sports Med 1986;3(6):447–60.
3. Lian ØB, Engebretsen L, Bahr R. Prevalence of jumper's knee among elite athletes from different sports: a cross-sectional study. Am J Sports Med 2005;33:561–7.
4. Warden SJ, Kiss ZS, Malara FA, et al. Comparative accuracy of magnetic resonance imaging and ultrasonography in confirming clinically diagnosed patellar tendinopathy. Am J Sports Med 2007; 35(3):427–36.
5. Warden SJ, Brukner P. Patellar tendinopathy. Clin Sports Med 2003;22(4):743–59.
6. Yu JS, Popp JE, Kaeding CC, et al. Correlation of MR imaging and pathologic findings in athletes undergoing surgery for chronic patellar tendinitis. AJR Am J Roentgenol 1995;165(1):115–8.
7. Sanders TG, Miller MD. A systematic approach to magnetic resonance imaging interpretation of sports medicine injuries of the knee. Am J Sports Med 2005;33(1):131–48.
8. Davies SG, Baudouin CJ, King JB, et al. Ultrasound, computed tomography and magnetic resonance imaging in patellar tendinitis. Clin Radiol 1991; 43(1):52–6.
9. El-Khoury GY, Wira RL, Berbaum KS, et al. MR imaging of patellar tendinitis. Radiology 1992; 184(3):849–54.
10. Karantanas AH, Zibis AH, Papanikolaou N. Increased signal intensity on fat-suppressed three-dimensional T1-weighted pulse sequences in patellar tendon: magic angle effect? Skeletal Radiol 2001;30(2): 67–71.
11. Reiff DB, Heenan SD, Heron CW. MRI appearances of the asymptomatic patellar tendon on gradient echo imaging. Skeletal Radiol 1995; 24(2):123–6.

12. Schmid MR, Hodler J, Cathrein P, et al. Is impingement the cause of jumper's knee? Dynamic and static magnetic resonance imaging of patellar tendinitis in an open-configuration system. Am J Sports Med 2002;30(3):388–95.

13. McLoughlin RF, Raber EL, Vellet AD, et al. Patellar tendinitis: MR imaging features, with suggested pathogenesis and proposed classification. Radiology 1995;197(3):843–8.

14. Kaufer H. Mechanical function of the patella. J Bone Joint Surg Am 1971;53(8):1551–60.

15. Fulkerson JP. Diagnosis and treatment of patients with patellofemoral pain. Am J Sports Med 2002; 30(3):447–56.

16. Christian SR, Anderson MB, Workman R, et al. Imaging of anterior knee pain. Clin Sports Med 2006;25(4):681–702.

17. McNally EG. Imaging assessment of anterior knee pain and patellar maltracking. Skeletal Radiol 2001;30(9):484–95.

18. Koskinen SK, Taimela S, Nelimarkka O, et al. Magnetic resonance imaging of patellofemoral relationships. Skeletal Radiol 1993;22(6):403–10.

19. McNally EG, Ostlere SJ, Pal C, et al. Assessment of patellar maltracking using combined static and dynamic MRI. Eur Radiol 2000;10(7):1051–5.

20. Shellock FG, Mink JH, Deutsch AL, et al. Kinematic MR imaging of the patellofemoral joint: comparison of passive positioning and active movement techniques. Radiology 1992;184(2):574–7.

21. Van Leersum M, Schweitzer ME, Gannon F, et al. Chondromalacia patellae: an in vitro study. Comparison of MR criteria with histologic and macroscopic findings. Skeletal Radiol 1996;25(8):727–32.

22. Outerbridge RE. Osteochondritis dissecans of the posterior femoral condyle. Clin Orthop Relat Res 1983;175:121–9.

23. Nakanishi K, Inoue M, Harada K, et al. Subluxation of the patella: evaluation of patellar articular cartilage with MR imaging. Br J Radiol 1992;65(776): 662–7.

24. Mosher TJ. MRI of osteochondral injuries of the knee and ankle in the athlete. Clin Sports Med 2006;25(4): 843–66.

25. Kendell SD, Helms CA, Rampton JW, et al. MRI appearance of chondral delamination injuries of the knee. AJR Am J Roentgenol 2005;184(5): 1486–9.

26. Stäbler A, Glaser C, Reiser M, et al. Knee. Eur Radiol 2000;10(2):230–41.

27. Mosher TJ, Pruett SW. Magnetic resonance imaging of superficial cartilage lesions: role of contrast in lesion detection. J Magn Reson Imaging 1999; 10(2):178–82.

28. Burstein D, Gray M. New MRI techniques for imaging cartilage. J Bone Joint Surg Am 2003; 85(Suppl 2):70–7.

29. Hargreaves BA, Gold GE, Beaulieu CF, et al. Comparison of new sequences for high-resolution cartilage imaging. Magn Reson Med 2003;49: 700–9.

30. Gold GE, Fuller SE, Hargreaves BA, et al. Driven equilibrium magnetic resonance imaging of articular cartilage: initial clinical experience. J Magn Reson Imaging 2005;21:476–81.

31. Kornaat PR, Doornbos J, van der Molen AJ, et al. Magnetic resonance imaging of knee cartilage using a water selective balanced steady-state free precession sequence. J Magn Reson Imaging 2004;20:850–6.

32. Weckbach S, Mendlik T, Horger W, et al. Quantitative assessment of patellar cartilage volume and thickness at 3.0 Tesla comparing a 3D-fast low angle shot versus a 3D-true fast imaging with steady-state precession sequence for reproducibility. Invest Radiol 2006;41:189–97.

33. Schmid MR, Pfirrmann CW, Koch P, et al. Imaging of patellar cartilage with a 2D multiple echo data image combination sequence. AJR Am J Roentgenol 2005; 184:1744–8.

34. Kornaat PR, Reeder SB, Koo S, et al. MR imaging of articular cartilage at 1.5T and 3.0T: comparison of SPGR and SSFP sequences. Osteoarthritis Cartilage 2005;13(4):338–44.

35. Rand T, Brossmann J, Pedowitz R, et al. Analysis of patellar cartilage: comparison of conventional MR imaging and MR and CT arthrography in cadavers. Acta Radiol 2000;41(5):492–7.

36. Peters TA, McLean ID. Osteochondritis dissecans of the patellofemoral joint. Am J Sports Med 2000; 28(1):63–7.

37. Muhle C, Ahn JM, Yeh L, et al. Iliotibial band friction syndrome: MR imaging findings in 16 patients and MR arthrographic study of six cadaveric knees. Radiology 1999;212(1):103–10.

38. Pecina MM, Bojanic I. Knee. In: Pecina MM, Bojanic I, editors. Overuse injuries of the musculoskeletal system. 2nd edition. London, UK: Informa Healthcare; 2003. p. 189–252.

39. Nishimura G, Yamato M, Tamai K, et al. MR findings in iliotibial band syndrome. Skeletal Radiol 1997; 26(9):533–7.

40. Murphy BJ, Hechtman KS, Uribe JW, et al. Iliotibial band friction syndrome: MR imaging findings. Radiology 1992;185(2):569–71.

41. Ekman EF, Pope T, Martin DF, et al. Magnetic resonance imaging of iliotibial band syndrome. Am J Sports Med 1994;22(6):851–4.

42. Kennedy JC, Hawkins R, Krissoff WB. Orthopaedic manifestations of swimming. Am J Sports Med 1978;6(6):309–22.

43. Stulberg SD, Shulman K, Stuart S, et al. Breaststroker's knee: pathology, etiology, and treatment. Am J Sports Med 1980;8(3):164–71.

44. Stevens MA, El-Khoury GY, Kathol MH, et al. Imaging features of avulsion injuries. Radiographics 1999;19(3):655–72.

45. Hirano A, Fukubayashi T, Ishii T, et al. Magnetic resonance imaging of Osgood-Schlatter disease: the course of the disease. Skeletal Radiol 2002;31(6): 334–42.

46. Jacobson JA, Lenchik L, Ruhoy MK, et al. MR imaging of the infrapatellar fat pad of Hoffa. Radiographics 1997;17(3):675–91.

47. Saddik D, McNally EG, Richardson M. MRI of Hoffa's fat pad. Skeletal Radiol 2004;33(8):433–44.

48. Magi M, Branca A, Bucca C, et al. Hoffa disease. Ital J Orthop Traumatol 1991;17(2):211–6.

49. Shabshin N, Schweitzer ME, Morrison WB. Quadriceps fat pad edema: significance on magnetic resonance images of the knee. Skeletal Radiol 2006;35: 269–74.

50. Chung CB, Skaf A, Roger B, et al. Patellar tendon-lateral femoral condyle friction syndrome: MR imaging in 42 patients. Skeletal Radiol 2001; 30(12):694–7.

51. Dupont JY. Synovial plicae of the knee: controversies and review. Clin Sports Med 1997;16(1): 87–122.

52. García-Valtuille R, Abascal F, Cerezal L, et al. Anatomy and MR imaging appearances of synovial plicae of the knee. Radiographics 2002;22(4):775–84.

53. Meier JL. Popliteal tenosynovitis in athletes apropos of 12 cases. Schweiz Z Sportmed 1986;34(3):109–12.

54. Yu JS, Petersilge C, Sartoris DJ, et al. MR imaging of injuries of the extensor mechanism of the knee. Radiographics 1994;14(3):541–51.

55. Janzen DL, Peterfy CG, Forbes JR, et al. Cystic lesions around the knee joint: MR imaging findings. AJR Am J Roentgenol 1994;163(1):155–61.

56. Beaman FD, Peterson JJ. MR imaging of cysts, ganglia, and bursae about the knee. Magn Reson Imaging Clin N Am 2007;15(1):39–52.

57. Tschirch FT, Schmid MR, Pfirrmann CW, et al. Prevalence and size of meniscal cysts, ganglionic cysts, synovial cysts of the popliteal space, fluid-filled bursae, and other fluid collections in asymptomatic knees on MR imaging. AJR Am J Roentgenol 2003;180(5):1431–6.

58. Gaeta M, Minutoli F, Scribano E, et al. CT and MR imaging findings in athletes with early tibial stress injuries: comparison with bone scintigraphy findings and emphasis on cortical abnormalities. Radiology 2005;235(2):553–61.

MR Imaging of Meniscal and Cartilage Injuries of the Knee

Steven Alatakis, MBBS, FRANZCR*, Parm Naidoo, MBBS, FRANZCR

KEYWORDS

- Meniscus • Meniscal tear • Meniscal trauma
- Chondral lesion • Knee injuries • Knee imaging

The meniscal fibrocartilages of the knee are important stabilizing structures commonly injured by sporting activities. This article addresses the role of MR imaging in the evaluation of meniscal injuries, with emphasis placed on the common meniscal injuries, including horizontal, longitudinal, radial, and flap tears. An understanding of typical meniscal postoperative findings, together with those factors responsible for the misinterpretation of meniscal abnormalities, is essential for the accurate assessment of MR imaging in the athlete. This article also reviews the common articular cartilage injuries identified in the knee. MR imaging is the imaging modality of choice for the assessment of the menisci and articular cartilage, with the ready availability of MR imaging allowing for the rapid assessment of the injured athlete.

MR IMAGING OF MENISCAL INJURIES OF THE KNEE

MR imaging is the imaging modality of choice for the assessment of meniscal pathology. The meniscal injuries seen in athletes are almost identical to meniscal abnormalities seen in the broader community, with degenerative change being less frequent in the acute setting, and acute traumatic pathologies seen more frequently. MR imaging provides valuable information regarding meniscal integrity in the athlete, and is accepted as being more accurate than physical examination. It also has the advantage of being noninvasive, in contrast to both arthrography and arthroscopy. The ready availability of MR imaging allows for the rapid assessment of the injured athlete, with availability on site at certain sporting events and arenas.

IMAGING PROTOCOLS FOR THE MR IMAGING ASSESSMENT OF THE MENISCI

Proton-density (PD) weighted sequences are optimal for the assessment of meniscal pathology because of their sensitivity for synovial fluid within meniscal tears.[1] Short TE sequences are more sensitive than high TE sequences in the detection of meniscal degeneration and tears.[2] Fast spin echo sequences are less sensitive to meniscal pathology than T2 spin echo sequences; however, they are useful in the assessment of meniscal morphology, especially complex meniscal tears and postoperative meniscal change, and their sensitivity for fluid allows for the demonstration of fluid within meniscal cysts. The administration of intra-articular gadolinium in selected cases may assist in differentiating between posttraumatic granulation tissue and subsequent tears in the postmeniscectomy or postmeniscal repair state.[3]

GENERAL MR IMAGING CHARACTERISTICS OF MENISCAL TEARS AND DEGENERATION

Normal menisci demonstrate homogeneous low signal intensity on all MR imaging pulse sequences. Meniscal tears and degenerative change result in synovial fluid being imbibed and accumulating within the meniscus, resulting in an

Department of Diagnostic Imaging, Southern Health, Monash Medical Centre, Locked Bag 29, Clayton South, Victoria 3169, Australia
* Corresponding author.
E-mail address: salatakis@connexus.net.au (S. Alatakis).

Magn Reson Imaging Clin N Am 17 (2009) 741–756
doi:10.1016/j.mric.2009.06.001

increase in signal intensity on standard pulse sequences.[1,2] If no joint effusion is present, meniscal signal abnormality may be associated with a relative reduction in signal abnormality on T2-weighted sequences. Gradient echo sequences are extremely sensitive in demonstrating increased signal abnormality. Fast spin echo sequences are not as sensitive in the detection of meniscal signal abnormality, and may underestimate the extent of meniscal injury.[4]

MR imaging–based grading systems for meniscal tears and degenerative change refer to the presence of abnormal signal relative to the meniscal articular surface, but not signal abnormality involving the nonarticular peripheral capsular margin of the meniscus.[1] MR imaging grade 1 signal abnormality consists of globular intrasubstance increased signal abnormality, which corresponds to meniscal mucinous degeneration.[5]

MR imaging grade 2 signal abnormality is defined as intrasubstance linear hyperintensity, which involves the meniscal capsular periphery, without directly involving the meniscal articular surface. There is no associated distinct cleavage plane or tear, although microscopy of such menisci may demonstrate microscopic clefts. Grade 2 signal abnormality is more extensive than grade 1 signal abnormality, representing a progression in the mucinous degeneration identified in grade 1 signal abnormality. Grade 2 signal abnormality is usually asymptomatic, does not necessarily progress to grade 3 signal abnormality, and is not a proved risk factor for the development of meniscal tears.[6] Grade 3 signal abnormality, however, usually occurs adjacent to or in continuity with grade 2 signal abnormality (**Fig. 1**). Grade 2 signal abnormality is most frequently seen in the posterior horn of the medial meniscus.

MR imaging grade 3 signal abnormality consists of linear intrasubstance increased signal, which extends to at least one articular surface. Grade 3 signal abnormality is always associated with tears of the meniscal fibrocartilage, at least at the microscopic level. This includes closed intrasubstance tears, which can only be accurately confirmed arthroscopically.[7]

MR imaging allows meniscal morphology to be accurately determined. Normal meniscal height measures 3 to 5 mm, with meniscal width being variable (eg, the anterior horn of the medial meniscus measures 6 mm in width, the posterior horn 12 mm, and the posterior horn of the lateral mensicus 10 mm).[8] On any given sagittal image, the posterior horn should always be wider than the anterior horn, and the width of the posterior horn should exceed its height.[9]

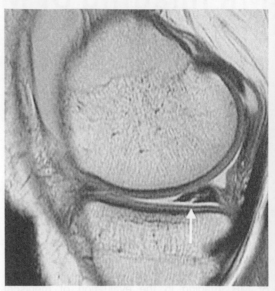

Fig. 1. Oblique meniscal tear adjacent to meniscal grade 2 signal abnormality. Sagittal proton-density (PD) image demonstrates subtle linear mildly T2 hyperintense signal involving the central aspect of posterior horn of medial meniscus, consistent with grade 2 signal abnormality. A further linear T2 hyperintense region extends from the region of grade 2 signal abnormality to the inferior edge (*arrow*), consistent with an associated oblique tear.

The sensitivity of MR imaging for the detection of meniscal tears is reported to be between 80% and 100%.[10–13] Meniscal tears are found in approximately 6% of asymptomatic patients, with lateral meniscal tears being twice as common as medial meniscal tears.[13] Diagnostic errors involving tears of the posterior horn of the lateral meniscus and the meniscal free edge are common.[14–16] False-negative diagnostic errors involving lateral meniscal tears are more common than false-positive diagnostic errors,[15,17] whereas false-negative and false-positive diagnostic errors are equally common in the medial meniscus.

CLASSIFICATION OF MENISCAL TEARS

The diagnosis of meniscal tears is based on the presence of intrameniscal signal abnormality and abnormal meniscal morphology. Meniscal tears are classified into two primary tear planes based on sagittal and coronal imaging (vertical and horizontal[18,19]), with further classification based on secondary tear patterns. Axial imaging may contribute to determining the primary and secondary tear pattern.[20]

Surface tear patterns occur secondary to the extension of a horizontal or vertical tear into a meniscal articular surface. Three surface tear patterns exist: (1) longitudinal; (2) radial; and (3) flap (oblique).[21,22] Horizontal cleavage tears extend into the meniscal apex, with no extension into the superior or inferior articular surfaces. Complex tears represent a combination of vertical and horizontal surface tear patterns.[23]

HORIZONTAL MENISCAL TEARS

Horizontal cleavage tears extend from the free edge of the meniscus to the peripheral capsular margin, resulting in the creation of two separate meniscal components. They are most commonly found in the posterior horn of the medial meniscus, and usually occur secondary to shear forces between the femoral condyle and tibial plateau.[23] Horizontal cleavage tears are usually clearly visualized on sagittal and coronal sequences, but are usually difficult to visualize in the axial plane. Extension to the peripheral capsular margin is not infrequently associated with the formation of meniscal cysts (**Fig. 2**). Symptoms commonly arise because of involvement of the vascularized periphery of the affected meniscus.[24]

LONGITUDINAL MENISCAL TEARS

Longitudinal tears represent vertical peripheral tears that develop along the meniscal longitudinal axis, and are best appreciated in the sagittal and coronal plane. Sagittal imaging may demonstrate vertical or horizontal morphology. Vertical tears

that involve the peripheral third of the meniscus are usually longitudinal, whereas vertical tears that involve the inner third of the meniscus are usually flap tears. They most frequently develop in the posterior horn of the meniscus, subsequently extending anteriorly into the body of the meniscus (**Fig. 3**), in a circumferential manner.[1]

Longitudinal tears commonly occur in younger patients secondary to acute trauma, including in sports-related injuries. They are frequently associated with injuries of the anterior cruciate ligament and medial collateral ligament. They are also frequently mistaken for normal anatomic structures, including the transverse intermeniscal ligament, the popliteus tendon sheath, and the meniscofemoral ligaments of Humphrey and Wrisberg. Longitudinal tears become complete when they extend from the superior to the inferior articular surfaces, or when a displaced fragment is present. The extent of longitudinal tear completeness, together with the length and position of the tear, determine the stability of the tear.[25]

Bucket-handle Longitudinal Tears

A bucket-handle longitudinal tear consists of a displaced central fragment, resembling the handle of a bucket, and most commonly involves the medial meniscus.[1] Various types of bucket-handle longitudinal tears exist, including vertical longitudinal bucket-handle tears, displaced bucket-handle tears, broken bucket-handle tears, and double or triple vertical longitudinal bucket-handle tears.[26] They frequently occur in younger patients and

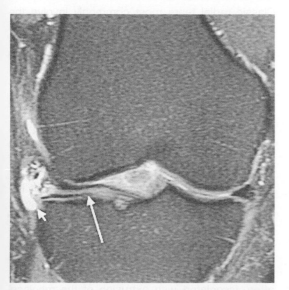

Fig. 2. Horizontal meniscal tear with associated parameniscal cyst. Coronal T2 fat-saturated (FS) image demonstrates a horizontal tear of the lateral meniscus (*long arrow*), associated with a multiseptated parameniscal cyst located in the lateral gutter (*short arrow*).

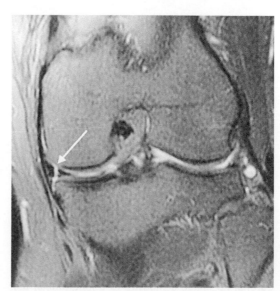

Fig. 3. Longitudinal meniscal tear. Coronal T2 FS image demonstrates a vertical longitudinal tear of the body of the medial meniscus (*arrow*).

are associated with significant trauma, including high-energy sports injuries.[27]

Bucket-handle longitudinal tears occur at least three times more frequently in the medial meniscus.[28] Coronal imaging can be used to demonstrate the displaced medial meniscal fragment to lie within the intercondylar notch (**Fig. 4**),[29] whereas sagittal imaging demonstrates the meniscal fragment to lie parallel and anterior to the posterior cruciate ligament within the inter-condylar notch (**Fig. 5**).[30] Axial imaging can be helpful in demonstrating the attachment of the dis-placed meniscal fragment to the remainder of the medial meniscus. The "double PCL sign" refers to the presence of the displaced meniscal frag-ment anterior to the posterior cruciate ligament within the intercondylar notch, giving the impres-sion of two separate posterior cruciate ligaments on sagittal imaging.[29–31] The "double delta sign" refers to the presence of the displaced medial fragment posterior to the anterior horn of the medial meniscus, giving the impression of two separate triangular structures.[31] This is best appreciated on sagittal sequences.

Bucket-handle meniscal tears are associated with anterior cruciate ligament injuries.[30] They frequently begin as longitudinal tears, followed by a secondary displaced radial tear pattern, which results in the bucket-handle morphology.

RADIAL TEARS

Radial (or transverse) tears are vertical tears that lie perpendicular to the meniscal free edge. They

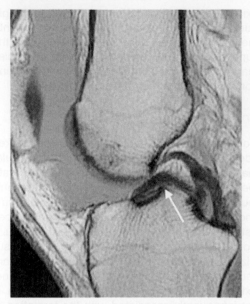

Fig. 5. Bucket-handle longitudinal meniscal tear. Sagittal PD image demonstrating a longitudinal tear of the medial meniscus, with a bucket-handle frag-ment (*arrow*) located anterior to the posterior cruciate ligament.

are subdivided into classic radial tears, which more commonly involve the lateral meniscus, and root tears, which more commonly involve the posterior horn of the medial meniscus.

Classic Radial Tears

Classic radial tears most commonly involve the junction of the anterior horn and the body of the lateral meniscus, producing blunting of the free edge.[21] Less commonly they involve the body of the lateral meniscus resulting in truncation of the free edge, or the junction of the body and posterior horn of the lateral meniscus. Classic radial tears are significant because of their resultant consider-able interruption of the tensile strength of the meniscus, which is caused by the tears being perpendicular to the longitudinal orientation of the meniscal fibers.

Sagittal imaging of classic radial tears of the junction of the anterior horn and body of the lateral meniscus demonstrates truncation of the anterior horn with relative elongation of the posterior horn.[32] Axial imaging often confirms the presence of a classic radial tear (**Fig. 6**). Extension of a classic radial tear into the meniscal periphery is often associated with extrusion of the meniscal body.[33] Classic radial tears of the lateral meniscus may be associated with secondary horizontal tears, resulting in the formation of complex tears. Incomplete classic radial tears are restricted to

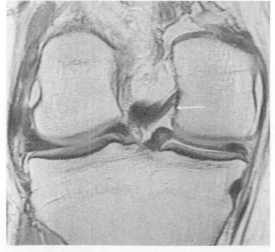

Fig. 4. Bucket-handle longitudinal meniscal tear. Coronal PD image demonstrates a longitudinal tear of the medial meniscus with a bucket-handle type dis-placed fragment within the intercondylar region (*arrow*).

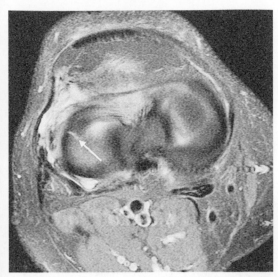

Fig. 6. Radial meniscal tear. Axial T2 FS image demonstrates a complete radial tear of the lateral meniscus (*arrow*).

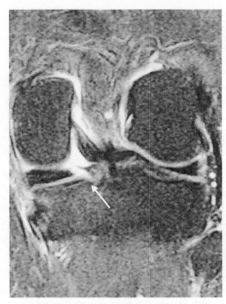

Fig. 7. Radial tear of meniscal root. Coronal T2 FS image showing a radial tear (*arrow*) involving the posterior meniscal root of the medial meniscus.

the free edge of the meniscus, whereas complete classic radial tears extend into the meniscal periphery. Radial tears that extend toward the periphery but change direction result in the formation of a flap tear.

Root Tears

Root tears represent a type of degenerative tear, and are more common in the medial meniscus.[23] They are located either at the level of the meniscotibial attachment of the posterior horn or at the junction of the meniscus and meniscal root (**Figs. 7** and **8**). Root tears are highly unstable meniscal injuries that result in a substantial loss of hoop strength within the meniscus. Coronal sequences demonstrate blunting of the meniscotibial attachment and truncation of the meniscus and meniscal extrusion. Given the loss of protective function of the meniscus, root tears have a high association with premature chondriomalacia and subchondral insufficiency fracture formation. Displacement of root tear fragments can result in the formation of a flipped fragment within the posterior aspect of the intercondylar notch or the coronal recess (**Figs. 9**A and B). Lateral meniscal root tears are associated with anterior cruciate ligament injuries.[34]

FLAP TEARS

Flap or oblique tears are the most common type of meniscal tear, representing a combination of longitudinal and radial tears that commence at the meniscal free edge and extend obliquely into

the meniscus. Findings on sagittal imaging include a vertical tear of the inner third of meniscus, blunting and truncation of the inferior leaf of torn meniscus, displacement of the meniscal fragment inferior to the periphery of the meniscus, and a change in angulation of the superior surface of

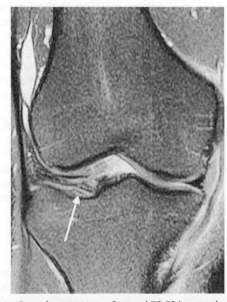

Fig. 8. Complex root tear. Coronal T2 FS image demonstrates poorly defined signal abnormality involving the root origin of the posterior horn of the lateral meniscus (*arrow*), consistent with a complex root tear.

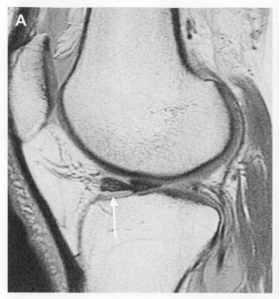
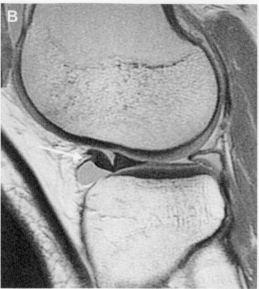

Fig. 9. (A, B) Meniscal root tear with flipped meniscal fragment. Sagittal PD image demonstrates a root tear of the lateral meniscus, with a flipped fragment consisting of the posterior horn of the lateral meniscus (arrow), which is now identified anterior to the anterior horn of the lateral meniscus.

the meniscus. Flap tears may be suspected when a meniscal tear extends to the superior or inferior articular surface on separate sagittal images and in different locations, because of the flap tear involving a change in the direction of the tear. Flap tears may result in extrusion of the flap fragment into the coronal recess below the level of the joint line (Fig. 10), and most commonly involve the posterior horn of the medial meniscus.[34] Flap fragments may rotate, resulting in the fragment overlying the source meniscus or within the meniscofemoral or meniscotibial recesses. Flap fragments may also displace into the intercondylar notch, especially when associated with an anterior cruciate ligament injury,[35] where the flap fragment in proximity to the anterior cruciate ligament produces a "double ACL sign."

Flap tears frequently occur after minimal meniscal trauma, especially on a background of meniscal degenerative change. The most common meniscal tear pattern is for the flap tear to involve the inferior meniscal leaflet. Complex meniscal tears may demonstrate both flap and radial components (Fig. 11).

DISCOID MENISCUS

A discoid meniscus is defined as a dysplastic meniscus that lacks normal semilunar morphology and possesses a disklike configuration, covering the central aspect of the tibial plateau instead of being confined to the periphery of the tibial plateau.[36,37] Discoid menisci more frequently

involve the lateral meniscus and are often bilateral. Discoid menisci are associated with an increased risk of meniscal tears and meniscal cyst formation (Figs. 12 and 13). They are subdivided into complete, incomplete, and Wrisberg ligament–type discoid menisci. The differentiation between complete and incomplete discoid menisci

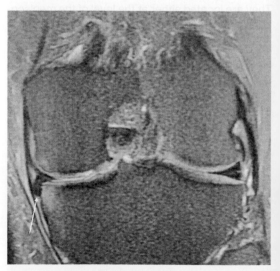

Fig. 10. Flap tear with displaced fragment. Coronal T2 FS image demonstrates a flap tear of the body of the medial meniscus with displacement of the meniscal flap fragment into the coronal recess (arrow). Additional findings include adjacent marrow stress response and chondral defect involving the medial femoral condyle.

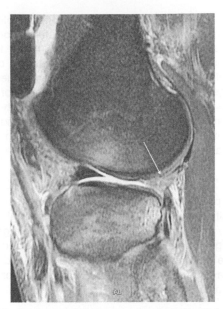

Fig. 11. Complex meniscal tear. Sagittal T2 FS image demonstrates poorly defined signal abnormality involving the posterior horn of the lateral meniscus (*arrow*), consistent with a complex tear, in the setting of an acute anterior cruciate ligament rupture (not shown).

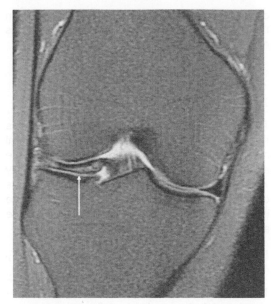

Fig. 12. Discoid meniscus with complex tear. Coronal T2 FS image demonstrates an enlarged lateral meniscus consistent with discoid morphology, associated with diffuse signal abnormality near the free edge (*arrow*) consistent with a complex tear.

depends on the extent to which the meniscus demonstrates discoid morphology,[2,38] with a complete discoid meniscus extending into the intercondylar notch.

Plain film radiographs may demonstrate increased joint space height, hypoplasia of the femoral condyle with squared morphology, superior migration of the femoral head, and cuplike deformity of the tibial plateau.[39] Sagittal MR imaging demonstrates a continuous bow-tie appearance of the meniscus with loss of central tapering.[39,40] Both sagittal and coronal MR imaging demonstrate an increase in height of a discoid meniscus relative to the normal adjacent meniscus.[41] Coronal MR imaging demonstrates extension of the apex of a discoid meniscus toward or into the intercondylar notch, with a coronal distance of 13 mm from the capsular margin to the free edge being highly suggestive of a discoid meniscus.[2]

Discoid menisci are prone to meniscal tears and degeneration because of their abnormal structure.[42] The frequency of all types of meniscal tears is higher in discoid menisci, with no increase in frequency of tears of the adjacent normal meniscus.[43] Undisplaced tears of a discoid meniscus are diagnosed using the same criteria as for normal menisci. Displaced meniscal tears may be misdiagnosed as bucket-handle tears

involving a normal meniscus. Furthermore, transverse and longitudinal tears of a discoid meniscus may be missed because the tears may lie parallel to the MR imaging plane.[44] Grade 2 signal abnormality corresponding with intrasubstance tears is more common in discoid menisci, and is more

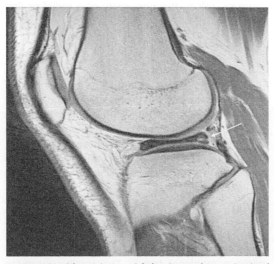

Fig. 13. Discoid meniscus with horizontal tear. Sagittal PD image demonstrates an enlarged lateral meniscus consistent with discoid morphology, associated with a horizontal tear of the posterior horn (*arrow*).

clinically significant in the discoid meniscus than in the morphologically normal meniscus, where it is more frequently symptomatic.

CAUSES OF MISINTERPRETATION OF MENISCAL ABNORMALITIES
Transverse Intermeniscal Ligament

The transverse intermeniscal ligament connects the anterior horns of the medial and lateral menisci, and can simulate an oblique tear of the anterior horn of the lateral meniscus, especially when a joint effusion is present.[45–49] Less commonly, the medial end of the transverse intermeniscal ligament may simulate a tear of the anterior horn of the medial meniscus.

Differences Between Grade 2 and Grade 3 Meniscal Signal Abnormality

The difference between grade 2 and grade 3 meniscal signal abnormality is defined as extension of the signal abnormality to the meniscal articular surface. The diagnosis of a meniscal tear is based on whether signal abnormality extends toward a meniscal articular surface, which is assessed in multiple planes. In cases where signal abnormality reaches a meniscal articular surface but is not as T2 hyperintense as fluid signal, an intrasubstance closed tear needs to be considered.[50]

Meniscal Fibrillation

Fibrillation of the free edge of the meniscus may result in the presence of signal abnormality but is seen in an otherwise morphologically normal meniscus.[51] The presence of meniscal truncation, however, raises the possibility of a radial or flap tear.

Attachment of Anterior Horn of the Lateral Meniscus

The ligamentous attachment of the anterior horn of the lateral meniscus frequently demonstrates punctate foci of signal abnormality, near the origin of the transverse intermeniscal ligament, which may mimic a tear of the ligamentous attachment. Careful assessment of the anterior horn on consecutive sagittal images avoids misinterpreting this as a tear.

Popliteus Tendon

The popliteus tendon is located adjacent to the posterior horn of the lateral meniscus and may mimic a meniscal tear.[49] The popliteus tendon sheath is located anterior to the popliteus tendon, and may distend with fluid when a joint effusion is present. Peripheral tears of the lateral meniscus

have an axis different to the axis of the popliteus tendon sheath, and tears of the posterior horn of the lateral meniscus can be distinguished from the adjacent popliteus tendon sheath by clear identification of the popliteus tendon on sequential images. Knowledge of the normal anatomy of this region enables the distinction to be made between a peripheral tear of the lateral meniscus and the normal cleft between the popliteus tendon and the lateral meniscus.

Partial Volume Averaging Artifact

The peripheral margin of a meniscus is concave, resulting in some sagittal images through the body of the meniscus appearing as at least grade 2 signal abnormality.[45,47] This phenomenon is more common in the medial meniscus, and can be avoided by cross-referencing with coronal and axial sequences.

Meniscal Flounce

A meniscal flounce is defined as a redundant meniscus that is not associated with a meniscal tear (Figs. 14 and 15). Meniscal flounce is more common in the medial meniscus and may mimic a peripheral tear.

Medial Collateral Ligament Bursa

The medial collateral ligament bursa is located between the periphery of the body of the medial meniscus and the medial collateral ligament. An

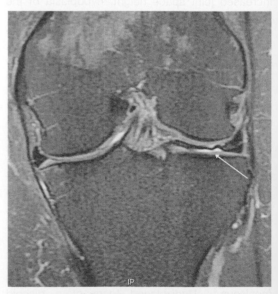

Fig. 14. Meniscal flounce. Coronal T2 FS image demonstrates a redundant lateral meniscus (*arrow*) consistent with a meniscal flounce, not associated with signal abnormality to suggest a meniscal tear.

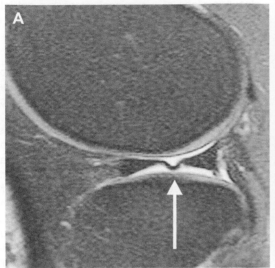
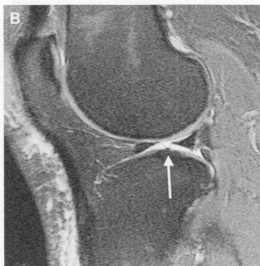

Fig. 15. (A, B) Meniscal flounce. Sagittal T2 FS images demonstrate a redundant body of the lateral meniscus (*arrows*) consistent with a meniscal flounce, with no associated signal abnormality to suggest an underlying meniscal tear.

enlarged medial collateral ligament bursa secondary to bursitis may mimic a peripheral meniscocapsular tear.[52]

Meniscofemoral Ligaments

The lateral aspect of the meniscofemoral ligament consists of the ligament of Humphrey, which is located anterior to the posterior cruciate ligament, and the posterior branch of the ligament of Wrisberg, which is located posterior to the posterior cruciate ligament. The meniscofemoral ligament is attached to the lateral meniscus and the medial femoral condyle. The meniscal attachment of the meniscofemoral ligament may mimic a vertical tear of the posterior horn of the lateral meniscus.

The oblique meniscomeniscal ligaments pass between the anterior and posterior cruciate ligaments, from the anterior horn of one meniscus to the posterior horn of the contralateral meniscus, and may be mistaken for flap or bucket-handle tears.[53]

Capsular Structures

Fat and vascular structures are located between the posterior horn of the medial meniscus and the joint capsule, and may mimic meniscocapsular separation, which can be excluded by clearly defining the margins of the meniscus.

MR IMAGING FEATURES OF THE POSTOPERATIVE MENISCUS
MR Imaging Features Postmeniscectomy

MR imaging allows for the accurate assessment of the residual meniscus post–partial meniscectomy.

Various classification systems have been created to characterize meniscal findings post–partial meniscectomy, depending on the appearance of the meniscus and the degree of associated degenerative changes.[54] Partial meniscectomy on MR imaging is seen as either sharp truncation of the meniscal apex or a contoured meniscal surface without blunting. Total meniscectomy is associated with complete loss of visualization of the meniscus. The postmeniscectomy state is frequently associated with articular cartilage loss and joint space narrowing, caused by direct contact between the femoral and tibial articular cartilage with secondary abnormal chondral load bearing.[55]

Accurate assessment of the postmeniscectomy state requires knowledge of the original meniscal tear pattern together with knowledge of the surgical findings and intervention. Intrameniscal signal conversion refers to residual grade 3 signal abnormality in the meniscal remnant postmeniscectomy. Localized fibrosis postmeniscectomy may mimic the meniscal fibrocartilage, but is usually smaller and of lower signal than the native meniscal substance. Postoperative meniscal remnants are at increased risk of further subsequent tears, which may demonstrate any type of meniscal tear morphology.[56] Fluid within meniscal tears involving meniscal remnants can be visualized with PD and T2* gradient recalled echo sequences, which are more specific than short TE sequences. MR arthrography improves the accuracy of the assessment of recurrent tears (**Fig. 16**) when more than 25% of the meniscus has been resected,[57] but is not necessary when a significant effusion is present or when a minimal quantity of meniscus has been

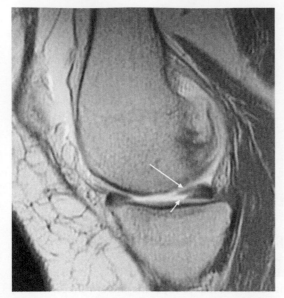

Fig. 16. Previous partial meniscectomy with recurrent meniscal tear. Sagittal PD image with intra-articular gadolinium, demonstrating mild T2 hyperintensity of the free edge of the posterior horn of the medial meniscus, consistent with a previous partial meniscectomy (*long arrow*). A further linear region of T2 hyperintensity extends from the inferior free edge of the posterior horn into the meniscal substance (*short arrow*), consistent with a recurrent tear.

resected.[58–60] The ability to diagnose a recurrent meniscal tear depends on the amount of residual meniscus present.[3,54]

MR Imaging Features Post–Meniscal Repair

Primary meniscal repair may be associated with variable signal intensity abnormality, ranging from grade 1 to grade 3 signal abnormality.[9,61–64] Grade 3 signal abnormality can convert into lower grades of signal abnormality over several months, because of healing of meniscal tears and regeneration of normal fibrocartilage.[61,63] Meniscal scarring and granulation tissue demonstrate intermediate signal on PD and T2 sequences, compared with higher signal for grade 3 signal abnormality associated with meniscal tears.

Secondary tears of repaired meniscal fibrocartilage can be determined using the same criteria as for secondary tears postmeniscectomy, including T2 or PD hyperintensity at the meniscal repair site, the presence of displaced meniscal fragments, and the development of signal abnormality at a location separate to the site of meniscal repair.[62,65] MR arthrography using intra-articular gadolinium can be used to assess meniscal tears post–meniscal repair, by determining the presence of extension of articular fluid into the cleavage plane of a meniscal retear, but not into the meniscal repair site.[3,66]

MENISCOCAPSULAR SEPARATION

Meniscocapsular separation refers to the avulsion of the meniscal periphery from the joint capsule, and usually involves the medial meniscus, which is less mobile.[67–69] The posterior horn of the medial meniscus is fixed to the tibia by the meniscotibial ligaments and is at risk of tears at the capsular attachment. Meniscocapsular tears can occur in the absence of grade 3 signal abnormality within the meniscus involved, and may heal spontaneously because of the vascularization of the meniscal periphery.[8] Features of meniscocapsular separation on sagittal sequences include displacement of the posterior horn of the medial meniscus from the joint capsule by over 5 mm, uncovering of the tibial articular cartilage, and the presence of a rim of fluid between the capsular margin of the meniscus and the capsule (**Fig. 17**). Disruption of the meniscotibial capsular ligament is associated with meniscal avulsion from the tibial plateau, resulting in a meniscus surrounded by fluid, which has been described as a "floating meniscus" (**Fig. 18**).[70]

MENISCAL CYSTS

Meniscal cysts are para-articular fluid collections associated with meniscal tears.[71,72] They are

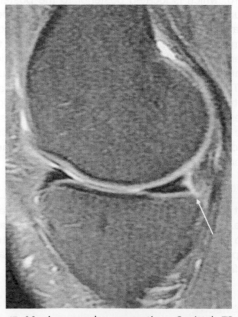

Fig. 17. Meniscocapsular separation. Sagittal T2 FS image demonstrates a linear region of T2 hyperintensity (*arrow*) between the posterior horn of the medial meniscus and the adjacent capsule.

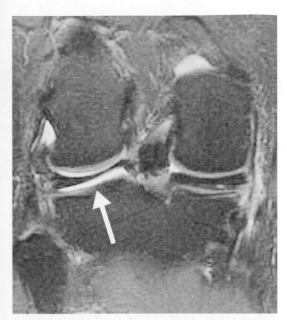

Fig. 18. Floating meniscus. Coronal T2 FS image demonstrates extensive fluid signal between the lateral meniscus and the tibial plateau (*arrow*), consistent with a "floating meniscus," a form of meniscocapsular separation.

classified into parameniscal, intrameniscal, and synovial cysts.[2] Parameniscal cysts are the most common type of meniscal cyst and consist of a fluid collection centered on the meniscal periphery, adjacent to a meniscal tear. Parameniscal cysts develop secondary to trauma, degenerative change, or post–partial meniscectomy, with synovial fluid expressed into the site of a horizontal meniscal tear, collecting at the meniscocapsular border.[72,73]

Lateral parameniscal cysts are more common than medial parameniscal cysts, and more commonly involve the central third of the meniscus.[71] They are usually associated with horizontal flap tears, horizontal cleavage tears, or complex tears with horizontal and radial components, and are usually located anterior to the lateral collateral ligament or between the lateral collateral ligament and the popliteus tendon (**Figs. 19** and **20**). Lateral parameniscal cysts are frequently larger than medial cysts because of the presence of less mass effect exerted on an expanding laterally positioned cyst by the surrounding soft tissues.

Medial parameniscal cysts may dissect through the adjacent soft tissues, resulting in a location away from the primary meniscal tear, often found deep to the medial collateral ligament or at the posteromedial corner. Parameniscal cysts arising from tears of the posterior horn of the medial meniscus

may dissect toward cruciate ligaments, resembling a ganglion cyst arising from the cruciate ligaments.[74] In all cases of parameniscal cyst dissection, a connecting channel between the cyst and the primary meniscal tear can usually be identified.

Meniscal cysts usually demonstrate central fluid signal characteristics, although variations in cyst content signal may vary if blood products or proteinaceous material is present. Septation and loculation are common, with progressive complexity as the cyst is located further away from the primary meniscal tear. Meniscal cysts typically demonstrate peripheral enhancement with intravenous gadolinium, which may be useful when attempting to differentiate between complex meniscal cysts and suspected mass lesions, such as soft tissue sarcomas.

MR IMAGING OF CARTILAGE INJURIES OF THE KNEE

MR imaging is ideally suited for the assessment of articular cartilage injuries of the knee. Hyaline cartilage demonstrates intermediate signal on T1-, PD-, and T2-weighted sequences. Fluid-sensitive sequences in the presence of a joint effusion create an arthrogram-like appearance, allowing for more sensitive assessment of cartilaginous pathology. T2-weighted sequences are associated with less contrast between articular

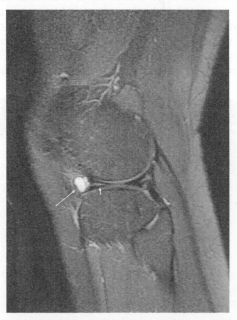

Fig. 19. Horizontal meniscal tear with parameniscal cyst. Sagittal T2 FS image demonstrating a horizontal tear of the anterior horn of the lateral meniscus (*short arrow*), with an adjacent parameniscal cyst (*long arrow*).

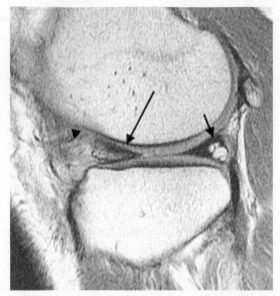

Fig. 20. Horizontal meniscal tear with associated intact and ruptured parameniscal cysts. Sagittal PD image demonstrates a horizontal tear of the lateral meniscus (*long arrow*), associated with an intact parameniscal cyst adjacent to the posterior horn (*short arrow*) and a ruptured parameniscal cyst adjacent to the anterior horn (*arrowhead*).

cartilage and subchondral bone, in the absence of a joint effusion.[52] T2*-weighted sequences demonstrate hyperintense signal in articular cartilage, but the lack of contrast between articular cartilage and joint effusion results in reduced sensitivity for articular cartilage pathology. Assessment of articular cartilage with spin echo, gradient recalled echo, and fast spoiled gradient

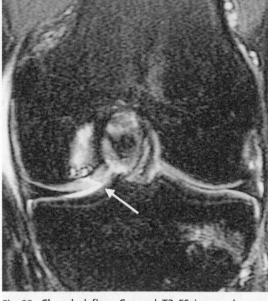

Fig. 22. Chondral flap. Coronal T2 FS image demonstrates a chondral flap arising from the medial femoral condyle (*arrow*), associated with subchondral cystic change and subjacent bone marrow edema.

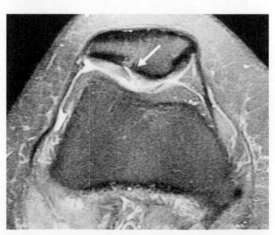

Fig. 21. Articular cartilage full-thickness cleft. Axial T2 FS image through patellofemoral joint demonstrating a full-thickness cleft of the lateral patellar articular cartilage (*arrow*), associated with chondral fissuring involving the patellar apex.

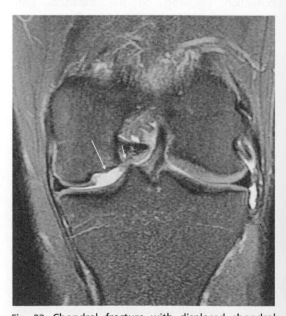

Fig. 23. Chondral fracture with displaced chondral fragment. Coronal T2 FS image demonstrating a full-thickness chondral defect involving the medial femoral condyle (*long arrow*), with a displaced chondral fragment within the intercondylar notch (*short arrow*).

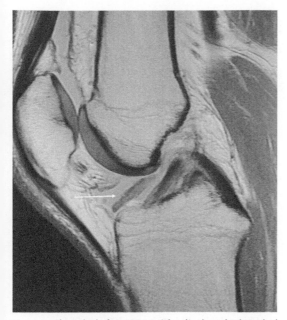

Fig. 24. Chondral fracture with displaced chondral fragment. Sagittal PD image demonstrating a loose chondral fragment (*arrow*) within the anterior aspect of the intercondylar notch.

echo sequences may demonstrate a trilaminar appearance, involving a hyperintense superficial layer, hypointense intermediate transitional zone, and deeper hyperintense radial zone.[52,75–77] Short tau inversion recovery sequences demonstrate hyperintense joint fluid, mildly hyperintense

articular cartilage, and subchondral marrow signal abnormality.[75] T1-weighted sequences with fat suppression and intra-articular gadolinium are useful in the identification of small chondral lesions, but not as useful in the assessment of pathology of the deeper cartilage layers.[78]

Chondral fractures involve a focal loss of integrity of the articular cartilage with no involvement of the underlying subchondral plate (Fig. 21). Adult articular cartilage is more likely to tear at the junction of the calcified and uncalcified zones, whereas traumatic shearing forces involving the immature osteochondral region directly involve the subchondral plate, resulting in osteochondral fractures.[66] Chondral lesions can be associated with hyperintense fluid or isointense fibrous tissue.[52] Chondral flaps are defined as fractures of the articular cartilage with insinuation of joint fluid into the articular cartilage (Figs. 22–24). Delamination is defined as a more extensive articular cartilage fracture, with joint fluid tracking between the cartilage and subchondral plate (Figs. 25A and B).

Articular cartilage lesions can be graded based on the depth of cartilage involvement. Grade 1 chondral lesions demonstrate superficial fissuring, grade 2 chondral lesions involve less than half of the depth of the articular cartilage (Fig. 26), grade 3 chondral lesions involve more than half of the depth of the articular cartilage without extension to the subchondral plate, and grade 4 chondral lesions extend to the subchondral plate.

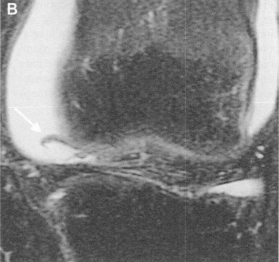
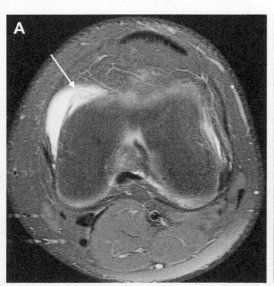

Fig. 25. (*A, B*) Chondral delamination. Axial T2 FS (Fig. 1A) and coronal T2 FS (Fig. 1B) images demonstrate a large elevated chondral fragment (*arrow*), arising from the medial femoral condyle and which continues to lie in continuity with the adjacent articular cartilage.

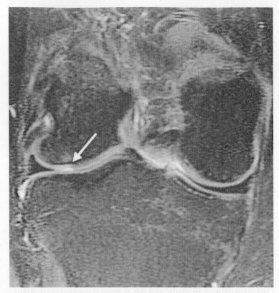

Fig. 26. Grade 2 chondral lesion. Coronal T2 FS image demonstrates a focal chondral abnormality of the weight-bearing surface of the lateral femoral condyle (*arrow*), demonstrating a partial reduction in thickness of under 50%, consistent with a grade 2 chondral lesion.

SUMMARY

MR imaging is highly accurate for the diagnosis of meniscal and articular cartilage abnormalities of the knee. Meniscal injuries and acute chondral pathology in athletes are almost identical to those seen in the general community, with degenerative changes being less frequent in the acute setting. Familiarity with the normal anatomy of the knee, together with an appreciation of the common causes of misinterpretation of meniscal abnormalities, maximizes diagnostic accuracy and allows meniscal pathology to be assessed and treated in an emergent manner. The nature of sports medicine is suitably matched to the highly accurate diagnostic abilities of MR imaging in the assessment of acute meniscal and articular cartilage injuries in athletes.

ACKNOWLEDGMENTS

The authors thank Dr. Daniel Saddik, Radiologist, Director of MRI, Northern Hospital, Epping, and Dr. Miranda Miocevic, Radiologist, Box Hill Hospital, Eastern Health Medical Imaging, for their assistance with the preparation of images for this article.

REFERENCES

1. Stoller DW, Martin C, Crues JV, et al. Meniscal tears: pathologic correlation with MR imaging. Radiology 1987;163:731–5.

2. Crues JV, Stoller DW. The menisci. In: Mink JH, Reicher MA, Crues JV, editors. MRI of the knee. New York: Raven Press; 1993. p. 91.

3. Applegate GR, Flannigan BD, Tolin BS, et al. MR diagnosis of recurrent tears in the knee: value of intraarticular contrast material. AJR AM J Roentgenol 1993;161:821–5.

4. Rubin DA, Kneeland JB, Listerud J, et al. MR diagnosis of meniscal tears of the knee: value of FSE vs conventional spin-echo pulse sequences. AJR Am J Roentgenol 1994;162:1131–5.

5. Ferrer-Roca O, Vilalta C. Lesions of the meniscus. I: macroscopic and histologic findings. Clin Orthop Relat Res 1980;146:289–300.

6. Kornick J, Trefelner E, McCarthy S, et al. Meniscal abnormalities in the asymptomatic population at MR imaging. Radiology 1990;177:463–5.

7. Smillie LS. Diseases of the knee joint. 2nd edition. London: Churchill-Livingstone; 1980. p. 340.

8. Mink JH. The knee. In: Mink JH, Deutsch A, editors. MRI of the musculoskeletal system: a teaching file. Philadelphia: JB Lippincott; 1990. p. 251.

9. Crues JV, Ryu R, Morgan FW. Meniscal pathology: the expanding role of magnetic resonance imaging. Clin Orthop Relat Res 1990;252:80–7.

10. Ruwe PA, Wright J, Randall RL, et al. Can MR imaging effectively replace diagnostic arthroscopy? Radiology 1992;183:335–9.

11. Mandelbaum BR, Finerman GA, Reicher MA, et al. Magnetic resonance imaging as a tool for evaluation of traumatic knee injuries. Anatomical and pathoanatomical correlations. Am J Sports Med 1986;14:361–70.

12. Warren RF, Levy IM. Meniscal lesions associated with anterior cruciate ligament injury. Clin Orthop Relat Res 1983;172:32–7.

13. LaPrade RF, Burnett QM, Veenstra MA, et al. The prevalence of abnormal magnetic resonance imaging findings in asymptomatic knees, with correlation of magnetic resonance imaging to arthroscopic findings in symptomatic knees. Am J Sports Med 1994;22:739–45.

14. De Smet AA, Graf BK. Meniscal tears missed on MR imaging: relationship to meniscal tear patterns and anterior cruciate ligament tears. AJR Am J Roentgenol 1994;162:905–11.

15. Justice WW, Quinn SF. Error patterns in the MR imaging evaluation of menisci of the knee. Radiology 1995;196:617–21.

16. Mink JH, Levy T, Crues JV. Tears of the anterior cruciate ligament and menisci of the knee: MR imaging evaluation. Radiology 1988;167:769–74.

17. Fischer SP, Fox JM, Del Pizzo W, et al. Accuracy of diagnosis from magnetic resonance imaging of the knee. A multi-center analysis of one thousand and fourteen patients. J Bone Joint Surg Am 1991;73:2–10.

18. Stoller DW. Three-dimensional rendering and classification of meniscal tears disarticulated from 3-D FT images. In: Abstracts of 9th Annual Meeting of the Society of Magnetic Resonance in Medicine. New York; 1990. p. 346.

19. Dandy DJ. The arthroscopic anatomy of symptomatic meniscal lesions. J Bone Joint Surg Br 1990; 72:628–33.

20. Tarhan NC, Chung CB, Mohana-Borges AV, et al. Meniscal tears: role of axial MRI alone and in combination with other imaging planes. AJR Am J Roentgenol 2004;183:9–15.

21. Tuckman GA, Miller WJ, Remo JW, et al. Radial tears of the menisci: MR findings. AJR Am J Roentgenol 1994;163:395–400.

22. Chernye S. Disorders of the knee. In: Deer S, editor, Principles of orthopaedic practise, vol. 2. New York: McGraw-Hill; 1989. p. 1283.

23. Insall JN, Scott WN. In: Surgery of the knee, vol. 1, 3rd edition. Philadelphia: Churchill Livingstone; 2001.

24. Zanetti M, Pfirrmann CW, Schmid MR, et al. Patients with suspected meniscal tears: prevalence of abnormalities seen on MRI of 100 symptomatic and 100 contralateral asymptomatic knees. AJR Am J Roentgenol 2003;181:635–41.

25. Newman AP, Daniels AU, Burks RT. Principles and decision making in meniscal surgery. Arthroscopy 1993;9:33–51.

26. Cannon WD, Vitton JM. Basic arthroscopy. In: Aichroth PM, Cannon WD, Disnitz M, editors. Knee surgery: current practise. London: Martin Dunitz; 1992. p. 54.

27. Rosenberg TO, Pavlos LE. Arthroscopic surgery of the knee. In: Chapman MW, editor. Operative orthopaedics. 2nd edition. Philadelphia: JB Lippincott; 1993. p. 2403.

28. Wright DH, De Smet AA, Norris M. Bucket-handle tears of the medial and lateral menisci of the knee: value of MR imaging in detected displaced fragments. AJR Am J Roentgenol 1995;165:621–5.

29. Singson RD, Feldman F, Staron R, et al. MR imaging of displaced bucket-handle tear of the medial meniscus. AJR Am J Roentgenol 1991;156:121–4.

30. Weiss KL, Morehouse HT, Levy IM. Sagittal MR images of the knee: a low-signal band parallel to the posterior cruciate ligament caused by a displaced bucket-handle tear. AJR Am J Roentgenol 1991;156:117–9.

31. Camacho MA. The double posterior cruciate ligament sign. Radiology 2004;233:503–4.

32. Helms CA. The meniscus: recent advances in MR imaging of the knee. AJR Am J Roentgenol 2002; 179:1115–22.

33. Costa RC, Morrison WB, Carrino JA. Medial meniscus extrusion on knee MRI: is extent associated with severity of degeneration or type of tear? AJR Am J Roentgenol 2004;183:17–23.

34. Voto S. A nomenclature system for meniscal lesions of the knee. Surgical Rounds for Orthopaedics 1989; 10:34–8.

35. Vande Berg BC, Malghem J, Poilvache P, et al. Meniscal tears with fragments displaced in notch and recesses of knee: MR imaging with arthroscopic comparison. Radiology 2005;234:842–50.

36. Dickason JM, Del Pizzo W, Blazina ME, et al. A series of ten discoid medial menisci. Clin Orthop 1982;168:75–9.

37. Weiner B, Rosenberg N. Discoid medial meniscus association with bone changes in the tibia. A case report. J Bone Joint Surg Am 1974;56:171–3.

38. Auge WK, Kaeding CC. Bilateral discoid medial menisci with extensive intrasubstance cleavage tears: MRI and arthroscopic correlation. Arthroscopy 1994;10:313–8.

39. Schonholtz GJ, Koenig TM, Prince A. Bilateral discoid medial menisci: a case report and literature review. Arthroscopy 1993;9:315–7.

40. Barnes CL, McCarthy RE, VanderSchilden JL, et al. Discoid lateral meniscus in a young child: case report and review of the literature. J Pediatr Orthop 1988;8:707–9.

41. Silverman JM, Mink JH, Deutsch AL. Discoid menisci of the knee: MR imaging appearance. Radiology 1989;173:351–4.

42. Araki Y, Ashikaga R, Fujii K, et al. MR imaging of meniscal tears with discoid lateral meniscus. Eur J Radiol 1998;27(2):153–60.

43. Rohren EM, Kosarek FJ, Helms CA. Discoid lateral meniscus and the frequency of meniscal tears. Skeletal Radiol 2001;30(6):316–20.

44. Ryu KN, Kim IS, Kim EJ, et al. MR imaging of tears of discoid lateral menisci. AJR Am J Roentgenol 1998; 171(4):963–7.

45. Mink JH. Pitfalls in interpretation. In: Mink JH, Reicher MA, Crues JV, editors. MRI of the knee. 2nd edition. New York: Raven Press; 1993. p. 433.

46. De Smet AA, Tuite MJ, Norris MA, et al. MR diagnosis of meniscal tears: analysis of causes of errors. AJR Am J Roentgenol 1994;163:1419–23.

47. Herman LJ, Beltran J. Pitfalls in MR imaging of the knee. Radiology 1988;167:775–81.

48. Vahey TN, Bennett HT, Arrington LE, et al. MR imaging of the knee: pseudotear of the lateral meniscus caused by the meniscofemoral ligament. AJR Am J Roentgenol 1990;154:1237–9.

49. Watanabe AT, Carter BC, Teitelbaum GP, et al. Normal variations in MR imaging of the knee: appearance and frequency. AJR Am J Roentgenol 1989;153:341–4.

50. Quinn SF, Brown TR, Szumowski J. Menisci of the knee: radial MR imaging correlated with arthroscopy in 259 patients. Radiology 1992;185:577–80.

51. Stoller DW, Li AE, Anderson LJ, et al. The knee. In: Stoller DE, Li AE, Bredella MA, editors, Magnetic

resonance imaging in orthopaedics and sports medicine, 3rd edition, vol. 1. Baltimore (MD): Lippincott Williams and Wilkins; 2007. p. 447.

52. Resnick D, Niwayama G. Internal derangements of joints. In: Diagnosis of bone and joint disorders, vol. 5, 2nd edition. Philadelphia: WB Saunders; 1988. 2899.

53. Sanders TG, Linares RC, Lawhorn KW, et al. Oblique meniscomeniscal ligament: another potential pitfall for a meniscal tear – anatomic description and appearance at MR imaging in three cases. Radiology 1999;213:213–6.

54. Smith DK, Totty WG. The knee after partial meniscectomy: MR imaging features. Radiology 1990; 176:141–4.

55. Cannon WD, Morgan CD. Meniscal repair: arthroscopic repair techniques. Instr Course Lect 1994; 43:77–96.

56. Magee T, Shapiro M, Williams D. Prevalence of meniscal radial tears of the knee revealed by MRI after surgery. AJR Am J Roentgenol 2004;182:931–6.

57. White L, Schweitzer M, Weishaupt D, et al. Diagnosis of recurrent meniscal tears: prospective evaluation of conventional MR imaging, indirect MR arthrography, and direct MR arthrography. Radiology 2002;222:421–9.

58. McCauley T. MR imaging evaluation of the postoperative knee. Radiology 2005;234:53–61.

59. Magee T, Shapiro M, Rodriguez J, et al. MR arthrography of postoperative knee: for which patients is it useful? Radiology 2003;229:159–63.

60. Recht M, Kramer J. MR imaging of the postoperative knee: a pictorial essay. Radiology 2002;22: 765–74.

61. Deutsch AL, Mink JH, Fox JM, et al. Peripheral meniscal tears: MR findings after conservative treatment or arthroscopic repair. Radiology 1990;176: 485–8.

62. Farley TE, Howell SM, Love KF, et al. Meniscal tears: MR and arthrographic findings after arthroscopic repair. Radiology 1991;180:517–22.

63. Arnoczky SP, Cooper TG, Stadelmaier DP, et al. Magnetic resonance signal in healing menisci: an experimental study in dogs. Arthroscopy 1994;10: 552–7.

64. Kent RH, Pope CF, Lynch JK, et al. Magnetic resonance imaging of the surgically repaired meniscus: six month follow-up. Magn Reson imaging 1991;9:335–41.

65. Lim P, Schweitzer M, Bhatia M, et al. Repeat tear of postoperative meniscus: potential MR imaging signs. Radiology 1999;210:183–8.

66. Drape JL, Thelen P, Gay-Depassier P, et al. Intraarticular diffusion of Gd-DOTA after intravenous injection in the knee: MR imaging evaluation. Radiology 1993;188:227–34.

67. Mink JH, Stoller DW, Martin C, et al. MR imaging of the knee: pitfalls in interpretation. Radiology 1986; 161:239.

68. Strobel M. Anatomy, proprioception and biomechanics. In: Diagnostic evaluation of the knee. Berlin: Springer-Verlag; 1990. p. 2.

69. Maeseneer MD, Roy FV, Lenchik L, et al. Three layers of the medial capsular and supporting structures of the knee: MR imaging-anatomic correlation. Radiographics 2000;20:S83–9.

70. Bikkina RS, Tujo CA, Schraner AB, et al. The floating meniscus: MRI in knee trauma and implications for surgery. AJR Am J Roentgenol 2005;184:200–4.

71. Bessette GC. The meniscus. Orthopedics 1992;15: 35–42.

72. Burk DL, Dalinka MK, Kanal E, et al. Meniscal and ganglion cysts of the knee: MR evaluation. AJR Am J Roentgenol 1988;150:331–6.

73. Gallimore GW, Harmes SE. Knee injuries: high-resolution MR imaging. Radiology 1986;160:457–61.

74. Lektrakul N, Skaf A, Yeh L, et al. Pericruciate meniscal cysts arising from tears of the posterior horn of the medial meniscus: MR imaging features that simulate posterior cruciate ganglion cysts. AJR Am J Roentgenol 1999;172:1575–9.

75. Recht MP, Resnick D. MR Imaging of articular cartilage: current status and future directions. AJR Am J Roentgenol 1994;163:283–90.

76. Recht MP, Kramer J, Marcelis S, et al. Abnormalities of articular cartilage in the knee: analysis of available MR techniques. Radiology 1993;187: 473–8.

77. Disler DG, Peters TL, Muscoreil SJ, et al. Fat-suppressed spoiled GRASS imaging of knee hyaline cartilage: technique optimization and comparison with conventional MR imaging. AJR Am J Roentgenol 1994;163:887–92.

78. Gylys-Morin VM, Hajek PC, Sortoris DJ, et al. Articular cartilage defects: detectability in cadaver knees with MR. AJR Am J Roentgenol 1987;148:1153–7.

MR Imaging of Muscle Injury

Martin J. Shelly, MD, MRCPI[a],*,
Philip A. Hodnett, MD, FFRRCSI, MRCPI, MMedSci[a],
Peter J. MacMahon, MD, MRCPI[a], Michael R. Moynagh, MD[a],
Eoin C. Kavanagh, MD, MB, FFRRCSI[a],
Stephen J. Eustace, MD, MSc, MB, FFRRCSI[a,b,c,d,e]

KEYWORDS

- MR imaging • Muscle injury • Muscle edema
- Myositis ossificans • Myotendinous junction
- Avulsion injury

Skeletal muscle is the single largest tissue in the body comprising 40% to 45% of an individual's total body mass.[1] Although most muscle injuries in the athlete are diagnosed clinically, MR imaging is an excellent noninvasive diagnostic adjunct to clinical examination, which allows the site and severity of muscle injury to be assessed accurately, influencing therapy and overall outcome.[2–4] There has been a rapid expansion in the clinical use of MR imaging during the past decade. MR imaging conveys unparalleled anatomic resolution and high sensitivity in the detection of acute and chronic muscle abnormalities.[5,6] Typical examples of muscle injuries include contusion, laceration, strains, and delayed-onset muscle soreness. In traumatic muscle conditions, such as chronic exertional compartment syndrome and acute denervation, the findings on clinical examination are often subtle or absent and MR imaging is essential in arriving at the correct diagnosis. In patients with known muscle trauma, MR imaging can detect complications, such as hematoma or seroma development, scarring, fibrosis, and myositis ossificans.[3] This article discusses the spectrum of muscle injuries, emphasizing the important role of MR imaging in their diagnosis and management.

MR IMAGING INDICATIONS AND TECHNICAL CONSIDERATIONS

Muscle and tendon disorders have a wide variety of causes, treatments, and prognoses. Clinical examination is often limited in its ability fully to evaluate a muscle injury and MR imaging is commonly used to identify the location, severity, and extent of injury (Box 1).

Although the exact MR imaging protocol used to image a muscle injury is specifically tailored to each patient, certain pulse sequences are commonly used and are helpful in designing an appropriate protocol. T1-weighted images provide a high signal-to-noise ratio and excellent anatomic detail, also allowing characterization of hemorrhagic lesions (eg, hematoma and hemorrhagic neoplasm) or abnormal fat deposition (eg, muscle atrophy or a lipoma).[1,7] Any protocol designed to highlight muscle injury must take advantage of T2 lengthening; most disease processes, traumatic or otherwise, cause an increase in the water content of muscle resulting in prolongation of the T2 relaxation time and hence signal hyperintensity.[8] Fat-suppressed T2-weighted and short tau inversion recovery (STIR) fast spin echo sequences are more sensitive to the presence of muscle edema and hemorrhage than longer time

[a] Department of Radiology, Mater Misericordiae University Hospital, Eccles Street, Dublin 7, Ireland
[b] Department of Radiology, Cappagh National Orthopaedic Hospital, Finglas, Dublin 11, Ireland
[c] University College Dublin, Belfield, Dublin 4, Ireland
[d] Institute of Radiological Sciences, University College Dublin, Dublin, Ireland
[e] Department of Radiology, Santry Sports Surgery Clinic, Santry Demense, Dublin 9, Ireland
* Corresponding author. 59 Belgrove Park, Clontarf, Dublin 3, Ireland.
E-mail address: martinshelly@gmail.com (M.J. Shelly).

Magn Reson Imaging Clin N Am 17 (2009) 757–773
doi:10.1016/j.mric.2009.06.012
1064-9689/09/$ – see front matter © 2009 Elsevier Inc. All rights reserved.

Box 1

Common indications for MR imaging in the management of muscle injury

- Rapid diagnosis of high-performance athletes
- Exclude superimposed injuries (eg, stress fracture)
- Provide a narrow clinical differential diagnosis
- Predict the prognosis or possible complications associated with a disorder
- Direct the type and location of an intervention (eg, biopsy or surgery)
- Monitor treatment response or complications

---

to echo (TE) sequences that are not fat suppressed.[7] Chronic hemorrhage is removed from muscle by macrophage phagocytosis of extracellular hemoglobin with macrophages subsequently accumulating hemosiderin. Gradient echo sequences exploit the paramagnetic effects of hemosiderin accumulation at the site of muscle injury and display "blooming" artifact, which can indicate the presence of hemorrhage.[8]

Intravenous contrast material is not generally necessary in the evaluation of muscle injury because areas affected by trauma or inflammation are well demonstrated on fat-suppressed T2-weighted and STIR imaging. Occasionally, fat-suppressed T1-weighted imaging post gadolinium administration can be helpful in difficult cases (eg, when evaluating for a cystic versus a solid mass).[8] After exercise, there is an acute increase in the T2 signal of muscle, a phenomenon known as "exercise enhancement." This is caused by an increased extracellular water content of muscle postexercise, which has a long T2 relaxation time when compared with the short T2 of intracellular water.[9] This phenomenon is exploited in the evaluation of patients with suspected chronic exertional compartment syndrome, because MR imaging pre-exercise and postexercise may be diagnostic. In addition to producing signal abnormality, conditions affecting the musculature commonly cause changes in muscle size and shape and this is best appreciated by comparison with the contralateral and presumably unaffected side.

MR IMAGING APPEARANCE OF NORMAL SKELETAL MUSCLE AND TENDON

The basic functional unit of skeletal muscle is the muscle fiber. Muscle fibers are grouped into fascicles, and the fascicles are grouped into muscles.[10] On MR imaging, skeletal muscle has an intermediate to long T1 and short T2 relaxation time, and

so it has signal intensity higher than water and lower than fat on T1-weighted imaging and much lower than water and fat on T2-weighted imaging.[1,7,11] Normal muscle fascicles are separated from one another by fat-containing septa; normal skeletal muscle has a subtle marbled appearance on non–fat-suppressed images.[8] The water molecules in the collagen fibers found in tendons are not freely mobile resulting in a short T2 relaxation time. Normal tendons display uniformly low signal intensity on all routine MR imaging sequences.[5,12,13]

PATTERNS OF ABNORMAL MR IMAGING SIGNAL INTENSITY IN SKELETAL MUSCLE

MR imaging facilitates the diagnostic process primarily by detecting changes in muscle size or signal intensity. Although these changes can be diagnostic in the appropriate clinical setting, a myriad of focal and systemic pathologic conditions affecting muscle may have a similar appearance and these must be borne in mind when arriving at a diagnosis. In addition to traumatic muscle injuries, common categories of disease affecting muscle include ischemia and necrosis, inflammation and infection, neoplasia, and iatrogenic injury. The recognition of one of three basic patterns on MR imaging simplifies the differential diagnosis approach to muscle injury:[14]

- Muscle edema: most commonly identified and associated with recent trauma (specifically strain injury), and with acute denervation, infectious or autoimmune myositis, vascular insult (diabetic muscle infarction, deep vein thrombosis), or recent iatrogenic insults (surgery, radiation therapy)
- Mass lesion: can been seen post traumatic injury (myositis ossificans), and with neoplasm and infection (bacterial myositis and abscess)
- Fatty infiltration: is observed in the chronic setting after myotendinous injury or chronic denervation

MUSCLE EDEMA PATTERN

Muscle edema can be broadly classified as being secondary to direct muscle injury (traumatic edema); impaired drainage of fluid from muscle (congestive edema); or increased delivery of fluid to the muscle (vasogenic edema).[7]

Traumatic Edema

Traumatic edema can be caused by several mechanisms ranging from a direct blow causing muscle contusion, to distraction or shearing forces causing muscle tears, and overuse injury seen in delayed-onset muscle soreness.[3,15] The underlying mechanism of injury is disruption of capillary vessels with subsequent hemorrhage eliciting an acute inflammatory response with increased permeability of undamaged capillaries and accumulation of interstitial fluid.

Muscle Contusion

This type of injury is caused by a direct blow to the muscle, usually by a blunt object, resulting in injury to the deep layers of the muscle belly as the muscle is compressed against the underlying bone.[13] MR imaging shows focal high signal intensity on fat-suppressed T2-weighted and STIR sequences that often has an indistinct, feathery appearance.[1,14] With sufficient force, focal edema is often accompanied by the development of an intramuscular hematoma, with myonecrosis and myositis ossificans being potential complications.[13] The MR imaging appearance of an intramuscular hematoma depends on the age of the lesion, with acute hematoma isointense to muscle on T1- and hypointense on T2-weighted sequences. As the hematoma becomes subacute, the proportion of extracellular methhemaglobin increases, which results in high signal on T1- and progressively increased signal on T2-weighted sequences. Chronic hematoma is characterized by hemosiderin deposition with consequent low signal on T1- and T2-weighted sequences and blooming artifact on gradient echo imaging.[16] There is often enlargement of the involved muscle but usually no evidence of muscle fiber discontinuity or laxity.[7]

Muscle Laceration

Muscle laceration is caused by a penetrating, sharp instrument, which results in focal, sharply demarcated discontinuity of muscle fibers and focal muscle edema with associated high signal intensity on T2-weighted sequences.[1] Because of the mechanism of injury, hematoma is often present at the site of injury.[17]

Muscle Strain

In the young skeletally mature athlete, the point of maximum weakness in normal skeletal muscle is the myotendinous junction and hence strains and tears arise at this site.[18–22] MR imaging is ideally suited for the evaluation of these injuries and it allows assessment of the entire myotendinous unit in multiple planes.[13] MR imaging has also been shown to be useful in determining the prognosis of muscle strains.[23,24] In one study of 23

injuries to the gastrocnemius, the myotendinous junction was involved in 96% of cases, with the medial head more frequently involved than the lateral head (86% and 14%, respectively).[25] Another study of 15 college athletes showed that acute hamstring injuries occurred at the myotendinous junction in diverse locations: the proximal myotendinous junction (33%); the intramuscular myotendinous junction (53%); and the distal myotendinous junction (13%).[26] Strains tend to occur in muscles that cross two joints; have a high proportion of fast twitch fibers; and undergo eccentric contraction (muscle fibers stretch during contraction).[27] The most commonly strained muscles in the extremities include the hamstrings, rectus femoris, and gastrocnemius muscles.[13,28] A muscle strain or tear is caused by excessive forceful muscle contraction and the degree of strain can be graded along a spectrum of injury from first- to third-degree strains. These grades are used to facilitate communication and to influence patient management.

First-degree strain

This is a mild strain with microscopic injury without identifiable muscle fiber disruption.[1] In the acute setting, MR imaging shows focal high signal intensity on T2-weighted and STIR sequences with muscle edema and hemorrhage at the myotendinous junction. Edema may track along muscle fascicles creating a feathery margin to the lesion (**Figs. 1 and 2**).[8,13,29]

Second-degree strain

This is a moderate strain with a partial-thickness macroscopic tear of the myotendinous junction (**Figs. 3–6**).[8] In the acute setting, this type of injury causes high signal intensity at the myotendinous junction on T2-weighted sequences and a focal hematoma at the myotendinous junction, which is diagnostic.[1,8] In young adults, most hamstring injuries are partial tears with complete hamstring tears or avulsions being relatively uncommon.[30] In another study of 65 patients with "tennis leg" (defined clinically as the sudden onset of sharp pain in the middle portion of the calf while participating in sport[31]), 51 partial and 14 complete tears were diagnosed.[32] Most first- and second-degree strains respond to conservative therapy but this type of injury has a high incidence and recurrence rate among athletes, often leading to a prolonged period out of competition. Early imaging to ascertain the severity of injury is important to guide clinicians as to the anticipated period of convalescence.[33]

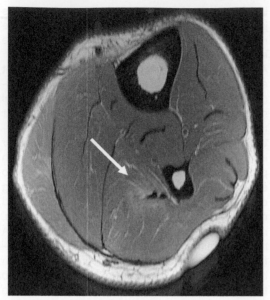

Fig. 1. Axial T1-weighted image of a grade 1 strain of the midbelly of the soleus muscle with characteristic feathery interstitial edema at the site of injury (*arrow*).

Third-degree strain

This is a severe strain with complete disruption of the myotendinous junction with or without muscle retraction (**Fig. 7**).[18] MR imaging shows discontinuity of muscle fibers and if muscle retraction is present, displays enlargement of the retracted muscle with a focal fluid collection filling the gap. Complete muscle tears are usually associated with significant hematoma formation.[8] MR imaging is useful for assessing the extent of tendon retraction for preoperative planning.[13] Third-degree strains usually require early surgical intervention to prevent permanent retraction and scar formation.

Tendon Injury

Tendinosis is a noninflammatory condition of collagen degeneration with disorientation of the collagen bundles, scattered vascular in-growth, and occasional local necrosis or calcification.[12] Athletes can suffer both acute tears and chronic tendon degeneration (tendinosis) secondary to overuse injury,[13] with most acute tears frequently occurring on a background of chronic tendinosis.[34] The most commonly injured tendons are the Achilles and quadriceps tendons.[5] As tendon degeneration progresses, partial or complete tears may occur, and it is at this stage that an inflammatory response may be seen if there is acute hemorrhage with vascular disruption.[35] The MR imaging features of tendinosis include tendon thickening and poorly or well-defined areas of increased signal intensity on short TE sequences (spin echo or gradient echo).[36] In a study of 118 patients with painful Achilles tendon, of the 21 cases of surgically confirmed tendinosis, 20 cases showed abnormally high signal intensity on T1-weighted gradient echo sequences.[37] It can be difficult to differentiate between tendinosis and partial tears on MR imaging; however, as the disease

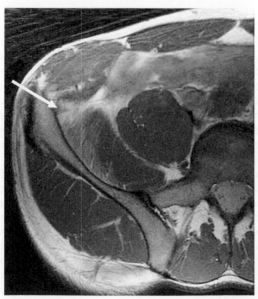

Fig. 2. Axial T1-weighted image showing a grade 1 strain with feathery interstitial edema at the myotendinous junction of the right iliacus (*arrow*).

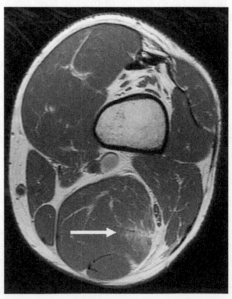

Fig. 3. Axial T1-weighted image of a grade 2 strain of the semimembranosus (*arrow*).

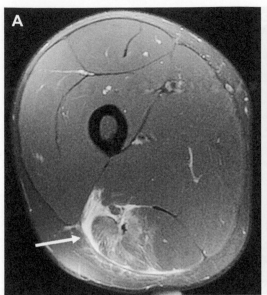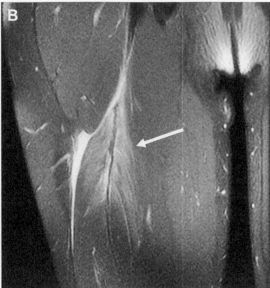

Fig. 4. Axial (*A*) and coronal (*B*) STIR images of a grade 2 strain of the proximal biceps femoris muscle (*arrows*).

progresses high signal on T2-weighted sequences matching the degree of signal intensity of free water is more indicative of a partial tear. Acute complete tendon ruptures are manifest by retraction of the tendon ends with associated intervening high signal hematoma, whereas chronic ruptures commonly display free water between the tendon ends.[38,39]

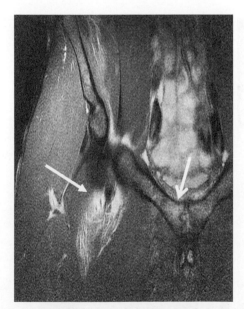

Fig. 5. Coronal STIR image showing a grade 2 strain of the right iliopsoas at the myotendinous junction (*solid arrowhead*). Incidental note is made of osteitis pubis (*pointed arrowhead*).

Delayed-onset of Muscle Soreness

This is a commonly encountered clinical entity characterized by muscle pain and mild swelling, which occurs several hours after unusually vigorous eccentric muscle contraction. The pain and swelling associated with delayed-onset muscle soreness is maximal 24 to 72 hours post-exercise and generally subsides gradually over the following 2 to 3 days.[1,8] It is thought to occur as a result of reversible structural damage at a cellular level in response to exercise with an increase in intracellular fluid secondary to an acute inflammatory reaction.[40–42] MR imaging shows high signal intensity on fat-suppressed T2-weighted and STIR sequences within the affected muscle group.[27] These imaging findings are similar to those seen in a first-degree muscle strain. The only reliable way to differentiate between delayed-onset muscle soreness and muscle strain is through clinical examination or imaging 2 to 3 days after the onset of symptoms when persistent high signal is indicative of a muscle strain.

Avulsion Injuries

Avulsion injuries occur at tendon attachment sites to bone after excessive muscle contraction or lengthening.[13] The age of a patient influences the location of injuries in the muscle-tendon-enthesis complex.[43] In children and adolescents (skeletally immature individuals), the point of maximal weakness in this chain tends to be the unfused apophysis, rather than the myotendinous junction.[44–47] Apophyseal avulsion injuries result from the same

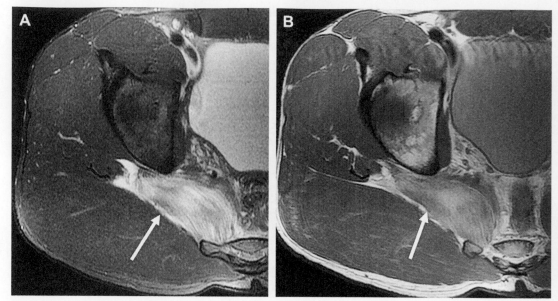

Fig. 6. Axial STIR (*A*) and axial T1-weighted (*B*) images of a grade 2 strain of the belly of the right piriformis (*arrows*).

mechanism of injury that results in a myotendinous injury in a skeletally mature athlete. Acute avulsion injuries result from extreme, unbalanced, and often eccentric muscle contractions and patients present with severe pain, swelling over the area, and loss of function with a definite history of a traumatic event.[13,43] In contrast, chronic avulsion injuries are the result of repetitive microtrauma or overuse and there is usually a lack of a single episode of trauma.[48] Healing chronic avulsion injuries can mimic an aggressive osseous lesion radiographically, with areas of osteolysis and heterotopic bone formation and are often mistaken for osteomyelitis, osteosarcoma, or Ewing sarcoma. A thorough clinical history and knowledge of the various tendon attachments and

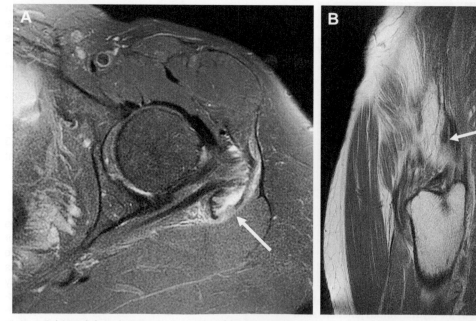

Fig. 7. Axial STIR (*A*) and sagittal T1-weighted (*B*) images showing a grade 3 strain of the distal attachment of the left gluteus medius (*arrows*).

common sites of chronic avulsion injury is necessary to avoid misinterpreting an old avulsion fracture as a more aggressive lesion and to avoid biopsy.[8,49,50]

The single most common site of apophyseal avulsion is the ischial tuberosity (attachment of the hamstring muscles and the hamstring portion of adductor magnus[51]); this injury tends to occur between the onset of puberty and age 25 years.[47,49] Radiographs are usually adequate to diagnose an apophyseal avulsion injury because they demonstrate displacement of the unfused apophysis; however, findings may be subtle and comparison with the opposite side may be helpful in confirming the diagnosis.[52] In the acute setting, MR imaging can be very useful in identifying minimally displaced or nondisplaced apophyseal injuries by showing

signal hyperintensity consistent with traumatic edema in the apophyseal marrow or between the apophysis and the parent bone, indicating a minimally displaced fracture. MR imaging also demonstrates the extent of soft tissue injury, such as muscle strain, which is recognized by the presence of fluid and traumatic edema tracking along the adjacent soft tissue planes near the level of muscle attachment (Figs. 8 and 9).[13,26,52,53] MR imaging of an older, healing avulsion injury may demonstrate a prominent osseous attachment site, callus formation, heterotopic bone formation, or possibly thickening of the tendon at the level of attachment; however, there should be no evidence of an osseous destructive lesion.[47,52] As such, T1 signal of the marrow should be normal, with no findings of a marrow infiltrative process.

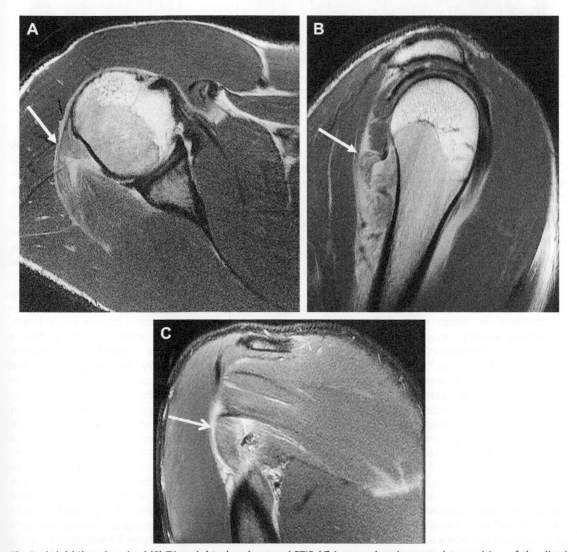

Fig. 8. Axial (A) and sagittal (B) T1-weighted and coronal STIR (C) images showing complete avulsion of the distal attachment of teres minor (arrow).

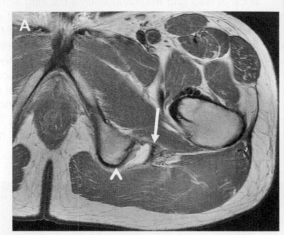
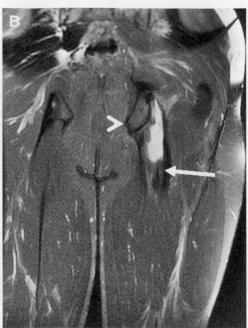

Fig. 9. Axial T1-weighted (*A*) and coronal STIR (*B*) images showing complete nonosseous avulsion (*arrow*) of the origin of the conjoint tendon (from which the semitendinosus and long head of biceps femoris arise) from the ischial tuberosity (*arrowhead*).

Congestive Edema

Congestive edema is caused by impaired exit of interstitial fluid from the muscle capillary bed and arises secondary to cellular swelling or venous hypertension. The net result is an accumulation of fluid in the extracellular space.[7] This form of muscle edema is a feature of compartment syndromes and traumatic denervation of muscle.

Compartment Syndromes

Compartment syndrome may be defined as a condition in which increased pressure in a confined anatomic space adversely affects the circulation and threatens the function and viability of the contained tissues.[54] Acute and less severe chronic subtypes are seen. Direct trauma, burns, excessive exercise, extrinsic compression, or intramuscular hemorrhage may initiate a vicious cycle of increased pressure within the containing fascia that leads to venous occlusion, muscle and nerve ischemia, arterial occlusion, and ultimately tissue necrosis.[55,56] Acute compartment syndrome usually occurs in young adults after an acute traumatic insult and is commonly, but not exclusively, seen associated with a fracture. The most important clinical symptoms of acute compartment syndrome are pain out of proportion to that expected from the traumatic injury and exacerbation of pain on passive stretching of the

affected muscle group.[57] The condition is a surgical emergency requiring surgical exploration and fasciotomy, and MR imaging is only indicated when the diagnosis is in doubt or to identify the involved muscle compartments to assist operative management.[8] The MR imaging findings are petechial hemorrhage in the affected muscles on T1-weighted images, diffuse muscle edema on T2-weighted images, and enlargement of the affected compartments.[1,57]

Chronic compartment syndrome may arise secondary to exertional causes (exercise or repetitive strain) or nonexertional causes (mass lesion or infection). Chronic exertional compartment syndrome is commonly encountered in athletes and the most frequently affected areas are the anterior and lateral compartments of the leg, with the thigh, forearm, and foot less commonly affected.[8,56] Clinically, patients present with pain that is throbbing or cramp-like in nature that is exacerbated by palpation or passive stretching of the affected muscles. Although clinical examination and direct intracompartmental pressure measurement remain the gold standard for the diagnosis of chronic exertional compartment syndrome, MR imaging is a very useful adjunct.[8,55,58,59] MR imaging shows transient increased signal intensity on T2-weighted imaging after exercise, which persists for at least 15 to 20 minutes after cessation of activity. The patient is asked to exercise until their symptoms are reproduced and they are imaged immediately. The increased signal intensity is confined to the musculature of the involved compartment and represents increased extracellular fluid with affected muscles becoming swollen when compared with the unaffected limb (**Fig. 10**).[14,56,59] In chronic compartment syndrome, affected muscles may develop fascial thickening, atrophy, and fibrosis leading to a loss of muscle bulk with fatty infiltration and a consequent increase in signal intensity on T1-weighted imaging.[56]

Acute and Subacute Muscle Denervation

The enhanced muscle bulk of the performance athlete may cause entrapment neuropathy with a sudden loss of muscle contractility in the acutely denervated muscle following nerve entrapment. An example of this type of injury is suprascapular nerve syndrome, which is commonly found in athletes who overuse their arm over their head, such as tennis and volleyball players, leading to atrophy of the supraspinatus and infraspinatus muscles.[60–63] Other common causes of nerve

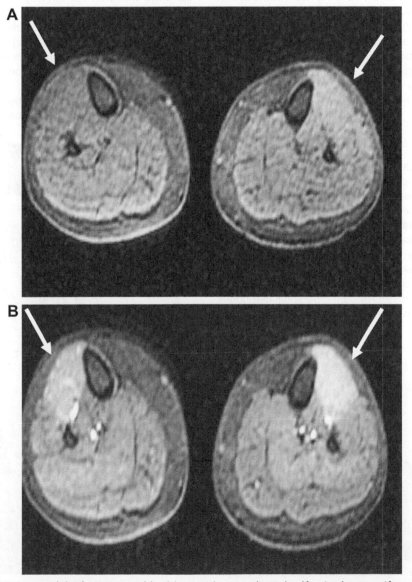

Fig. 10. Axial STIR images (*A*) of a 26-year-old athlete with anterolateral calf pain shows uniform muscle signal pre-exercise (*arrows*). Axial STIR images (*B*) of the same patient postexercise showing high signal intensity in the peroneal compartment indicating chronic exertional compartment syndrome (*arrows*).

injury include traumatic laceration; iatrogenic insult; or neural inflammation (neuritis). The absence of contractility impedes extracellular fluid egression and ultimately leads to congestive muscle edema with high signal intensity on T2- and normal signal intensity on T1-weighted sequences (**Fig. 11**).[64,65] This MR imaging appearance develops within days to weeks of neural injury and is the characteristic imaging feature of acutely denervated muscle.[65–67] There are three distinct imaging features that may help distinguish the high signal on T2-weighted sequences associated with acute and subacute denervation from that seen with strained muscles:[68] (1) unlike strain injury, high signal on T2-weighted sequences in denervated muscle is not associated with perifascial edema; (2) the pattern of muscle involvement may suggest a specific nerve distribution responsible for the denervation changes; and (3) abnormally high signal in a peripheral nerve suggests a nerve injury rather than a muscle strain as the etiology of the abnormal signal change.

Vasogenic Edema

Vasogenic edema is caused by increased local blood flow and permeability of capillaries caused by the presence of inflammatory chemokines released in response to inflammation or infection.[69] This leads to an accumulation of extracellular fluid in muscle with resultant signal hyperintensity on T2-weighted sequences. Although inflammatory myopathies and bacterial myositis are uncommon in the athlete, they are considered here as relevant differential diagnoses for sudden-onset muscle pain, tenderness, and weakness.[70]

Polymyositis and dermatomyositis are idiopathic inflammatory myopathies caused by an autoimmune cell-mediated (type 4) hypersensitivity reaction to skeletal muscle in the affected individual.[71] Patients present with gradual muscle weakness initially affecting the muscles of the thighs and pelvic girdle and progressing to involve the upper extremities, neck flexors, and pharyngeal musculature.[72] MR imaging at presentation is characterized by bilateral, symmetric high signal intensity on fat-suppressed T2-weighted sequences within the involved musculature and perimuscular edema.[73–75] The magnitude of abnormal signal intensity has been shown to correlate well with the severity of the underlying disease.[76] Individuals in whom dermatomyositis is the underlying disorder display conspicuous subcutaneous edema on T2-weighted sequences in addition to muscle edema; this is in contrast to patients with polymyositis in whom subcutaneous edema is absent (**Fig. 12**).[76]

Bacterial myositis can occur in healthy individuals partaking in strenuous physical exercise.[70,77]

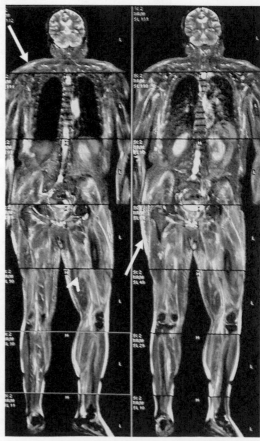

Fig. 12. Whole-body fat-suppressed MR imaging showing diffuse subcutaneous (*arrows*) and muscle edema (*arrowhead*) typical of dermatomyositis.

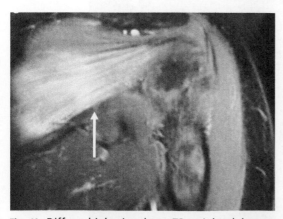

Fig. 11. Diffuse high signal on T2-weighted images consistent with congestive edema throughout the infraspinatus muscle (*arrow*) secondary to acute brachial neuritis or Parsonage Turner syndrome.

Bacterial myositis may result from direct spread of infection from adjacent tissues, such as osteomyelitis or a subcutaneous abscess, with *Staphylococcus aureus* the likely causative organism.[77,78] The lower limb is typically affected, with the most common pattern of disease being a solitary abscess in the quadriceps musculature.[79] The presence of an infective agent leads to the release of inflammatory chemokines with subsequent increased blood flow and capillary permeability in the affected muscles with resultant extracellular fluid accumulation. The MR imaging appearance of early stage bacterial myositis is of high signal intensity on T2-weighted sequences; however, progression to abscess formation with involvement of adjacent soft tissues and bone is frequent. In this setting the high T1 signal of normal bone marrow is lost and postgadolinium T1-weighted sequences display a rim-enhancing mass with high signal intensity in the surrounding soft tissues and marrow.[79] Because there is often a significant delay in establishing the diagnosis and in view of the high morbidity associated with this condition, early MR imaging to detect, localize, and define the extent of disease is essential to a successful outcome.[77–79]

Necrosis of skeletal muscle is commonly associated with diabetes and alcoholism; however, its pathogenesis remains unknown and it is often considered idiopathic.[80–82] Myonecrosis usually presents with sudden onset of a focal, tender mass in skeletal muscle in the absence of a causative insult, such as ischemia, trauma, infection, or neoplasia.[83] Management involves conservative treatment with rest and immobilization. Early diagnosis is essential to avoid unnecessary

interventions, such as excision biopsy (to exclude neoplasia) or debridement.[81,82] MR imaging is the diagnostic imaging modality of choice because of its excellent soft tissue contrast. T1-weighted imaging of myonecrosis demonstrates isointense swelling of the involved muscles with mildly displaced fascial planes and a loss of muscle fiber definition, whereas fat-suppressed T2-weighted imaging demonstrates diffuse, heterogenous high signal intensity in the muscle indicative of edema with postcontrast imaging demonstrating a mass with peripheral enhancement and central nonenhancing areas consistent with necrotic muscle.[83,84]

MASS LESION PATTERN

In the mass lesion pattern, a localized mass with morphology and signal intensity different than those of normal muscle is found on all sequences, also demonstrating enhancement following contrast administration. This pattern, however, is nonspecific and hence may be seen in a wide range of conditions, such as neoplasia,[85] intramuscular abscess,[74] traumatic injury,[3,15] and myositis ossificans. It is beyond the scope of this article to discuss the tumors that may occur in skeletal muscle.

Tumor-induced Edema

Tumor-induced edema is caused by an acute inflammatory response elicited in adjacent muscle by both benign and malignant lesions, which may reflect muscle edema, tumor invasion, or both (Fig. 13).[86] MR imaging displays high signal intensity on T2-weighted sequences; however, the presence or absence of this finding does not allow

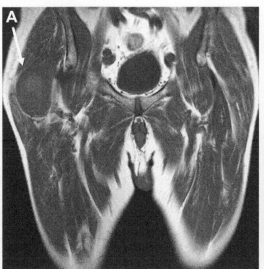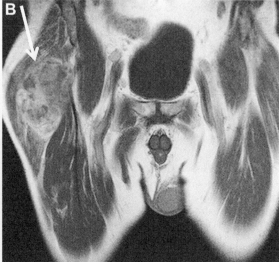

Fig. 13. Coronal T1-weighted images precontrast (*A*) and postcontrast (*B*) showing heterogenous enhancement of a rhabdomyosarcoma of the proximal right thigh musculature (*arrows*).

reliable distinction between benign and malignant lesions, nor does it allow assessment of the true location of the tumor margins (**Fig. 14**).[85] Where extensive edema is associated with a muscle mass, then abscess, hematoma, and myositis ossificans should be strongly considered in the differential diagnosis.[87]

Myositis Ossificans

Myositis ossificans is a form of heterotopic ossification that occurs in muscle. Common predisposing factors include trauma (contusion, burns, or surgery); neural injury (paraplegia or traumatic denervation); and bleeding dyscrasias (hemophilia).[88,89] There are three distinct phases of evolution of myositis ossificans: (1) an acute or pseudoinflammatory phase, (2) a subacute or pseudotumoral phase, and (3) a chronic self-limited phase that often undergoes spontaneous resolution.[90] In the acute and subacute phases of maturation, MR imaging findings are nonspecific because the involved muscle is enlarged and exhibits intermediate signal intensity on T1- and high signal intensity on T2-weighted sequences with rim enhancement of the lesion and high signal intensity in adjacent muscle on postcontrast T1-weighted sequences, appearances similar to abscess or

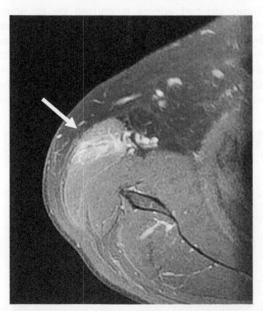

Fig. 14. Postgadolinium T1-weighted image showing diffuse high signal intensity in the right latissimus dorsi muscle (*arrow*), which was initially thought to be caused by a muscle strain; however, the clinical history of a rapidly enlarging mass was not supportive of this diagnosis and a malignant lesion was suspected. Subsequent percutaneous biopsy yielded the diagnosis of nodular fasciitis. (*Courtesy of* Dr. Peter Dunn, Exact Radiology, Qld, Australia.)

necrotic tumor.[91–94] In the chronic phase of maturation, there is fatty change within a well-defined, sharply marginated mass visible on T1-weighted sequences with a thin rim of calcification surrounding the lesion.[93,95] As the lesion matures, the rim of calcification becomes considerably thickened and the lesion appears heterogeneous with areas of T2 hyperintensity and contrast enhancement progressively decreasing and a corresponding increase in areas of signal intensity equivalent to fat and cortical bone.[96,97]

Hematoma

Hematomas are a common occurrence after a muscle strain or laceration and are predominantly intramuscular in location. They are typically heterogeneous in appearance and subacute hematomas display moderately increased signal intensity on T1- and high signal intensity on T2-weighted sequences because of the presence of methemaglobin.[1] Muscle hematomas typically resolve completely in 6 to 8 weeks; however, after the blood products have resorbed, a seroma with fluid signal intensity may develop and persist.[27] An intramuscular hematoma has a masslike appearance and differentiation on MR imaging between a simple hematoma and a hemorrhagic tumor can be difficult.[3,98] The administration of intravenous gadolinium aids diagnosis by displaying a lack of enhancement of the lesion on T1-weighted sequences, making tumor less likely.[99] It is important to remember, however, that the absence of central enhancement does not allow the exclusion of a neoplasm because central necrosis or an avascular tumor may be present.[85] It is important to image the patient promptly after contrast administration because gadolinium may slowly diffuse into a fluid-filled space, such as a hematoma, and give the false impression of a solid enhancing mass.[14,100]

FATTY INFILTRATION PATTERN

Fatty infiltration involves the abnormal deposition of fat within a muscle. It is the final common pathway in many pathologic conditions that affect skeletal muscle, such as chronic disuse, chronic denervation, and chronic tendon tear, and it is usually seen in association with muscle atrophy.[14,101] The MR imaging features of muscle atrophy are increased signal on T1-weighted sequences because of fatty degeneration or muscle volume loss.[65] Muscle fibrosis is a recognized sequela of myotendinous injury and displays low signal intensity on T2- and high signal intensity on T1-weighted sequences after a subacute insult.[102–104] Common sites of muscle fibrosis include the deltoid (in association with intramuscular injections)[103,104] and the vastus lateralis muscles (associated with recurrent patellar dislocation).[102] Chronic denervation results in fatty infiltration with consequent high signal intensity on T1-weighted sequences and loss of muscle bulk.[65,101] Although the signal intensity changes of acute and subacute denervation are reversible, the profound atrophic changes seen late in the course of denervation are typically irreversible.[101,105]

Phosphorus MR Spectroscopy in the Evaluation of Muscle Injury

Phosphorus MR spectroscopy (^{31}P-MRS) is a noninvasive and reproducible test that can be used to determine concentrations of various chemical compounds in skeletal muscle. ^{31}P-MRS measurements of skeletal muscle can be used to obtain intracellular concentrations of ATP, phosphocreatine (PCr), and inorganic phosphate (Pi).

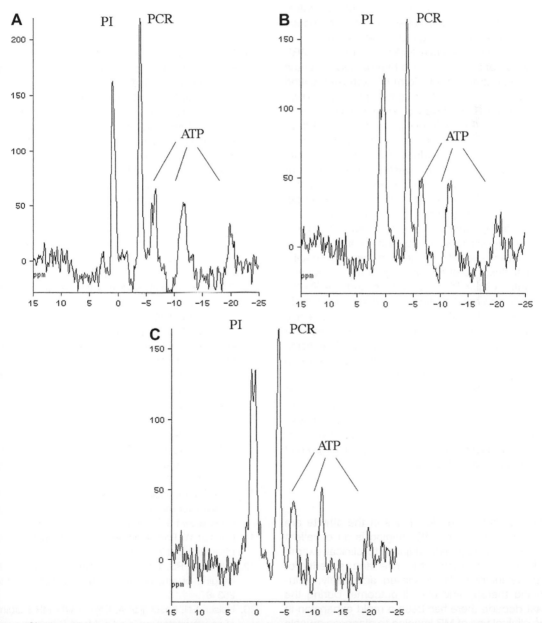

Fig. 15. ^{31}P-MR spectroscopy of skeletal muscle pre-exercise (*A*), after 3 minutes (*B*), and 5 minutes (*C*) exercise. As exercise progresses there is a reduction in the intracellular concentration of phosphocreatine (PCR), with an increase in the intracellular concentration of inorganic phosphate (Pi). The intracellular concentration of adenosine triphosphate (ATP) remains stable throughout exercise.

ATP is the universal energy source in skeletal muscle and the intracellular concentration of ATP is maintained by the breakdown of PCr; as exercise progresses, the concentration of Pi increases and PCr decreases (**Fig. 15**).[106,107] In resting skeletal muscle, the ratio of Pi/PCr is very low, but with increasing levels of activity the Pi/PCr ratio increases as ATP is consumed (with a consequent increase in intracellular Pi concentrations) to provide energy for oxidative metabolism.[106] This ratio provides a simple reflection of the level of oxidative metabolism in muscle.[108] Muscle intracellular pH can be calculated from the frequency shift of the Pi peak using PCr as reference.[106]

Several studies have looked at the ^{31}P-MRS response of skeletal muscle to repeated eccentric muscle contraction; this form of exercise resulted in mild muscle pain that lasted for several days and ^{31}P-MRS displayed a sustained increase in the resting Pi/PCr ratio that lasted for several days postexercise, eventually returning to pre-exercise levels.[106,107,109–111] This indicates that muscle injury caused a small increase in resting muscle metabolism.[106] A recent study performed ^{31}P-MRS, three-dimensional MR imaging, and isometric strength testing on healthy subjects and patients with an ankle fracture after 7 weeks of immobilization and during physical rehabilitation. After immobilization, there was a significant decrease in the specific plantar flexor torque and a significant increase in the intracellular Pi concentration and the Pi/PCr ratio. During rehabilitation, both the intracellular Pi content and the Pi/PCr ratio decreased and specific torque increased, approaching control values after 10 weeks of physical rehabilitation. Regression analysis showed an inverse relationship between the intracellular Pi concentration and specific torque.[112] ^{31}P-MRS affords the sports medicine physician the ability to monitor noninvasively the metabolism of injured and recovering muscle, providing a valuable tool to understand exercise-induced muscle injury better and objectively predict when return to play is appropriate.

SUMMARY

Although most muscle injuries in the athlete are diagnosed clinically, MR imaging is an excellent noninvasive diagnostic adjunct to clinical examination, which allows the site and severity of muscle injury to be assessed accurately, influencing therapy and overall outcome. During the past decade there has been a rapid expansion in the clinical use of MR imaging to diagnose muscle injuries. MR imaging conveys unparalleled anatomic resolution and high sensitivity in the detection of acute and chronic muscle abnormalities. In traumatic muscle conditions, such as chronic exertional compartment syndrome and acute denervation, the findings on clinical examination are often subtle or absent and MR imaging is essential in arriving at the correct diagnosis. This article describes the spectrum of exercise-induced muscle injury and emphasizes the central role that MR imaging and MR spectroscopy play in the diagnosis and management of acute and chronic muscle injury.

REFERENCES

1. Elsayes KM, Lammle M, Shariff A, et al. Value of magnetic resonance imaging in muscle trauma. Curr Probl Diagn Radiol 2006;35(5):206–12.
2. Linklater J, Potter HG. Emergent musculoskeletal magnetic resonance imaging. Top Magn Reson Imaging 1998;9(4):238–60.
3. Palmer WE, Kuong SJ, Elmadbouh HM. MR imaging of myotendinous strain. AJR Am J Roentgenol 1999;173(3):703–9.
4. Koulouris G, Connell D. Hamstring muscle complex: an imaging review. Radiographics 2005; 25(3):571–86.
5. Ahn JM, El-Khoury GY. Role of magnetic resonance imaging in musculoskeletal trauma. Top Magn Reson Imaging 2007;18(3):155–68.
6. Bencardino JT, Rosenberg ZS, Brown RR, et al. Traumatic musculotendinous injuries of the knee: diagnosis with MR imaging. Radiographics 2000; 20(Spec No):S103–20.
7. Napier N, Shortt C, Eustace S. Muscle edema: classification, mechanisms, and interpretation. Semin Musculoskelet Radiol 2006;10(4):258–67.
8. Rybak LD, Torriani M. Magnetic resonance imaging of sports-related muscle injuries. Top Magn Reson Imaging 2003;14(2):209–19.
9. Warfield SK, Mulkern RV, Winalski CS, et al. An image processing strategy for the quantification and visualization of exercise-induced muscle MRI signal enhancement. J Magn Reson Imaging 2000;11(5):525–31.
10. Snell RS. Introduction. In: Snell RS, editor. Clinical anatomy for medical students. 5th edition. Boston: Little, Brown & Company; 1995. p. 1–45.
11. Dahnert W. Radiology review manual. 6th edition. Philadelphia: Lippincott Williams & Wilkins; 2007.
12. Campbell RS, Grainger AJ. Current concepts in imaging of tendinopathy. Clin Radiol 2001;56(4): 253–67.
13. Nelson EN, Kassarjian A, Palmer WE. MR imaging of sports-related groin pain. Magn Reson Imaging Clin N Am 2005;13(4):727–42.
14. May DA, Disler DG, Jones EA, et al. Abnormal signal intensity in skeletal muscle at MR imaging:

patterns, pearls, and pitfalls. Radiographics 2000; 20(Spec No):S295–315.

15. De Smet AA. Magnetic resonance findings in skeletal muscle tears. Skeletal Radiol 1993;22(7): 479–84.

16. Bencardino JT, Kassarjian A, Palmer WE. Magnetic resonance imaging of the hip: sports-related injuries. Top Magn Reson Imaging 2003;14(2):145–60.

17. Bordalo-Rodrigues M, Rosenberg ZS. MR imaging of the proximal rectus femoris musculotendinous unit. Magn Reson Imaging Clin N Am 2005;13(4): 717–25.

18. Speer KP, Lohnes J, Garrett WE Jr. Radiographic imaging of muscle strain injury. Am J Sports Med 1993;21(1):89–95 [discussion: 96].

19. Noonan TJ, Garrett WE Jr. Muscle strain injury: diagnosis and treatment. J Am Acad Orthop Surg 1999;7(4):262–9.

20. Noonan TJ, Garrett WE Jr. Injuries at the myotendinous junction. Clin Sports Med 1992;11(4): 783–806.

21. Kirkendall DT, Garrett WE Jr. Clinical perspectives regarding eccentric muscle injury. Clin Orthop Relat Res 2002;(403 Suppl):S81–9.

22. Hasselman CT, Best TM, Seaber AV, et al. A threshold and continuum of injury during active stretch of rabbit skeletal muscle. Am J Sports Med 1995;23(1):65–73.

23. Pomeranz SJ, Heidt RS Jr. MR imaging in the prognostication of hamstring injury. Work in progress. Radiology 1993;189(3):897–900.

24. Koulouris G, Connell D. Evaluation of the hamstring muscle complex following acute injury. Skeletal Radiol 2003;32(10):582–9.

25. Weishaupt D, Schweitzer ME, Morrison WB. Injuries to the distal gastrocnemius muscle: MR findings. J Comput Assist Tomogr 2001;25(5):677–82.

26. De Smet AA, Best TM. MR imaging of the distribution and location of acute hamstring injuries in athletes. AJR Am J Roentgenol 2000;174(2):393–9.

27. El-Khoury GY, Brandser EA, Kathol MH, et al. Imaging of muscle injuries. Skeletal Radiol 1996; 25(1):3–11.

28. Koulouris G, Ting AY, Jhamb A, et al. Magnetic resonance imaging findings of injuries to the calf muscle complex. Skeletal Radiol 2007;36(10): 921–7.

29. Nguyen B, Brandser E, Rubin DA. Pains, strains, and fasciculations: lower extremity muscle disorders. Magn Reson Imaging Clin N Am 2000;8(2): 391–408.

30. Kujala UM, Orava S, Jarvinen M. Hamstring injuries: current trends in treatment and prevention. Sports Med 1997;23(6):397–404.

31. Delgado GJ, Chung CB, Lektrakul N, et al. Tennis leg: clinical US study of 141 patients and anatomic investigation of four cadavers with MR imaging and US. Radiology 2002;224(1):112–9.

32. Bianchi S, Martinoli C, Abdelwahab IF, et al. Sonographic evaluation of tears of the gastrocnemius medial head (tennis leg). J Ultrasound Med 1998; 17(3):157–62.

33. Koulouris G, Connell D. Imaging of hamstring injuries: therapeutic implications. Eur Radiol 2006; 16(7):1478–87.

34. Maffulli N, Khan KM, Puddu G. Overuse tendon conditions: time to change a confusing terminology. Arthroscopy 1998;14(8):840–3.

35. Khan KM, Maffulli N, Coleman BD, et al. Patellar tendinopathy: some aspects of basic science and clinical management. Br J Sports Med 1998; 32(4):346–55.

36. Weatherall PT, Crues III JV. Musculotendinous injury. Magn Reson Imaging Clin N Am 1995;3(4): 753–72.

37. Karjalainen PT, Soila K, Aronen HJ, et al. MR imaging of overuse injuries of the Achilles tendon. AJR Am J Roentgenol 2000;175(1):251–60.

38. Ohashi K, El-Khoury GY, Albright JP, et al. MRI of complete rupture of the pectoralis major muscle. Skeletal Radiol 1996;25(7):625–8.

39. Kijowski R, Tuite M, Sanford M. Magnetic resonance imaging of the elbow. Part II: abnormalities of the ligaments, tendons, and nerves. Skeletal Radiol 2005;34(1):1–18.

40. Cheung K, Hume P, Maxwell L. Delayed onset muscle soreness: treatment strategies and performance factors. Sports Med 2003;33(2):145–64.

41. MacIntyre DL, Reid WD, McKenzie DC. Delayed muscle soreness: the inflammatory response to muscle injury and its clinical implications. Sports Med 1995;20(1):24–40.

42. Smith LL. Acute inflammation: the underlying mechanism in delayed onset muscle soreness? Med Sci Sports Exerc 1991;23(5):542–51.

43. EL-Khoury GY, Daniel WW, Kathol MH. Acute and chronic avulsive injuries. Radiol Clin North Am 1997;35(3):747–66.

44. Fernbach SK, Wilkinson RH. Avulsion injuries of the pelvis and proximal femur. AJR Am J Roentgenol 1981;137(3):581–4.

45. Anderson K, Strickland SM, Warren R. Hip and groin injuries in athletes. Am J Sports Med 2001; 29(4):521–33.

46. Kocher MS, Tucker R. Pediatric athlete hip disorders. Clin Sports Med 2006;25(2):241–53, viii.

47. Stevens MA, El-Khoury GY, Kathol MH, et al. Imaging features of avulsion injuries. Radiographics 1999;19(3):655–72.

48. Micheli LJ, Fehlandt AF Jr. Overuse injuries to tendons and apophyses in children and adolescents. Clin Sports Med 1992;11(4):713–26.

49. Sanders TG, Zlatkin MB. Avulsion injuries of the pelvis. Semin Musculoskelet Radiol 2008;12(1):42–53.

50. Metzmaker JN, Pappas AM. Avulsion fractures of the pelvis. Am J Sports Med 1985;13(5):349–58.

51. Snell RS. The lower limb. In: Snell RS, editor. Clinical anatomy for medical students. 5th edition. Boston: Little, Brown & Company; 1995. p. 509–630.

52. Pisacano RM, Miller TT. Comparing sonography with MR imaging of apophyseal injuries of the pelvis in four boys. AJR Am J Roentgenol 2003; 181(1):223–30.

53. Slavotinek JP, Verrall GM, Fon GT. Hamstring injury in athletes: using MR imaging measurements to compare extent of muscle injury with amount of time lost from competition. AJR Am J Roentgenol 2002;179(6):1621–8.

54. Stedman TL. Stedman's medical dictionary. 27th edition. Philadelphia: Lippincott, Williams & Wilkins; 2000.

55. Wood GW. General principles of fracture treatment. In: Canale ST, editor. Campbell's operative orthopedics. 11th edition. Philadelphia: Mosby; 2007. 2669–724.

56. Verleisdonk EJ. The exertional compartment syndrome: a review of the literature. Ortop Traumatol Rehabil 2002;4(5):626–31.

57. Elliott KG, Johnstone AJ. Diagnosing acute compartment syndrome. J Bone Joint Surg Br 2003;85(5):625–32.

58. van den Brand JG, Nelson T, Verleisdonk EJ, et al. The diagnostic value of intracompartmental pressure measurement, magnetic resonance imaging, and near-infrared spectroscopy in chronic exertional compartment syndrome: a prospective study in 50 patients. Am J Sports Med 2005; 33(5):699–704.

59. Verleisdonk EJ, van Gils A, van der Werken C. The diagnostic value of MRI scans for the diagnosis of chronic exertional compartment syndrome of the lower leg. Skeletal Radiol 2001; 30(6):321–5.

60. Bredella MA, Tirman PF, Fritz RC, et al. Denervation syndromes of the shoulder girdle: MR imaging with electrophysiologic correlation. Skeletal Radiol 1999;28(10):567–72.

61. Beltran J, Rosenberg ZS. Nerve entrapment. Semin Musculoskelet Radiol 1998;2(2):175–84.

62. Beltran J, Rosenberg ZS. Diagnosis of compressive and entrapment neuropathies of the upper extremity: value of MR imaging. AJR Am J Roentgenol 1994;163(3):525–31.

63. Rosenberg ZS, Bencardino J, Beltran J. MR features of nerve disorders at the elbow. Magn Reson Imaging Clin N Am 1997;5(3):545–65.

64. Helms CA, Martinez S, Speer KP. Acute brachial neuritis (Parsonage-Turner syndrome): MR imaging appearance–report of three cases. Radiology 1998;207(1):255–9.

65. Kamath S, Venkatanarasimha N, Walsh MA, et al. MRI appearance of muscle denervation. Skeletal Radiol 2008;37(5):397–404.

66. Misamore GW, Lehman DE. Parsonage-Turner syndrome (acute brachial neuritis). J Bone Joint Surg Am 1996;78(9):1405–8.

67. Kikuchi Y, Nakamura T, Takayama S, et al. MR imaging in the diagnosis of denervated and reinnervated skeletal muscles: experimental study in rats. Radiology 2003;229(3):861–7.

68. Fritz RC, Boutin RD. Magnetic resonance imaging of the peripheral nervous system. Phys Med Rehabil Clin N Am 2001;12(2):399–432.

69. Acute and chronic inflammation. In: Cotran R, editor. Robbin's pathologic basis of disease. 6th edition. Philadelphia: WB Saunders; 1998. p. 50–88.

70. Meehan J, Grose C, Soper RT, et al. Pyomyositis in an adolescent female athlete. J Pediatr Surg 1995; 30(1):127–8.

71. Creus KK, De Paepe B, De Bleecker JL. Idiopathic inflammatory myopathies and the classical NF-kappaB complex: current insights and implications for therapy. Autoimmun Rev 2009;8(7):627–31.

72. Rheumatology and bone disease. In: Kumar P, editor. Clinical medicine. 6th edition. London: Saunders; 2005.

73. Reimers CD, Schedel H, Fleckenstein JL, et al. Magnetic resonance imaging of skeletal muscles in idiopathic inflammatory myopathies of adults. J Neurol 1994;241(5):306–14.

74. Fleckenstein JL, Reimers CD. Inflammatory myopathies: radiologic evaluation. Radiol Clin North Am 1996;34(2):427–39, xii.

75. Hernandez RJ, Keim DR, Chenevert TL, et al. Fat-suppressed MR imaging of myositis. Radiology 1992;182(1):217–9.

76. Hernandez RJ, Sullivan DB, Chenevert TL, et al. MR imaging in children with dermatomyositis: musculoskeletal findings and correlation with clinical and laboratory findings. AJR Am J Roentgenol 1993;161(2):359–66.

77. Block AA, Marshall C, Ratcliffe A, et al. Staphylococcal pyomyositis in a temperate region: epidemiology and modern management. Med J Aust 2008; 189(6):323–5.

78. Tsirantonaki M, Michael P, Koufos C. Pyomyositis. Clin Rheumatol 1998;17(4):333–4.

79. Theodorou SJ, Theodorou DJ, Resnick D. MR imaging findings of pyogenic bacterial myositis (pyomyositis) in patients with local muscle trauma: illustrative cases. Emerg Radiol 2007;14(2):89–96.

80. Bjornskov EK, Carry MR, Katz FH, et al. Diabetic muscle infarction: a new perspective on pathogenesis and management. Neuromuscul Disord 1995; 5(1):39–45.

81. Khoury NJ, EL-Khoury GY, Kathol MH. MRI diagnosis of diabetic muscle infarction: report of two cases. Skeletal Radiol 1997;26(2):122–7.

82. Kiers L. Diabetic muscle infarction: magnetic resonance imaging (MRI) avoids the need for biopsy. Muscle Nerve 1995;18(1):129–30.

83. Kattapuram TM, Suri R, Rosol MS, et al. Idiopathic and diabetic skeletal muscle necrosis: evaluation by magnetic resonance imaging. Skeletal Radiol 2005;34(4):203–9.

84. Jelinek JS, Murphey MD, Aboulafia AJ, et al. Muscle infarction in patients with diabetes mellitus: MR imaging findings. Radiology 1999;211(1): 241–7.

85. May DA, Good RB, Smith DK, et al. MR imaging of musculoskeletal tumors and tumor mimickers with intravenous gadolinium: experience with 242 patients. Skeletal Radiol 1997;26(1):2–15.

86. Beltran J, Simon DC, Katz W, et al. Increased MR signal intensity in skeletal muscle adjacent to malignant tumors: pathologic correlation and clinical relevance. Radiology 1987;162(1 Pt 1): 251–5.

87. Weatherall P. Imaging of muscle tumors. Semin Musculoskelet Radiol 2000;4(4):435–58.

88. Beiner JM, Jokl P. Muscle contusion injury and myositis ossificans traumatica. Clin Orthop Relat Res 2002;(403 Suppl):S110–9.

89. McCarthy EF, Sundaram M. Heterotopic ossification: a review. Skeletal Radiol 2005;34(10):609–19.

90. Gould CF, Ly JQ, Lattin GE Jr, et al. Bone tumor mimics: avoiding misdiagnosis. Curr Probl Diagn Radiol 2007;36(3):124–41.

91. Shirkhoda A, Armin AR, Bis KG, et al. MR imaging of myositis ossificans: variable patterns at different stages. J Magn Reson Imaging 1995;5(3):287–92.

92. De Smet AA, Norris MA, Fisher DR. Magnetic resonance imaging of myositis ossificans: analysis of seven cases. Skeletal Radiol 1992;21(8):503–7.

93. Kransdorf MJ, Meis JM, Jelinek JS. Myositis ossificans: MR appearance with radiologic-pathologic correlation. AJR Am J Roentgenol 1991;157(6): 1243–8.

94. Crundwell N, O'Donnell P, Saifuddin A. Non-neoplastic conditions presenting as soft-tissue tumours. Clin Radiol 2007;62(1):18–27.

95. McKenzie G, Raby N, Ritchie D. Non-neoplastic soft-tissue masses. Br J Radiol 2008.

96. Ledermann HP, Schweitzer ME, Morrison WB. Pelvic heterotopic ossification: MR imaging characteristics. Radiology 2002;222(1):189–95.

97. Parikh J, Hyare H, Saifuddin A. The imaging features of post-traumatic myositis ossificans, with emphasis on MRI. Clin Radiol 2002;57(12):1058–66.

98. Temple HT, Kuklo TR, Sweet DE, et al. Rectus femoris muscle tear appearing as a pseudotumor. Am J Sports Med 1998;26(4):544–8.

99. Kransdorf MJ, Murphey MD. The use of gadolinium in the MR evaluation of soft tissue tumors. Semin Ultrasound CT MR 1997;18(4):251–68.

100. Kransdorf MJ, Murphey MD. Radiologic evaluation of soft-tissue masses: a current perspective. AJR Am J Roentgenol 2000;175(3):575–87.

101. Fleckenstein JL, Watumull D, Conner KE, et al. Denervated human skeletal muscle: MR imaging evaluation. Radiology 1993;187(1):213–8.

102. Lai KA, Shen WJ, Lin CJ, et al. Vastus lateralis fibrosis in habitual patella dislocation: an MRI study in 28 patients. Acta Orthop Scand 2000;71(4): 394–8.

103. Ogawa K, Takahashi M, Naniwa T. Deltoid contracture: MR imaging features. Clin Radiol 2001;56(2): 146–9.

104. Chen CK, Yeh L, Chen CT, et al. Contracture of the deltoid muscle: imaging findings in 17 patients. AJR Am J Roentgenol 1998;170(2):449–53.

105. Steinbach LS, Fleckenstein JL, Mink JH. Magnetic resonance imaging of muscle injuries. Orthopedics 1994;17(11):991–9.

106. McCully K, Shellock FG, Bank WJ, et al. The use of nuclear magnetic resonance to evaluate muscle injury. Med Sci Sports Exerc 1992;24(5):537–42.

107. McCully KK, Argov Z, Boden BP, et al. Detection of muscle injury in humans with 31-P magnetic resonance spectroscopy. Muscle Nerve 1988;11(3): 212–6.

108. Chance B, Eleff S, Leigh JS Jr, et al. Mitochondrial regulation of phosphocreatine/inorganic phosphate ratios in exercising human muscle: a gated 31P NMR study. Proc Natl Acad Sci U S A 1981;78(11):6714–8.

109. McCully KK, Kent JA, Chance B. Application of 31P magnetic resonance spectroscopy to the study of athletic performance. Sports Med 1988;5(5): 312–21.

110. McCully KK, Kent JA, Chance B. Muscle injury and exercise stress measured with 31-P magnetic resonance spectroscopy. Prog Clin Biol Res 1989;315: 197–207.

111. Raymer G, Green HJ, Ranney D, et al. Muscle metabolism and acid-base status during exercise in forearm work-related myalgia measured with 31P-MRS. J Appl Phys 2008.

112. Pathare N, Walter GA, Stevens JE, et al. Changes in inorganic phosphate and force production in human skeletal muscle after cast immobilization. J Appl Phys 2005;98(1):307–14.

MR Imaging of Ankle Impingement Lesions

James Linklater, MBBS, FRANZCR

KEYWORDS
- Ankle • Ankle impingement • Ankle injuries
- Ankle abnormalities • Ankle MR imaging
- Dancer injuries • Athlete injuries

Impingement is defined as a painful limitation of motion. Impingement lesions as identified on MR imaging of the ankle may relate to a range of soft tissue or bony pathologies that can be interpreted as predisposing to painful limitation of motion, accepting that the diagnosis of impingement remains clinical and not radiological. Typically, impingement lesions are classified according to their location and whether the underlying pathology is osseous or soft tissue in nature. Most commonly, impingement lesions relate to posttraumatic synovitis and intra-articular fibrous bands–scar tissue, capsular scarring, or bony prominences, the latter either developmental or acquired. Well-recognized sites of impingement around the ankle include the anterolateral, centroanterior, anteromedial, posteromedial, and posterior sites. This article briefly reviews the anatomy in these regions and focuses on common causes of impingement around the ankle; their pathogenesis, clinical features, and management; the approach to imaging of these lesions with MR imaging and their imaging features; and the relevant imaging differential diagnoses.

ANTEROLATERAL IMPINGEMENT
Anatomy of the Anterolateral Gutter

The anterolateral gutter or recess of the ankle is the area bounded by the anterolateral border of the talar dome-body, the anterior border of the lateral malleolus, and the inferior margin of the anterior inferior tibiofibular ligament (AITFL) (**Fig. 1**). There is some variation in the degree of inferior extension of the inferior fascicle of the AITFL into the anterolateral gutter. The anterior talofibular ligament (ATFL) lies at the superficial margin of the anterolateral gutter. The calcaneofibular ligament lies at the inferior margin of the anterolateral gutter. The normal recess often contains a small amount of simple joint fluid. During ankle dorsiflexion, the anterolateral border of the talus protrudes somewhat into the anterolateral gutter, narrowing it and displacing any native joint fluid.

Pathogenesis of Anterolateral Impingement

Anterolateral soft tissue impingement most commonly occurs as a complication of a plantar flexion-inversion sprain, with associated tear of the ATFL. There is often an associated hemarthrosis, with fibrinous debris in the joint and subsequently a posttraumatic synovitis in the anterolateral gutter.[1] In the weeks to months after the initial injury, the synovitis may impinge on the anterolateral talar dome during dorsiflexion, causing pain and restriction of dorsiflexion. Over time, the synovitis may coalesce and undergo hyalinized fibrosis,[2,3] marginating around the intra-articular inferior fascicle of the AITFL, the anterolateral talar dome, and the anterior margin of the lateral malleolus. The hyalinized fibrotic tissue may become triangular or meniscoid in shape.[4] During ankle dorsiflexion, the meniscoid lesion may impinge on the anterolateral margin of the talar dome, causing pain and limiting sports activity.[5] Repetitive abrasion may result in a chondral lesion on the anterolateral talar dome.[6]

Syndesmotic ligament complex injuries may also be complicated by anterolateral impingement because of hypertrophic scar response and

Castlereagh Sports Imaging, North Sydney Orthopaedic and Sports Medicine Centre, 286 Pacific Highway, Crows Nest, NSW 2065, Australia
E-mail address: jameslinklater@casimaging.com.au

Magn Reson Imaging Clin N Am 17 (2009) 775–800
doi:10.1016/j.mric.2009.06.006
1064-9689/09/$ – see front matter © 2009 Published by Elsevier Inc.

A   **B**

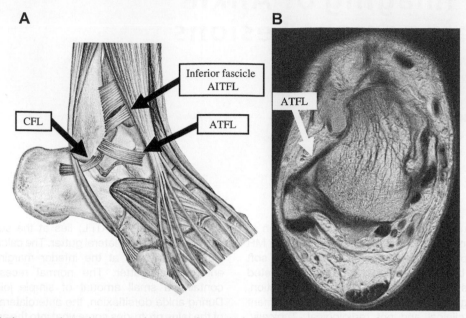

Fig. 1. (A) The anterolateral gutter is demarcated superiorly by the inferior fascicle of the AITFL and inferiorly by the lateral gutter articular facet of the talar dome and anterior border of the lateral malleolus, with the antero-lateral gutter capsule and anterior talofibular ligament (ATFL) at the superficial margin. (B) Axial proton density–weighted MR image through a normal anterolateral gutter, containing a small amount of synovial fluid with an intact ATFL at the superficial margin. CFL, calcaneofibular ligament.

synovitis at the inferior margin of the AITFL, some-times forming a meniscoid lesion. Scar response associated with syndesmotic injuries may also protrude into the syndesmotic recess, causing impingement symptoms[7,8] that may mimic a soft tissue impingement lesion in the anterolateral gutter. Occasionally, ganglia may arise from the anterolateral gutter capsule and cause anterolat-eral impingement symptoms. A low-lying fibular attachment of the AITFL may predispose to ante-rolateral impingement.[9] Laxity of the ATFL may also predispose to anterolateral impingement because of increased anterior translation of the talus in relation to the tibial plafond and resultant impingement by the inferior fascicle of the AITFL.[10] *Arthrofibrosis* is a term used to describe a thick-ened scarred joint capsule, which may result in joint stiffness, pain, and impingement symptoms. Arthrofibrosis occurs because of excessive prolif-eration of fibrous tissue, usually following trauma or surgery.[11] Trauma or surgery results in an influx of inflammatory cells and initiation of the clotting cascade within the damaged tissue. Subsequent fibroblastic and myofibroblastic proliferation ensues with exuberant collagen synthesis, which results in fibrosis clinically and pathologically. Immobilization, especially following trauma or surgery, can facilitate the proliferation of fibrous tissue and is a recognized risk factor.[12] The severity of the initiating injury is also related to

arthrofibrosis development, with several reports demonstrating increasing incidence of arthrofibro-sis following multiple ligament injuries or when multiple procedures are performed.[13]

Anterolateral ankle bony impingement lesions consist of bony spurs at the anterior border of the tibial plafond, lateral of midline, often not ex-tending to the anterolateral border of the tibial pla-fond. To explain the pathogenesis of these spurs, several theories have been proposed, but little scientific evidence supports any of them. The theory that the spurs relate to recurrent traction at the anterior capsular insertion has been discredited, given that at arthroscopy the spurs are consistently visualized as an intra-articular structure, separate to the anterior ankle capsule.[14,15] While anterolateral osteophytes are commonly seen in patients with established ankle osteoarthrosis, a large proportion of patients with anterolateral impingement spurs do not have significant osteoarthrosis. Repetitive impaction on the anterior rim of the tibial plafond has been suggested as a factor in the pathogenesis of ante-rolateral plafond spurs.[16] It has been noted that these lesions are more commonly seen in the sporting population[17] and are not always symp-tomatic.[18] It has been hypothesized that the cause of pain with anterior ankle bony impingement spurs is not the spur itself but rather entrapment of or impingement on the adjacent anterior capsule.[15] Occasionally, fracture of impingement spurs can be a cause of anterior ankle pain (**Fig. 13**). In addition, if the plafond spur demonstrates inferior prolongation, it may impinge on the talar dome articular cartilage, causing a tram-track–type chondral lesion. Small chondral delamination lesions are often present at the tibial plafond adjacent to an impingement spur and may be a cause of anterolateral ankle pain. Ossicles in the anterolateral gutter may also cause anterolateral impingement symptoms. These ossicles often relate to a remote avulsive injury at the fibular origin of the ATFL, with subsequent growth of a small avulsed flake of periosteum.

Clinical Features, Differential Diagnosis, and Management of Anterolateral Impingement

Anterolateral gutter synovitis and meniscoid lesions represent a common cause of persistent anterolateral pain and tenderness, impingement symptoms, and functional instability in the absence of objective evidence of lateral ligament complex insufficiency. Typically, anterolateral impingement is seen after an ankle sprain. A 1.2% incidence of anterolateral impingement was reported in one series of 5000 ankle sprains.[19] Frequently, scar remodeling of the torn ATFL is sufficient to prevent ongoing mechanical instability symptoms. Pain is typically precipitated by single-leg squatting and dorsiflexion and eversion. However, this maneuver can give false-negative results.[20] Pain on palpation has been reported to be a more reliable clinical finding.[20] Clinical examination has been reported to be highly accurate.[21] Occasionally, it may be

difficult clinically to differentiate anterolateral impingement from an anterolateral talar dome chondral or osteochondral lesion. The impingement pathology is amenable to arthroscopic debridement if there is not an adequate response to a rehabilitation program and corticosteroid injection.[3,22] Athletes are usually able to return to their preinjury level of sports activity at a mean of 6 weeks postarthroscopy.[22] Debridement of anterolateral osteophytes in the setting of significant osteoarthrosis may result in exacerbation of the patient's osteoarthritic symptoms because of the increased range of motion afforded by the osteophyte excision.

MR Imaging of Anterolateral Impingement

On high-resolution proton density–weighted and fat-suppressed proton density– or T2-weighted MR sequences, posttraumatic synovitis is manifest as either linear or conglomerate foci of intermediate signal intensity on both axial and coronal series and sometimes on sagittal imaging (**Figs. 2** and **3**). The synovitis may marginate around the inferior fascicle of the AITFL, becoming confluent, representing the early stages of a meniscoid lesion (**Fig. 4**). As the meniscoid lesion matures, signal intensity falls (**Figs. 5** and **6**). The ATFL usually appears scarred if there has been prior ATFL tear. Sometimes a meniscoid lesion will abut a scarred AITFL, indicating prior syndesmotic ligament complex injury (**Fig. 6**). Following arthroscopy, postsurgical scarring of the anterolateral gutter capsule can mimic a meniscoid lesion on MR imaging, even though clinically

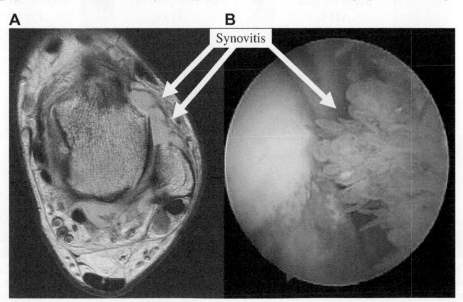

Fig. 2. (*A*) Axial proton density–weighted MR image demonstrating several foci of posttraumatic synovitis in the anterolateral gutter. (*B*) Corresponding arthroscopic image demonstrating anterolateral gutter synovitis.

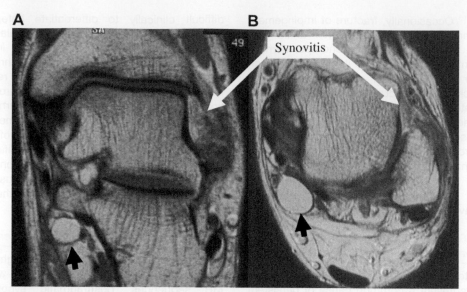

Fig. 3. Coronal (*A*) and axial (*B*) proton density–weighted MR images demonstrating posttraumatic synovitis in the anterolateral gutter. Note the tarsal tunnel ganglion cyst (*black arrowheads*).

such focal scarring is rarely symptomatic (**Fig. 7**). More generalized scarring of the anterior capsule (arthrofibrosis) may be seen, with capsular thickening in symptomatic cases usually over 3 mm, with lower (darker) signal intensity on all pulse sequences correlating with longstanding cases (**Fig. 8**) (James Linklater, MBBS, FRANZCR, unpublished data, 2005). Small ganglia arising

from the anterolateral ankle capsule may occasionally be a cause of anterolateral soft tissue impingement. Often these ganglia are small and may appear inconspicuous on MR imaging, easily mistaken for joint fluid or a pericapsular vein (**Fig. 9**). Occasionally, scar response associated with prior syndesmotic ligament complex injury may protrude into the syndesmotic recess

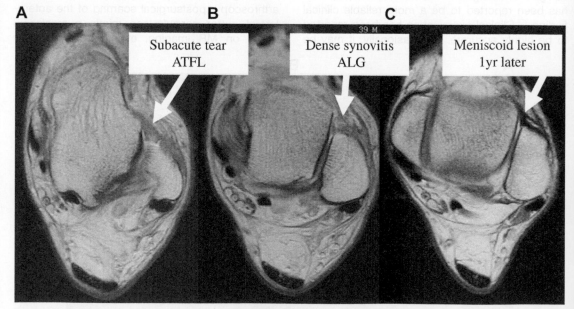

Fig. 4. Thirty-nine-year-old recreational surfer with anterolateral impingement symptoms. (*A*) Axial proton density–weighted MR image demonstrating subacute tear of the ATFL with immature scar response. (*B*) Axial proton density–weighted MR image through the anterolateral gutter, superior to the ATFL, demonstrates dense posttraumatic synovitis. (*C*) Axial proton density–weighted MR image performed 1 year later demonstrates a meniscoid lesion having formed at the site of previously demonstrated synovitis. ALG, anterolateral gutter.

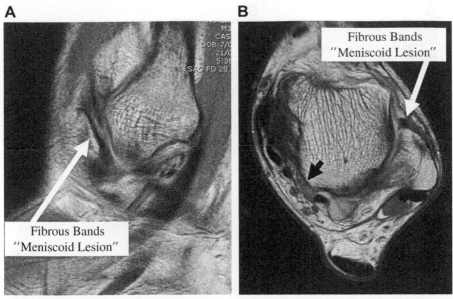

Fig. 5. Sagittal (*A*) and axial (*B*) proton density–weighted MR images through the anterolateral gutter demonstrating a thick fibrous band in the anterolateral gutter extending inferiorly from the inferior margin of the inferior fascicle of the AITFL, consistent with a meniscoid lesion. Note mild scarring of the posteromedial gutter capsule (*short black arrow*).

between the distal tibia and fibula and cause impingement symptoms (**Fig. 10**).

Anterolateral bony tibial plafond impingement spurs and ossicles are readily visualized on MR imaging (**Figs. 11–14**). Careful inspection of the adjacent plafond chondral surface is required to detect the commonly associated small

delamination chondral lesions on the tibial plafond (see **Fig. 13**), which often demonstrate subchondral bone marrow edema, rendering the lesions more conspicuous on MR imaging. The adjacent talar dome chondral surface should also be carefully inspected for subtle tram-track sagittally oriented superficial chondral fissures (see

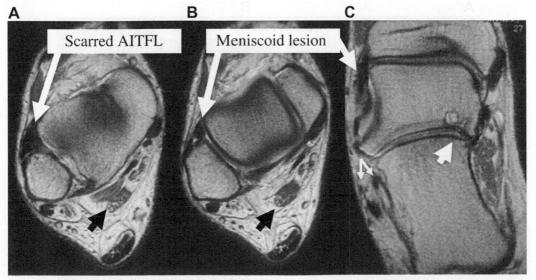

Fig. 6. Twenty-seven-year-old motorcyclist with anterolateral impingement symptoms. Sequential axial (*A* and *B*) and coronal (*C*) proton density–weighted MR images demonstrating a mature meniscoid lesion in the anterolateral gutter and intimately related to a densely scarred, thickened inferior fascicle of the AITFL, reflecting remote syndesmotic injury. Note accessory flexor muscle (*black arrowheads*), complete longitudinal split-tear peroneus brevis tendon (*white arrows*) and posterior talar facet osteochondral lesion (*white arrowhead*).

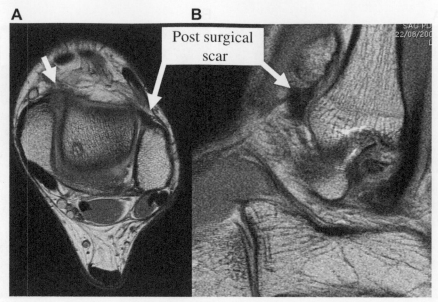

Fig. 7. Postsurgical scarring anterolateral gutter mimics meniscoid lesion (*A, B*). Note postsurgical scarring of the anteromedial ankle capsule at the site of prior anteromedial arthroscopic portal (*A, short white arrow*).

Fig. 13), usually seen in the setting of significant inferior prolongation of the plafond spur, resulting in impingement on the talar dome during plantar flexion.

There have been variable reports in the literature as to the accuracy of MR imaging in the diagnosis of anterolateral impingement lesions. Ferkel and colleagues[22] reported that MR imaging was the most useful diagnostic screening test. Rubin and colleagues[23] used as MR imaging criterion the presence of "abnormal soft tissue in the antero-lateral gutter separate to the ATFL" to retrospectively diagnose an anterolateral impingement lesion in 8 of 9 patients with ankle joint effusions and surgically confirmed lesions. They were unable to identify an anterolateral impingement

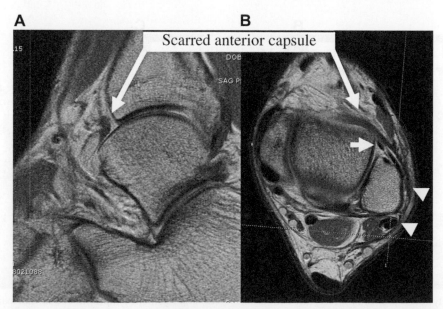

Fig. 8. Arthrofibrotic change of the anterior ankle capsule causing anterior impingement symptoms. Sagittal (*A*) and axial (*B*) proton density–weighted MR images demonstrating thickening and scarring of the anterior ankle capsule lateral of midline. Note separate, small fibrous band in the anterolateral gutter (*short white arrow*), avulsion of the superior peroneal retinaculum, and scarring of the extensor retinaculum (*white arrowheads*).

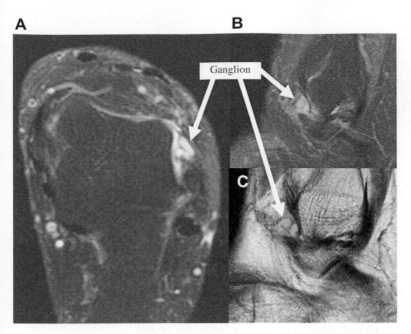

Fig. 9. Oblique axial fat-suppressed T2-weighted image (A), sagittal proton density–weighted image with fat suppression (B), and sagittal proton density–weighted image without fat suppression (C). Each image demonstrates a small ganglion cyst at the superficial margin of the anterolateral gutter capsule. The ganglion was aspirated under ultrasound guidance, with resolution of the patient's symptoms.

lesion in 9 patients who did not have an effusion. Axial images were most helpful, while coronal and sagittal images sometimes provided confirmatory evidence. Liu and colleagues,[21] in a study of 22 athletes, found that MR imaging had a sensitivity for an anterolateral impingement lesion of 39% and a specificity of 50%, while clinical examination had a sensitivity of 94% and specificity of 75%, using arthroscopy as a gold standard. Farooki and colleagues[24] identified the somewhat subjective finding of anterolateral gutter fullness in 7 of 12 patients with anterolateral impingement and 7 of 20 patients who had undergone surgery for other pathologies and did not have anterolateral impingement. This highlights the fact that pathology demonstrated on MR imaging within the ankle may not necessarily be symptomatic. A reasonable approach when reporting these findings is to describe them and state that they predispose to impingement symptoms.

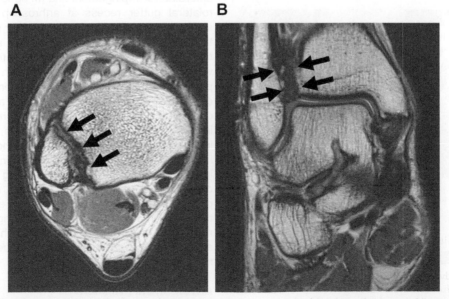

Fig. 10. Axial (A) and coronal (B) proton density–weighted MR images demonstrating extensive scar response (arrows) within the syndesmotic recess in a patient who had sustained prior syndesmotic injury and was experiencing impingementlike ankle pain laterally with dorsiflexion.

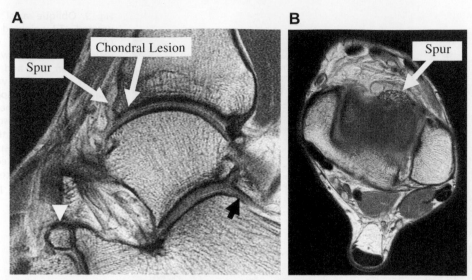

Fig. 11. (*A*) Sagittal proton density–weighted MR image demonstrating an anterolateral plafond impingement spur, with moderate inferior prolongation and adjacent in situ, unstable full-thickness chondral flap on the tibial plafond. (*B*) Axial proton density–weighted MR image demonstrating the anterolateral position of the bony spur. Note an os trigonum (*short black arrow*) and calcaneus secundarius (*white arrowhead*).

The use of intravenous contrast has been advocated as a means of making soft tissue impingement lesions more conspicuous. The basis of this proposal is that posttraumatic synovitis and vascularized scar tissue will undergo contrast enhancement. Bagnolesi and colleagues[25] demonstrated mild to moderate contrast enhancement of the abnormal synovium in 8 of 14 patients with synovial impingement lesions. In patients with a mature meniscoid lesion, the hyalinized fibrosis

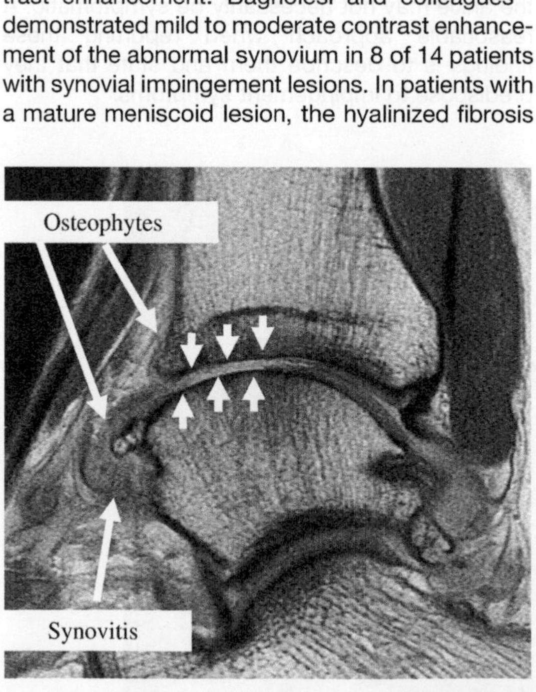

Fig. 12. Advanced ankle-joint osteoarthrosis with extensive full-thickness cartilage loss (*short arrows*), anterolateral tibial plafond and talar dome osteophytes, and degenerative synovitis in the anterior recess of the ankle.

is relatively avascular and may not enhance. This may account for the findings of a recent study that found indirect MR arthrography less accurate than conventional MR imaging of the ankle.[26]

Direct MR arthrography has been reported to have greater levels of accuracy than conventional MR imaging.[27] Robinson and colleagues[27] prospectively performed MR arthrography to assess the anterolateral gutter/recess in 32 patients. All 12 patients with clinical evidence of anterolateral impingement and an abnormal anterolateral gutter recess at arthroscopy demonstrated either focal or irregular nodular soft tissue thickening in the anterolateral gutter at MR arthrography. Interestingly, the anterolateral gutter was abnormal at MR arthrography in 11 of 19 patients without anterolateral impingement. This correlated with scarring or synovitis at arthroscopy. The study again illustrates that anterolateral impingement is a clinical diagnosis and that imaging is able to demonstrate pathology that may render the individual at risk of anterolateral impingement symptoms, without being predictive of them. MR arthrography is, however, not widely practiced and it is the author's clinical experience that MR imaging of the ankle using a high-resolution nonarthrographic approach provides a satisfactory assessment for soft tissue impingement lesions.

ANTERIOR IMPINGEMENT

While anterolateral impingement is relatively common, some pathologies may involve the

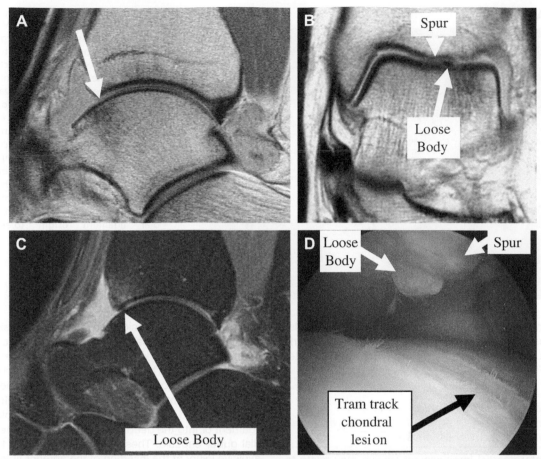

Fig. 13. Sagittal proton density–weighted MR image (*A*) demonstrating a subtle tram-track–type sagittally oriented superficial chondral lesion on the talar dome (*arrow*), with focal loss of the thin layer of low signal intensity (lamina splendens) at the superficial margin of the chondral surface. Corresponding small anterior tibial plafond spur and loose body demonstrated on (*B*) coronal proton density–weighted and (*C*) sagittal fat-suppressed proton density–weighted MR images. Arthroscopic image (*D*) from the same patient demonstrating the spur, loose body, and tram-track chondral lesion.

central aspect of the anterior recess of the ankle. These pathologies include fibrinous debris in the acute setting after an ankle sprain (**Fig. 15**). This debris may subsequently undergo hyalinized fibrosis and form fibrous bands, often extending from the medial to lateral margin of the anterior recess. These fibrous bands may impinge on the talar dome during dorsiflexion, causing pain. The bands may also cause pain during plantar flexion because of traction on the anterior capsule (**Fig. 16**). Anterior plafond impingement spurs may arise in the midline and cause anterior impingement symptoms. Loose bodies may also lodge in the central aspect of the anterior recess of the ankle (**Fig. 17**). The talus is a well-recognized site for osteoid osteoma in the hindfoot and occasionally these lesions may present with impingementlike symptoms (**Fig. 18**).

ANTEROMEDIAL ANKLE IMPINGEMENT
Anatomy of the Anteromedial Gutter and Deltoid Ligament Complex

The anteromedial recess or gutter of the ankle lies anterior to the medial malleolus and medial to the anteromedial margin of the talar dome, body, and neck. This recess or gutter is demarcated superficially by the anteromedial ankle capsule. The deltoid ligament complex can be subdivided into deep and superficial components on the basis of its distal insertions. The deltoid can be further subdivided into anterior and posterior tibiotalar ligaments. The posterior tibiotalar ligament fibers extend from the medial malleolus to the posterior aspect of the talar body, posteroinferior to the talar articular surface for the medial malleolus. The fibers are normally multifascicular in appearance

A   B

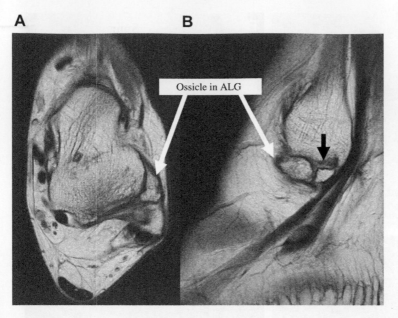

Ossicle in ALG

Fig. 14. Axial (A) and sagittal (B) proton density–weighted MR images demonstrating a large longstanding ossicle in the anterolateral gutter (ALG). The ossicle served as the point of proximal attachment of the ATFL and was related to remote fibular avulsion ATFL, with subsequent growth of a small avulsed fragment and fibrous nonunion. The ossicle was causing impingement symptoms. Note the separate avulsion fragment more posterior. This fragment is related to remote avulsive injury at the calcaneofibular ligament origin (*black arrow*).

on MR imaging (**Fig. 19**). The anterior tibiotalar fascicle of the deltoid ligament lies more anteriorly at the inferior margin of the anteromedial gutter (**Fig. 20**).

Pathogenesis of Anteromedial Impingement Lesions, Clinical Features, and Differential Diagnosis

Anteromedial impingement lesions may relate to bony spurs arising from the dorsomedial talar neck, anteromedial plafond, or the anterior margin of the medial malleolus. Similar to anterolateral plafond spurs, these lesions have a pathogenesis that is thought to relate to recurrent low-grade impaction associated with sporting activities, such as soccer.[28] These spurs are not necessarily indicative of osteoarthritis. Sometimes anteromedial impingement may relate to a posttraumatic ossicle scarred into the deep fibers of the deltoid ligament or into the deep margin of the anteromedial gutter capsule. These ossicles may relate to avulsive injury at the insertion of the anterior tibiotalar ligament or anteromedial capsule, to dystrophic ossification following prior ligamentous injury, or to fracture of an impingement spur.

A   B

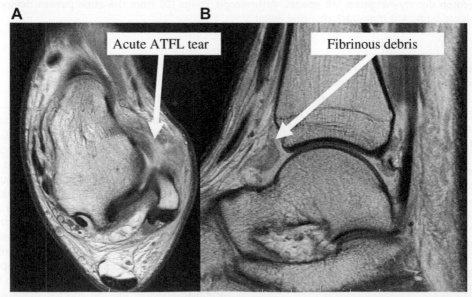

Acute ATFL tear   Fibrinous debris

Fig. 15. Acute ATFL tear on an axial proton density–weighted MR image (A), with globular fibrinous debris in the anterior recess of the ankle, also evident on the corresponding sagittal proton density–weighted sequence (B).

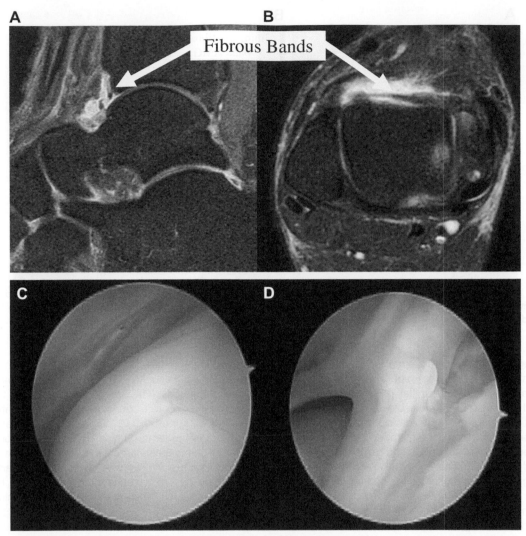

Fig. 16. Fibrous bands in the anterior recess of the ankle. (*A*) Sagittal fat-suppressed proton density–weighted MR image demonstrating two transversely oriented fibrous bands in the anterior recess of the ankle. (*B*) Axial fat-suppressed T2-weighted MR image demonstrates one of the fibrous bands, which extends from medial to lateral. (*C*) Arthroscopic image from same patient with the ankle in dorsiflexion demonstrates the fibrous band impinging on the talar dome. (*D*) Arthroscopic image with the ankle in plantar flexion demonstrates the fibrous band clear of the talar dome. The fibrous band is partially tethered to the anterior capsule medially and laterally, resulting in the fibrous band being under tension due to capsular traction.

Soft tissue pathology may cause anteromedial impingement symptoms in the absence of underlying anteromedial impingement spurs. Plantar flexion inversion ankle injuries are often associated with a medial rotational impaction component, resulting in contusional injury to the posterior and sometimes anterior tibiotalar ligaments, and microtrabecular injury to the medial malleolus and medial talar body-neck (medial kissing-bone contusions). These injuries may be associated with persistent anteromedial pain, which may relate to bone contusions, deltoid ligament edema and immature scarring, and adjacent synovitis in the anteromedial gutter, which may subsequently form intra-articular fibrous bands and adjacent capsular scar, causing impingement symptoms.[29,30] Patients with anteromedial impingement typically report chronic anteromedial ankle pain and localized tenderness exacerbated by ankle dorsiflexion. Snapping or popping may occur with dorsiflexion.[29]

MR Imaging of Anteromedial Impingement

Anteromedial impingement spurs are readily diagnosed at plain radiography, usually best

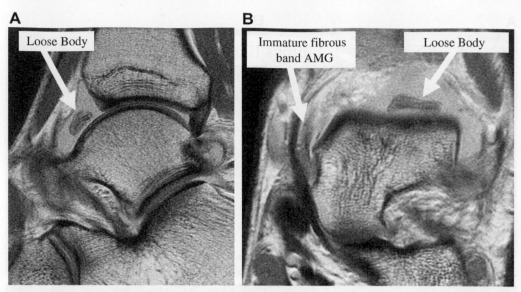

Fig. 17. Osteochondral loose body in the anterior recess of the ankle, just lateral of midline, demonstrated on sagittal (*A*) and coronal (*B*) proton density–weighted MR images. Note also the immature fibrous band in the medial gutter anteriorly, predisposing to anteromedial impingement symptoms. AMG, anteromedial gutter.

seen on an oblique radiograph of the foot.[31] Anteromedial impingement spurs are also usually clearly evident on sagittal MR images (**Fig. 21**) and may also be appreciable on coronal imaging. MR imaging may provide additional diagnostic information by demonstrating bone marrow edema within the spur and adjacent synovitis and capsular thickening in the anteromedial gutter (**Fig. 21**), often present in the setting of symptomatic impingement spurs.[20]

Injury to the anterior tibiotalar ligament is usually evident on sagittal and sometimes coronal proton density–weighted images, manifest as ligament thickening and edema (**Fig. 22**). Adjacent synovitis and fibrous bands in the anteromedial gutter can at times be difficult to appreciate, usually being evident on axial and sagittal proton density–weighted images. Initial reports of anteromedial impingement in the surgical literature suggested that MR imaging had been unhelpful in cases diagnosed at surgery.[29] MR arthrography has been reported to improve the conspicuity of pathology related to injury to the anterior tibiotalar ligament.[32] However, the pathology can be also demonstrated on high-resolution, nonarthrographic proton density–weighted MR sequences (**Figs. 22** and **23**). Contusional injury to the posterior tibiotalar ligament and adjacent medial kissing-bone contusions are also common causes of medial ankle pain that occurs after an inversion sprain but is not necessarily associated with an ongoing impingement lesion (**Fig. 24**). Avulsion fracture fragments and foci of dystrophic

ossification related to prior deltoid ligament trauma are usually appreciable on most pulse sequences (**Fig. 25**). Correlation with fat-suppressed proton density– or T2-weighted imaging is important to assess for associated bone marrow edema (**Fig. 26**). Medial talar dome lesions can mimic anteromedial impingement symptoms (**Fig. 27**), as can injury to the anterior aspect of the flexor retinacular insertion on the medial malleolus, also known as the laciniate ligament (**Fig. 28**).

POSTEROMEDIAL IMPINGEMENT
Anatomy of the Posteromedial Gutter

The posteromedial gutter is a recess defined anteriorly by the posterior border of the medial malleolus and the posterior tibiotalar ligament. The posteromedial border of the talar dome-body and posteromedial process of the talus lie at the deep margin while the posteromedial capsule lies at the superficial and posterior margin. The posteromedial gutter is normally evident as a small recess containing minimal fluid, with a thin overlying capsular layer. It is readily identified on axial images as the recess lying deep to the interval between the flexor digitorum longus and flexor hallucis longus (FHL) tendons.

Pathogenesis of Posteromedial Impingement, Clinical Features, and Differential Diagnosis

Posteromedial impingement usually complicates an acute plantar flexion inversion injury in which

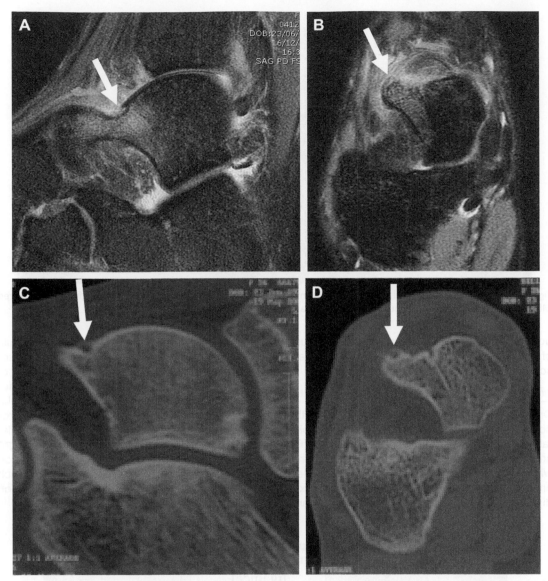

Fig. 18. Twenty-six-year-old principal ballerina with persistent anterior impingement–like symptoms due to talar neck osteoid osteoma. (A) Sagittal fat-suppressed proton density–weighted MR image and (B) coronal fat-suppressed proton density–weighted MR image demonstrating bone marrow edema in the talar neck dorsally, adjacent soft tissue edema, mild synovitis in the anterior recess of the ankle, and focal periosteal deformity (*arrows*), which was confirmed on multislice CT with sagittal (C) and coronal (D) reconstructions. The lesion was excised with resolution of the patient's symptoms and histopathologic confirmation of the diagnosis.

there is a medial rotational impaction injury to the posterior tibiotalar ligament that is usually contusional in nature and usually without ligament fiber discontinuity. Initially there is edema and subsequently immature scarring of the posterior tibiotalar ligament, with some protrusion into the posteromedial gutter, and an overlying posttraumatic synovitis with thickening of and displacement of the posteromedial ankle capsule.[33] The clinical course is variable. With appropriate rehabilitation, there may be resolution of the synovitis and remodeling and thinning of any scar tissue. In some cases, dense mature scar tissue may form in the posteromedial gutter and cause ongoing posteromedial impingement symptoms, sometimes requiring surgical debridement.[33,34] The typical clinical finding is localized tenderness to palpation of the posteromedial gutter, becoming worse with plantar flexion and inversion.[33] Avulsion fractures of the posteromedial process of the talus at the insertion of the posterior tibiotalar ligament can also cause

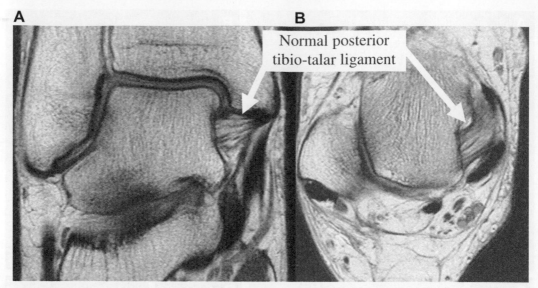

Fig. 19. Normal posterior tibiotalar ligament demonstrated on coronal (*A*) and axial (*B*) proton density–weighted MR images. Note the normal multifascicular appearance.

posteromedial impingement symptoms because of the avulsion fracture fragment and adjacent scar tissue.

MR Imaging of Posteromedial Impingement

On axial MR imaging, there is usually loss of the normal striated appearance of the posterior tibiotalar ligament and protrusion of scar response and synovitis into the medial gutter posteriorly, with loss of the normal clear space in the posteromedial gutter between the levels of the flexor digitorum longus and FHL tendons and thickening of the posteromedial ankle capsule (**Fig. 29**). Concurrent injury to the flexor retinaculum may result in partial scar encasement of the posterior tibial tendon between the retinaculum and the scarred posterior tibiotalar ligament.[35,36] Avulsion fractures of the posteromedial process of the talus can have a similar appearance to a typical posteromedial impingement lesion on MR imaging, with the avulsion fragment often being difficult to identify, such that CT scan may be required for confirmation (**Fig. 30**).

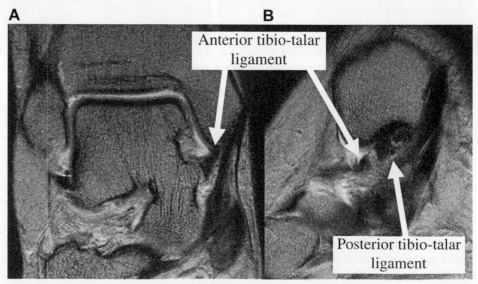

Fig. 20. Anterior tibiotalar ligament demonstrated on coronal (*A*) and sagittal (*B*) proton density–weighted cadaveric 3-T MR arthrographic images. The anterior tibiotalar ligament is mildly thickened because of scarring. Note on the sagittal image the relationship to the posterior tibiotalar ligament.

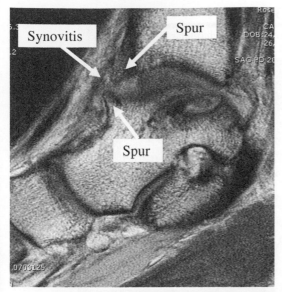

Fig. 21. Sagittal proton density–weighted MR image demonstrating prominent anteromedial plafond and dorsomedial talar neck bony spurs with adjacent synovitis in the anteromedial gutter.

POSTERIOR ANKLE IMPINGEMENT AND FLEXOR HALLUCIS LONGUS TENOSYNOVITIS

Posterior ankle pain is common in athletes who perform in the equinus position, most commonly female dancers and, to a lesser extent, soccer players, cricket fast bowlers, javelin throwers, divers, figure skaters, and gymnasts.[37] The pain may be due to one or both of two distinct, commonly coexistent clinical entities: posterior ankle impingement and FHL tenosynovitis. In one series of dancers undergoing surgery for posterior ankle pain, combined clinical diagnoses of posterior impingement and FHL tendinosis were present in 26 of 41 patients.[38]

Pathogenesis of Posterior Ankle Impingement, Clinical Features, and Differential Diagnosis

Posterior ankle impingement may complicate an acute traumatic hyper–plantar flexion event, such as an ankle sprain, or may relate to repetitive low-grade trauma associated with hyper–plantar flexion, the prototype of which is the female dancer performing *en pointe*. In general, the prognosis in the latter setting is better than that for posterior ankle impingement–complicating trauma,[39] in part because of other injuries that may be associated with an acute traumatic event.[20] The underlying mechanism for the impingement symptoms is a failure to accommodate the reduced interval between the posterosuperior aspect of the calcaneus and the adjacent posterior margins of the talus and tibial plafond during plantar flexion.

Variations in the bony anatomy of the posterior aspect of the talus, such as the presence of an os trigonum or prominence of the posterolateral process, can predispose to posterior ankle impingement. Hamilton and colleagues[38] reported on a series of 32 dancers undergoing surgery for posterior ankle impingement, 24 of whom had an os trigonum excised. Given that the prevalence of an os trigonum in cadaver studies is 2% to 7%,[40] Hamilton's findings indicate that the presence of an os trigonum does

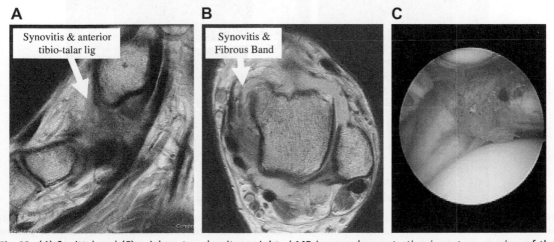

Fig. 22. (*A*) Sagittal and (*B*) axial proton density–weighted MR images demonstrating immature scarring of the anterior tibiotalar ligament, manifesting as ligament thickening and hyperintensity signal abnormality, with adjacent synovitis and immature fibrous band in the anteromedial gutter. (*C*) Arthroscopic image from the same patient demonstrating the synovitis in the anteromedial gutter.

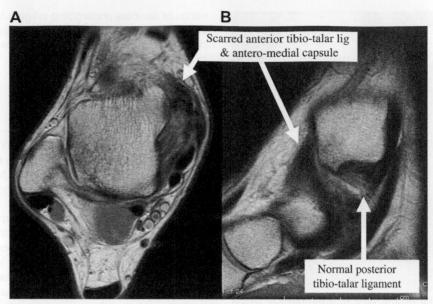

Fig. 23. Patient with anteromedial impingement symptoms. (*A*) Axial and (*B*) sagittal proton density–weighted MR images demonstrating mature scarring of the anterior tibiotalar ligament, anteromedial gutter capsule, anterior aspect of the superficial deltoid ligament, and overlying anterior aspect of the flexor retinaculum at the medial malleolar insertion.

predispose to posterior ankle impingement. However, the presence of an os trigonum in itself is not sufficient to produce the syndrome. Van Dijk and colleagues[41] reported on a group of 19 retired dancers who had been dancing *en pointe* for an average of 45 hours per week. An os trigonum or prominent posterolateral process was present in 18 of the 38 ankles and yet

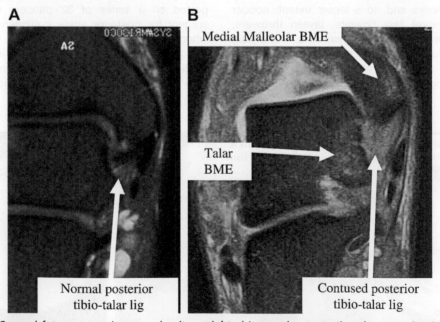

Fig. 24. (*A*) Coronal fat-suppressed proton density–weighted image demonstrating the normal striated appearance of the posterior tibiotalar ligament, with high-signal fibrovascular tissue interspersed between the ligament fascicles. (*B*) Coronal fat-suppressed proton density–weighted MR image demonstrating contusional injury to the posterior tibiotalar ligament, manifesting as ligament edema with loss of normal striated morphology. Note adjacent bone marrow edema (BME) in the medial talar body and medial malleolus, reflecting medial kissing-bone contusions.

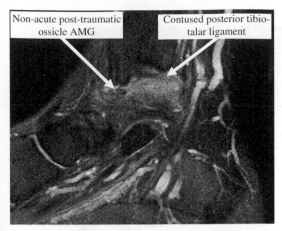

Fig. 25. Sagittal fat-suppressed proton density–weighted MR image demonstrating subacute contusional injury to the posterior tibiotalar ligament, with resultant ligament edema and loss of normal striated morphology. Note small rounded nonacute ossicle scarred into the anteromedial gutter (AMG) in the region of the anterior tibiotalar ligament.

none of the dancers had experienced posterior ankle impingement symptoms and, importantly, none had sustained ankle macrotrauma. Van Dijk and colleagues[41] concluded that an os trigonum must be combined with a traumatic event, such as a supination trauma, dancing on hard

surfaces, or pushing beyond anatomic limits, before there is complicating posterior ankle impingement.

Posterior ankle impingement symptoms may relate to destabilization of the cartilaginous synchondrosis of an os trigonum, compression between the os trigonum and tibia, or compression between os trigonum and calcaneus.[20] When osseous abutment occurs at the posterior aspect of the ankle, there may be entrapment of the adjacent soft tissues and a secondary synovitis may develop, often centered on the posterior talofibular ligament (PTFL). Synovitis may extend to involve the posterior recess of the ankle or the subtalar joint and the FHL tendon sheath. Occasionally, a localized proliferative synovitis in the posterior recess of the ankle or subtalar joint may cause posterior impingement symptoms.

Acute fractures of the posterolateral process of the talus have been described eponymously as a Shepherd fracture[42] and may result in acute posterior impingement symptoms. Such fractures are particularly common in soccer players.[43] Nonunion of such a fracture can result in chronic posterior impingement symptoms. Hamilton and colleagues[38] reported that nonunion of a fracture was present in 4 of 32 dancers undergoing surgery for posterior impingement.

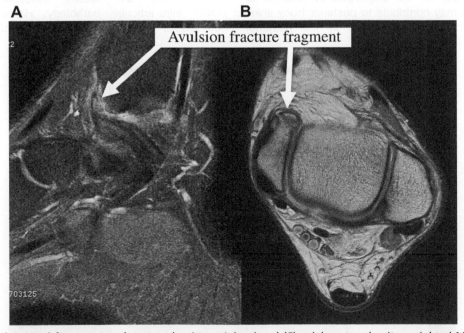

Fig. 26. (A) Sagittal fat-suppressed proton density–weighted and (B) axial proton density–weighted MR images from a patient presenting with anteromedial impingement symptoms. Images demonstrate a small avulsion fracture fragment at the anterior margin of the medial malleolus. The fragment serves as the point of attachment of the anterior tibiotalar ligament and anterior margin of the superficial deltoid ligament. Note the bone marrow edema in the fragment (A) and adjacent synovitis in the anteromedial gutter.

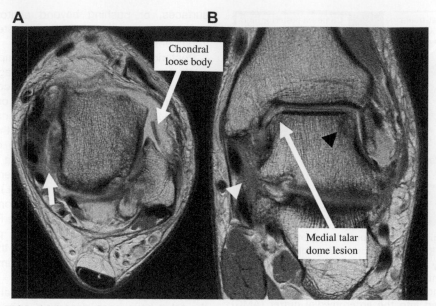

Fig. 27. (*A*) Axial and (*B*) coronal proton density–weighted MR images from a professional rugby league football player. Images demonstrate subacute complete tear of the posterior tibiotalar fibers of the deltoid ligament, with moderate adjacent posttraumatic synovitis in the posteromedial gutter (*short white arrow*). Note the subacute interstitial tear of the tibiocalcaneal component of the superficial deltoid (*white arrowhead*), the medial talar dome lesion with full-thickness chondral defect, the displaced chondral fragment in the anterolateral gutter, and the chronic lateral talar dome lesion (*black arrowhead*). As this case shows, athletes with posttraumatic ankle pain frequently have pathology at multiple sites.

Bony spurs at the posterior margin of the tibial plafond and posteroinferiorly directed bony spurs off the posterolateral process of the talus may contribute to posterior bony ankle impingement. Loose bodies in the posterior recesses of the ankle or posterior subtalar joint may also cause posterior impingement symptoms. They are usually associated with other intra-articular pathology. Hamilton and colleagues[38] reported that loose bodies were

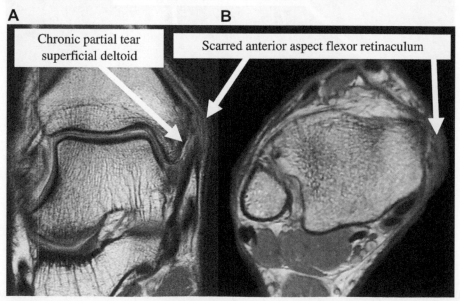

Fig. 28. (*A*) Coronal and (*B*) axial proton density–weighted MR images from a professional rugby league player with chronic anteromedial ankle pain related to chronic partial tear at the medial malleolar origin of the superficial fibers of the deltoid ligament and overlying anterior aspect of the flexor retinaculum. The findings were confirmed at the time of surgical exploration and repair.

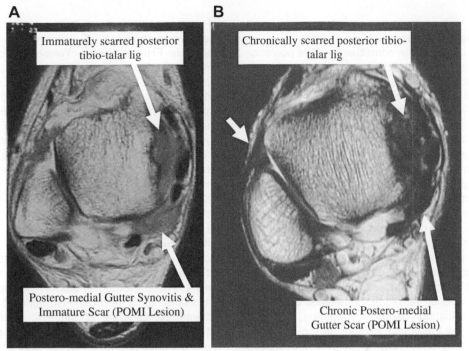

Fig. 29. (A) Axial proton density–weighted MR image of a rugby player with posteromedial impingement symptoms following subacute plantar flexion inversion injury. Image demonstrates immature scarring of the posterior tibiotalar ligament, exuberant posttraumatic synovitis, and immature scar response in the posteromedial gutter. (B) Axial T2-weighted image from a motorcyclist with chronic posteromedial impingements due to dense, mature, hypointense scarring of the posterior tibiotalar ligament with protrusion of scar response into the posteromedial gutter. Note the meniscoid lesion in the anterolateral gutter (short white arrow).

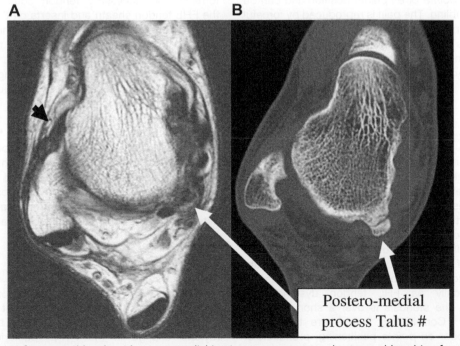

Fig. 30. Thirty-four-year-old male with posteromedial impingement symptoms due to an old avulsion fracture at the posteromedial process talus insertion of the posterior tibiotalar ligament. The avulsion fracture fragment is difficult to appreciate on an axial proton density–weighted MR image because of similar signal intensity of the fragment and adjacent scar tissue (A). However, the fragment was confirmed on CT (B). Note the scarred ATFL on the MR image (arrowhead).

present in 5 of 32 dancers undergoing surgery for posterior impingement.

Tears of one of the constituents of the posterior ankle ligament complex and subsequent chronic synovitis and scar response represent another potential cause of posterior impingement symptoms.[38,44,45] Hamilton and colleagues[38] reported a "posterior slip of the tibial branch of the posterior talo-fibular ligament" in 5 of 32 dancers undergoing surgery for posterior ankle impingement. The investigators speculated that this posterior slip might have contributed to the posterior impingement symptoms. Presumably, this represents a scarred intermalleolar ligament, a reported potential cause of posterior impingement.[46] Laxity of the lateral ankle ligament complex may also predispose to posterior impingement.

Myxoid change may develop in the PTFL, with resultant ligament thickening and infiltration of the pericapsular fat plane. Sometimes there may be complicating ganglion formation, typically occurring at the fibular insertion of the PTFL decompressing posteriorly. Both of these entities may cause posterior impingement symptoms. Ganglionic change may also occur within the FHL tendon sheath.

Posterior ankle impingement is typically associated with pain at the posterior aspect of the ankle on plantar flexion. The pain usually has a lateral predominance. In ballet dancers, this occurs in the *demi pointe* or *en pointe* position and can be quite disabling. The pain is reproduced by forceful passive plantar flexion. The clinical differential diagnosis includes peroneal tendon pathology, retrocalcaneal bursitis, and Achilles tendon pathology.

Pathogenesis of Flexor Hallucis Longus Tenosynovitis

There is little published systematic analysis of the pathogenesis of FHL tenosynovitis. It is presumed that repetitive overload of the FHL tendon in dancers is an important factor.[47] Repetitive irritation and thickening of the retinaculum that forms the roof of the fibro-osseous tunnel for the FHL may result in focal narrowing of the tunnel and limit gliding of the tendon within the tendon sheath, referred to as a stenosing tenosynovitis, presenting clinically as FHL tendon dysfunction.[48] Typically, the stenosis is over a short segment (5 mm).[49] Contributing factors are thought to include poor *en pointe* positioning, pronation of the foot, and poor turn-out (external rotation) at the hips. A low-lying FHL muscle-tendon junction may also predispose to FHL tenosynovitis.

Hamilton and colleagues[38] reported on the operative treatment of 35 dancers with a clinical diagnosis FHL tendinitis. Twenty-six of these dancers also had a clinical diagnosis of posterior impingement. Their operative diagnoses included FHL tenosynovitis in 13 patients, longitudinal FHL tendon tear in 5 patients, focal nodular FHL tendinosis in 2 patients, low-lying junction of FHL muscle and tendon in 7 patients, flexor hallucis accessorius in 5 patients, and a ganglion in 3 patients. An os trigonum was present in many of these patients.

Kolettis and colleagues[47] reported a series of 13 female ballet dancers who had operative release of the FHL tendon for isolated stenosing FHL tenosynovitis. Their operative findings included thickening and stenosis of the FHL tendon sheath in 13 patients, synovial hypertrophy in 10 patients, adhesions in 9 patients, mucoid tendon degeneration in 8 patients, focal nodular FHL tendinosis in 3 patients, partial tears of the FHL tendon in 3 patients, and tear of the distal muscle in 2 patients. There are case reports of partial tears of the FHL tendon at the level of the knot of Henry where there is a fibrous band connecting the FHL and flexor digitorum longus tendons. The tears are thought to relate to a hyperextension injury to the great toe.[50]

Rarely, the tendon of the accessory flexor muscle, peroneocalcaneus internus, may result in posterior impingement or FHL tendinitis symptoms.[51] This accessory tendon courses within the FHL tendon sheath and inserts on the medial aspect of the calcaneus at the level of the sustentaculum. In the vast majority of cases, the peroneocalcaneus internus is asymptomatic.

FHL tenosynovitis often has a stenosing component.[38] It is characterized by posteromedial ankle pain and swelling, pain with passive or active movement of the great toe, limited range of great-toe motion, and tenderness over the fibro-osseous tunnel for the FHL. There may be associated palpable crepitus or triggering. The clinical differential diagnosis includes a deltoid ligament sprain, posterior tibial tenosynovitis, posteromedial tarsal coalition and posteromedial talar dome osteochondral lesion, plantar fasciitis, and tarsal tunnel syndrome.

MR Imaging of Posterior Ankle Impingement

The MR imaging protocol employed for investigating posterior ankle impingement should adequately demonstrate a small os trigonum, myxoid change in the PTFL, posterior ankle ganglia, FHL tendon pathology, and synovitis. The protocols vary according to the MR imaging unit and personal preference.

An os trigonum is usually readily identified on MR imaging. The synchondrosis may vary in orientation from coronal to oblique sagittal, the latter often not evident on sagittal images and only appreciable on straight axial images. When present, the synchondrosis should be evaluated for fluid signal intensity, indicating destabilization. Assessment should also be made for the presence of bone marrow edema at the synchondrosis margins and adjacent synovitis in the posterior recesses of the ankle and posterior subtalar joint. When present, these findings are suggestive of active posterior impingement, without being totally specific (**Fig. 31**). Sclerosis and cystic change at the synchondrosis margins indicates a degree of chronic stress across the synchondrosis. Sometimes a small os trigonum can be extremely subtle on an MR image, only being evident on a single axial or sagittal sequence. It is important to look for bone marrow signal on T1- or proton density–weighted sequences and to assess for corticated margins. Sometimes a small sclerotic os trigonum may not demonstrate a central fatty marrow component. Pericapsular fat may occasionally mimic an os trigonum.

Assessment of the posterolateral process of the talus is best done on sagittal MR images. The posterolateral process is considered prominent if it extends posterior to the arc of curvature of the talar dome in the sagittal plane (**Fig. 32**). Fractures of the posterolateral process are usually readily demonstrated on MR image (**Fig. 33**).

Assessment of the PTFL requires review of sagittal, axial, and coronal images. Myxoid change in the PTFL is manifest as mild signal hyperintensity on all pulse sequences, together with mild thickening of the ligament (**Fig. 34**). There may be adjacent capsulosynovial thickening. Ganglionic change is manifest as a discrete area of fluid signal intensity, often decompressing posteriorly (**Fig. 34**). There may be a small component of intraosseous decompression into the digital fossa of the lateral malleolus. A fluid-distended recess of the ankle or subtalar joint may mimic a posterior ankle ganglion. Sometimes the distinction can be difficult. Occasionally, correlative dynamic ultrasound may be required to provide clarification.

Fluid distension of the posterior recesses of the ankle and subtalar joints is a relatively nonspecific finding that may be seen in the setting of active posterior impingement. Ancillary supporting signs of the latter include associated synovial thickening and edema in the adjacent fat planes. Enhancement with intravenous contrast can provide confirmatory evidence of a localized synovitis.

The posterior ankle ligament complex is best assessed on coronal and axial scans with the ankle in neutral. In plantar flexion, the intermalleolar ligament usually cannot be identified as a separate structure. Oh and colleagues[52] demonstrated the presence of an intermalleolar ligament in 26 out of 26 cadaver ankles, with substantial variation being seen in ligament morphology. The key findings in the setting of posterior impingement due to

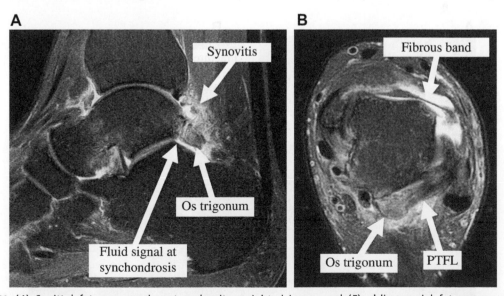

Fig. 31. (*A*) Sagittal fat-suppressed proton density–weighted image and (*B*) oblique axial fat-suppressed T2-weighted image demonstrating moderate bone marrow edema within a moderate-size os trigonum, with adjacent fluid signal intensity at the synchondrosis, indicating at least partial destabilization. Moderate adjacent synovitis in the posterior recesses of the ankle and subtalar joint is consistent with a degree of active posterior impingement. Note the separate calcaneal articular facet for the os trigonum and fibrous band in the anterior recess of the ankle.

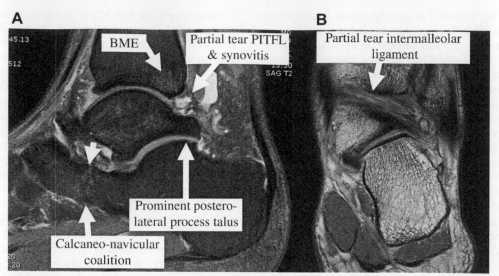

Fig. 32. Twenty-eight-year-old elite cricketer with posterior impingement symptoms. (A) Sagittal fat-suppressed proton density–weighted MR image and (B) coronal proton density–weighted image demonstrating a prominent posterolateral process talus, partial tear of the posterior inferior tibiofibular ligament (PITFL) and posterior inter-malleolar ligament with adjacent synovitis in the posterior recess of the ankle, and bone marrow edema (BME) in the posterior aspect of the tibial plafond. Note the cartilaginous calcaneonavicular coalition (arrowhead).

intermalleolar ligament pathology are altered ligament morphology and adjacent synovial thick-ening, manifest as intermediate signal intensity tissue with ill-defined margins on proton density–weighted or fat-suppressed proton density–weighted sequences (Figs. 32 and 37). Frequently, this will be the only sign of a nonacute tear. In the acute setting, redundancy of the torn ligament and focal ligament fiber discontinuity may be seen.

Loose bodies are frequently small. Their presence should be confirmed in three planes. The deep fibers of the posteroinferior tibiofibular ligament may mimic a loose body on sagittal scans, as may a fibrous band. Pericapsular fat may also mimic a loose body. Other unusual causes of posterior impingement symptoms may include a displaced distal tear of the calcaneofibular ligament, with protrusion of the ligament stump into the posterior

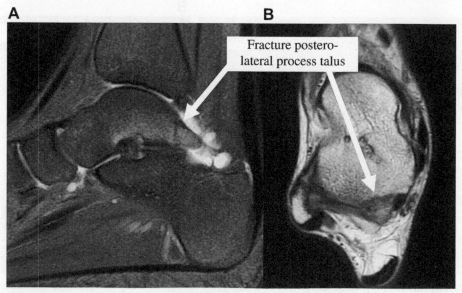

Fig. 33. Sagittal fat-saturated proton density–weighted MR image (A) and axial proton density–weighted MR image (B) in an athlete with posterior ankle impingement symptoms. Images show late subacute undisplaced fracture posterolateral process talus with extensive bone marrow edema at the margins, adjacent fluid distension of the posterior recesses of the ankle and subtalar joints, and associated synovitis.

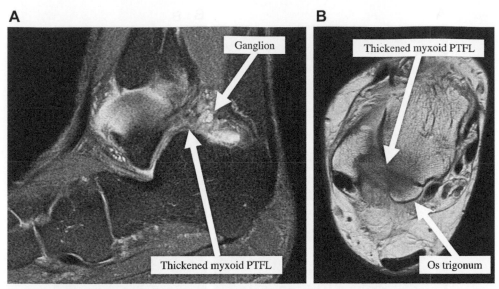

Fig. 34. (*A*) Sagittal fat-suppressed proton density–weighted MR image and (*B*) axial proton density–weighted MR image demonstrating PTFL thickening and signal hyperintensity, consistent with myxoid change. Complicating ganglionic change is evident, decompressing posteriorly. Note the moderate-size os trigonum.

recess of the posterior subtalar joint (**Fig. 35**) and a focal proliferative synovitis in the posterior recess of the ankle or subtalar joint (**Fig. 36**).

MR Imaging of Flexor Hallucis Longus Tendon Pathology

FHL tendon pathology may mimic or accompany posterior impingement symptoms. The diagnosis of FHL tendon pathology on MR imaging can be difficult because of the relatively common presence of fluid distension of the FHL tendon sheath in asymptomatic ankles. Schweitzer and colleagues[53] found an FHL tendon sheath effusion in 31% of a heterogeneous group of asymptomatic volunteers and patients who clinically did not have FHL tendon pathology. Although this may reflect fluid decompression from an ankle or subtalar joint effusion, Schweitzer and colleagues[53] found no correlation between the presence of an ankle or subtalar joint effusion and an FHL tendon sheath effusion.

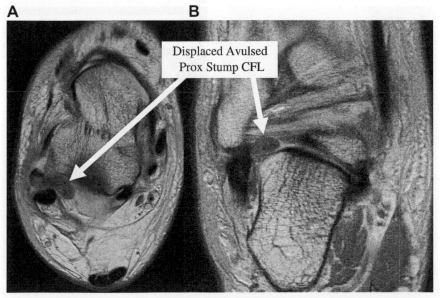

Fig. 35. Elite rugby league player with posterior impingement symptoms due to displaced tear of the calcaneofibular ligament, with the ligament stump displaced into the posterior recess of the subtalar joint, demonstrated on axial (*A*) and coronal (*B*) proton density–weighted MR images. CFL, calcaneofibular ligament.

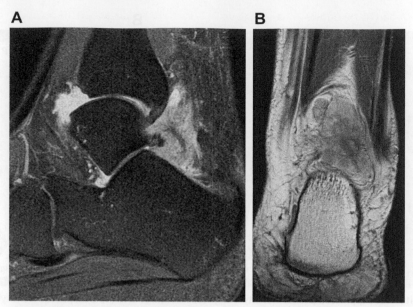

Fig. 36. Twenty-five-year-old beach sprinter with posterior impingement symptoms. (*A*) Sagittal fat-suppressed proton density–weighted MR image and (*B*) coronal proton density–weighted MR image demonstrating a proliferative synovial mass in the posterior recess of the ankle, separate to the PTFL, accounting for the patient's symptoms. The patient underwent surgical excision and the subsequent histopathologic diagnosis of granulomatous synovitis.

Features suggestive of an FHL tenosynovitis include synovial thickening within the tendon sheath, thickening of the retinaculum for the FHL at the fibro-osseous tunnel level, tendon thickening, and intratendon signal hyperintensity. An FHL tendon sheath effusion in the absence of an ankle or posterior subtalar joint effusion is also more suggestive of an FHL tenosynovitis, but is still nonspecific. Enhancement within the tendon sheath after intravenous contrast is also suggestive of FHL tenosynovitis and is a relatively specific finding.

Ganglionic change within the FHL tendon sheath can also mimic posterior impingement. Internal septation and mass effect on the distal

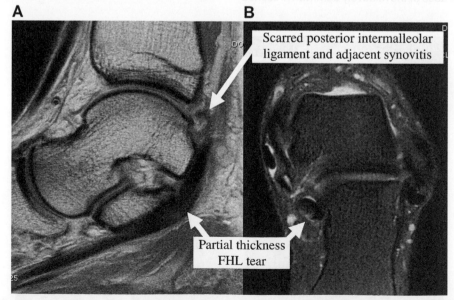

Fig. 37. Thirty-six-year-old elite dancer with persistent posterior impingement symptoms. (*A*) Sagittal proton density–weighted MR image and (*B*) oblique axial fat-suppressed T2-weighted MR image demonstrating partial-thickness FHL tendon tear at fibro-osseous tunnel level and thickened scarred posterior intermalleolar ligament with adjacent synovitis in the posterior recess of the ankle.

FHL muscle support a diagnosis of a ganglion. Loose bodies are occasionally seen in the FHL tendon sheath and are frequently asymptomatic.

FHL tendinosis may manifest as mild intratendinous signal hyperintensity on any pulse sequence, usually at the fibro-osseous tunnel. Magic angle phenomenon on short echo time (T1- or proton density–weighted) sequences can mimic tendinosis. Using operative findings as a gold standard, the author's personal experience has been that MR imaging is of limited sensitivity in depicting tendinosis. FHL tendon tears may be occasionally seen. These are usually incomplete longitudinal split tears, manifest as a focal abnormality in tendon surface contour (**Fig. 37**). A "frenulum" within the FHL tendon sheath should not be mistaken for a longitudinal split tear. The FHL muscle tendon junction usually does not enter the fibro-osseous tunnel when the ankle is in neutral flexion.

SUMMARY

As illustrated, there are multiple potential sites and causes of impingement symptoms in the athlete. Most commonly, impingement lesions relate to posttraumatic synovitis and intra-articular fibrous bands–scar tissue, capsular scarring, or bony prominences, the latter either developmental or acquired. Sites of impingement around the ankle include anterolateral, centroanterior, anteromedial, posteromedial, and posterior sites. These pathologies are readily identified on MR imaging and, when present, should be interpreted as predisposing to impingement symptoms, accepting that the diagnosis of impingement remains clinical and not radiological.

ACKNOWLEDGMENTS

The author thanks Dr. Dzung Vu, University of New South Wales, for his expert skills as a medical illustrator, and Dr. HK Slater for kindly providing the arthroscopic images in this article.

REFERENCES

1. Guhl JF. Soft tissue (synovial) pathology. In: Ankle Arthroscopy, editor. Pathology and surgical techniques. 2nd edition. Thorofare (NJ): Slack Publishing; 1993. p. 93–135.
2. Brostrum L, Sundelin P. Histologic changes in recent and "chronic" ligament ruptures. Acta Chir Scand 1966;132(3):248–53.
3. Meislin RJ, Rose DJ, Parisien JS, et al. Arthroscopic treatment of synovial impingement of the ankle. Am J Sports Med 1993;21(2):186–9.
4. Wolin I, Glassman F, Sideman S, et al. Internal derangement of the talo-fibular component of the ankle. Surg Gynecol Obstet 1950;91:193–200.
5. Lahm A, Erggelet C, Steinwachs M, et al. Arthroscopic management of osteochondral lesions of the talus: results of drilling and usefulness of magnetic resonance imaging before and after treatment. Arthroscopy 2000;16(3):299–304.
6. Bassett F, Gates H, Billys J, et al. Talar impingement by the anteroinferior tibiofibular ligament. J Bone Joint Surg Am 1990;72:55–9.
7. Ferkel RD, Scranton PE. Current concepts review: arthroscopy of the ankle and foot. J Bone Joint Surg Am 1993;75:1233–45.
8. Shaffler GJ, Tirman PFJ, Stoller DW, et al. Impingement syndrome of the ankle following supination external rotation trauma: MR imaging findings with arthroscopic correlation. Eur Radiol 2003;13:1357–62.
9. Akseki D, Pinar H, Yaldiz K, et al. The anterior inferior tibiofibular ligament and talar impingement: a cadaveric study. Knee Surg Sports Traumatol Arthrosc 2002;10:321–6.
10. Golano P, Vega J, Pérez-Carro L, et al. Ankle anatomy for the arthroscopist. Part II: Role of the ankle ligaments in soft tissue impingement. Foot Ankle Clin N Am 2006;11:275–96.
11. Lindenfeld TN, Wojtys EM, Husain A. Operative treatment of arthrofibrosis of the knee. J Bone Joint Surg Am 1999;81(12):1772–84.
12. Enneking WF, Horowitz M. The intra-articular effects of immobilization on the human knee. J Bone Joint Surg Am 1972;54(5):973–85.
13. Noyes FR, Barber-Westin SD. Reconstruction of the anterior and posterior cruciate ligaments after knee dislocation: use of early protected postoperative motion to decrease arthrofibrosis. Am J Sports Med 1997;25(6):769–78.
14. Van Dijk CN, Tol JL, Verheyen CC. A prospective study of prognostic factors concerning the outcome of arthroscopic surgery for anterior ankle impingement. Am J Sports Med 1997;25:737–45.
15. Tol JL, Verheyen CP, van Dijk CN. Arthroscopic treatment of anterior impingement in the ankle. J Bone Joint Surg Br 2001;83:9–13.
16. O'Donoghue DH. Impingement exostoses of the talus and tibia. J Bone Joint Surg Am 1957;39:835–52.
17. Hawkins RB. Arthroscopic treatment of sports-related anterior osteophytes in the ankle. Foot Ankle 1988;9:87–90.
18. Cheng JC, Ferkel RD. The role of arthroscopy in ankle and subtalar degenerative joint disease. Clin Orthop 1998;349:65–72.
19. De Berardino TM, Arciero RA, Taylor DC. Arthroscopic treatment of soft-tissue impingement of the ankle in athletes. Arthroscopy 1997;13(4):492–8.
20. van Dijk CN. Anterior and posterior ankle impingement. Foot Ankle Clin N Am 2006;11:663–83.

21. Liu SH, Nuccion SL, Finerman G. Diagnosis of ante-rolateral ankle impingement. Comparison between magnetic resonance imaging and clinical examination. Am J Sports Med 1997;25(3):389–93.

22. Ferkel RD, Karzel RP, Del Pizzo W, et al. Arthroscopic treatment of anterolateral impingement of the ankle. Am J Sports Med 1991;19(5):440–6.

23. Rubin DA, Tishkoff NW, Britton CA, et al. Anterolateral soft-tissue impingement in the ankle: diagnosis using MR imaging. Am J Roentgenol 1997;169(3): 829–35.

24. Farooki S, Yao L, Seeger LL. Anterolateral impingement of the ankle: effectiveness of MR imaging. Radiology 1998;207(2):357–60.

25. Bagnolesi P, Carafoli D, Ortori S, et al. Anterolateral fibrous impingement of the ankle: discrepancy between MRI findings and arthroscopy [abstract]. Eur Radiol 1998;8:1295.

26. Haller J, Bernt R, Seeger T, et al. MR-imaging of anterior tibiotalar impingement syndrome: agreement, sensitivity and specificity of MR-imaging and indirect MR-arthrography. Eur J Radiol 2006;58: 450–60.

27. Robinson P, White LM, Salonen DC, et al. Anterolateral ankle impingement: MR arthrographic assessment of the anterolateral recess. Radiology 2001; 221(1):186–90.

28. Tol JL, van Dijk CN. Etiology of the anterior ankle impingement syndrome: a descriptive anatomical study. Foot Ankle Int 2004;25:382–6.

29. Mosier-La Clair SM, Monroe MT, Manoli A. Medial impingement syndrome of the anterior tibiotalar fascicle of the deltoid ligament on the talus. Foot Ankle Int 2000;21:385–91.

30. Egol KA, Parisien JS. Impingement syndrome of the ankle caused by a medial meniscoid lesion. Arthroscopy 1997;13:522–5.

31. van Dijk CN, Wessel RN, Tol JL, et al. Oblique radiograph for the detection of bone spurs in anterior ankle impingement. Skeletal Radiol 2002;31: 214–21.

32. Robinson P, White LM, Salonen D, et al. Anteromedial impingement of the ankle: MR arthrography assessment of the anteromedial recess. AJR Am J Roentgenol 2002;178:601–4.

33. Paterson RS, Brown JN. The posteromedial impingement lesion of the ankle. A series of six cases. Am J Sports Med 2001;29(5):550–7.

34. Liu SH, Mirzayan R. Postero-medial impingement. Arthroscopy 1993;9(6):709–11.

35. Koulouris G, Connell D, Schneider T, et al. Posterior tibiotalar ligament injury resulting in the posteromedial impingement. Foot Ankle Int 2003;24:575–83.

36. Messiou C, Robinson P, O'Connor PJ, et al. Subacute posteromedial impingement of the ankle in athletes: MR imaging evaluation and ultrasound-guided therapy. Skeletal Radiol 2006;35:88–94.

37. DeAsla R, O'Malley M, Hamilton WG. Flexor hallucis tendonitis and posterior ankle impingement in the athlete. Foot Ankle Surg 2002;1(2):123–30.

38. Hamilton WG, Geppert MJ, Thompson FM. Pain in the posterior aspect of the ankle in dancers. Differential diagnosis and operative treatment. J Bone Joint Surg Am 1996;78(10):1491–500.

39. Stibbe AB, Van Dijk CN, Marti RK. The os trigonum syndrome. Acta Orthop Scand 1994;(Suppl 262):60–1.

40. Sarrafian SH. Anatomy of the ankle: descriptive, topgraphic and functional. Philadelphia: JB Lippincott; 1993.

41. van Dijk CN, Lim LS, Poortman A, et al. Degenerative joint disease in female ballet dancers. Am J Sports Med 1995;23:295–300.

42. Shepherd FJ. A hitherto undescribed fracture of astragalus. J Anat Physiol 1882;17:79–81.

43. Dunfee WR, Dalinka MK, Kneeland JB. Imaging of athletic injuries to the ankle and foot. Radiol Clin North Am 2002;40(2):289–312.

44. Rosenberg Z, Cheung Y, Beltran J, et al. Posterior intermalleolar ligament of the ankle: normal anatomy and MR imaging features. Am J Roentgenol 1995; 165(2):387–90.

45. Petty DR, Gibbon WW. MR imaging of professional soccer players presenting with persistent acute onset posterolateral ankle pain. ARRS Annual Meeting. New Orleans, AJR Am J Roentgenol; 174(s):40. 2001.

46. Fiorella D, Helms CA, Nunley JA 2nd. The MR imaging features of the posterior intermalleolar ligament in patients with posterior impingement syndrome of the ankle. Skeletal Radiol 1999;28(10):573–6.

47. Kolettis GJ, Micheli LJ, Klein JD. Release of the flexor hallucis longus tendon in ballet dancers. J Bone Joint Surg Am 1996;78(9):1386–90.

48. Hamilton WG. Stenosing tenosynovitis of the flexor hallucis longus tendon and posterior impingement upon the os trigonum in ballet dancers. Foot Ankle 1982;3(2):74–80.

49. Na JB, Bergman AG, Oloff LM, et al. The flexor hallucis longus: tenographic technique and correlation of imaging findings with surgery in 39 ankles. Radiology 2005;236(3):974–82.

50. Boruta PM, Beauperthuy GD. Partial tear of the flexor hallucis longus at the knot of Henry: presentation of three cases. Foot Ankle Int 1997;18(4):243–6.

51. Seipel R, Linklater J, Pitsis G, et al. The peroneocalcaneus internus muscle: an unusual cause of posterior ankle impingement. Foot Ankle Int 2005;26(10):890–3.

52. Oh CS, Won HS, Hur MS, et al. Anatomic variations and MRI of the intermalleolar ligament. AJR 2006; 186:943–7.

53. Schweitzer ME, van Leersum M, Ehrlich SS, et al. Fluid in normal and abnormal ankle joints: amount and distribution as seen on MR images. AJR Am J Roentgenol 1994;162(1):111–4.

Index

Note: Page numbers of article titles are in **boldface** type.

mri.theclinics.com

United States Postal Service

Statement of Ownership, Management, and Circulation
(All Periodicals Publications Except Requestor Publications)

1. Publication Title	2. Publication Number	3. Filing Date
Magnetic Resonance Imaging Clinics of North America	0 1 1 - 9 0 0 9	9/ _/09

4. Issue Frequency	5. Number of Issues Published Annually	6. Annual Subscription Price
Feb, May, Aug, Nov	4	$276.00

7. Complete Mailing Address of Known Office of Publication (Not printer) (Street, city, county, state, and ZIP+4®)

Elsevier Inc.
360 Park Avenue South
New York, NY 10010-1710

Contact Person: Stephen Bushing
Telephone (Include area code): 215-239-3688

8. Complete Mailing Address of Headquarters or General Business Office of Publisher (Not printer)

Elsevier Inc., 360 Park Avenue South, New York, NY 10010-1710

9. Full Names and Complete Mailing Addresses of Publisher, Editor, and Managing Editor (Do not leave blank)

Publisher (Name and complete mailing address)

John Schrefer, Elsevier, Inc., 1600 John F. Kennedy Blvd. Suite 1800, Philadelphia, PA 19103-2899

Editor (Name and complete mailing address)

Joanne Husovski, Elsevier, Inc., 1600 John F. Kennedy Blvd. Suite 1800, Philadelphia, PA 19103-2899

Managing Editor (Name and complete mailing address)

Catherine Bewick, Elsevier, Inc., 1600 John F. Kennedy Blvd. Suite 1800, Philadelphia, PA 19103-2899

10. Owner (Do not leave blank. If the publication is owned by a corporation, give the name and address of the corporation immediately followed by the names and addresses of all stockholders owning or holding 1 percent or more of the total amount of stock. If not owned by a corporation, give the names and addresses of the individual owners. If owned by a partnership or other unincorporated firm, give its name and address as well as those of each individual owner. If the publication is published by a nonprofit organization, give its name and address.)

Full Name	Complete Mailing Address
Wholly owned subsidiary of	4520 East-West Highway
Reed/Elsevier, US holdings	Bethesda, MD 20814

11. Known Bondholders, Mortgagees, and Other Security Holders Owning or Holding 1 Percent or More of Total Amount of Bonds, Mortgages, or Other Securities. If none, check box ☐ None

Full Name	Complete Mailing Address
N/A	

12. Tax Status (For completion by nonprofit organizations authorized to mail at nonprofit rates) (Check one)
The purpose, function, and nonprofit status of this organization and the exempt status for federal income tax purposes:
☐ Has Not Changed During Preceding 12 Months
☐ Has Changed During Preceding 12 Months (Publisher must submit explanation of change with this statement)

PS Form 3526, September 2007 (Page 1 of 3 (Instructions Page 3)) PSN 7530-01-000-9931 PRIVACY NOTICE: See our Privacy policy in www.usps.com

---

13. Publication Title	14. Issue Date for Circulation Data Below
Magnetic Resonance Imaging Clinics of North America	August 2009

15. Extent and Nature of Circulation		Average No. Copies Each Issue During Preceding 12 Months	No. Copies of Single Issue Published Nearest to Filing Date
a. Total Number of Copies (Net press run)		3625	3700
b. Paid Circulation (By Mail and Outside the Mail)	(1) Mailed Outside-County Paid Subscriptions Stated on PS Form 3541. (Include paid distribution above nominal rate, advertiser's proof copies, and exchange copies)	1952	1844
	(2) Mailed In-County Paid Subscriptions Stated on PS Form 3541 (Include paid distribution above nominal rate, advertiser's proof copies, and exchange copies)		
	(3) Paid Distribution Outside the Mails Including Sales Through Dealers and Carriers, Street Vendors, Counter Sales, and Other Paid Distribution Outside USPS®	682	621
	(4) Paid Distribution by Other Classes Mailed Through the USPS (e.g. First-Class Mail®)		
c. Total Paid Distribution (Sum of 15b (1), (2), (3), and (4))	▲	2634	2465
d. Free or Nominal Rate Distribution (By Mail and Outside the Mail)	(1) Free or Nominal Rate Outside-County Copies Included on PS Form 3541	93	86
	(2) Free or Nominal Rate In-County Copies Included on PS Form 3541		
	(3) Free or Nominal Rate Copies Mailed at Other Classes Through the USPS (e.g. First-Class Mail)		
	(4) Free or Nominal Rate Distribution Outside the Mail (Carriers or other means)		
e. Total Free or Nominal Rate Distribution (Sum of 15d (1), (2), (3) and (4))	▲	93	86
f. Total Distribution (Sum of 15c and 15e)	▲	2727	2551
g. Copies not Distributed (See instructions to publishers #4 (page #3))	▲	898	1149
h. Total (Sum of 15f and g)	▲	3625	3700
i. Percent Paid (15c divided by 15f times 100)		96.59%	96.63%

16. Publication of Statement of Ownership
☑ If the publication is a general publication, publication of this statement is required. Will be printed ☐ Publication not required
in the November 2009 issue of this publication.

17. Signature and Title of Editor, Publisher, Business Manager, or Owner | Date

Stephen R. Bushing | September 15, 2009

Stephen R. Bushing – Subscription Services Coordinator

I certify that all information furnished on this form is true and complete. I understand that anyone who furnishes false or misleading information on this form or who omits material or information requested on the form may be subject to criminal sanctions (including fines and imprisonment) and/or civil sanctions (including civil penalties).

PS Form 3526, September 2007 (Page 2 of 3)

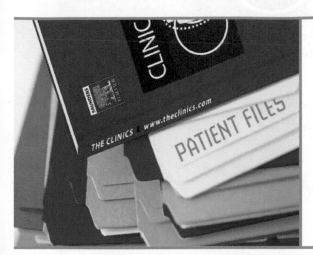
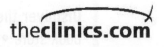

Our issues help you manage *yours.*

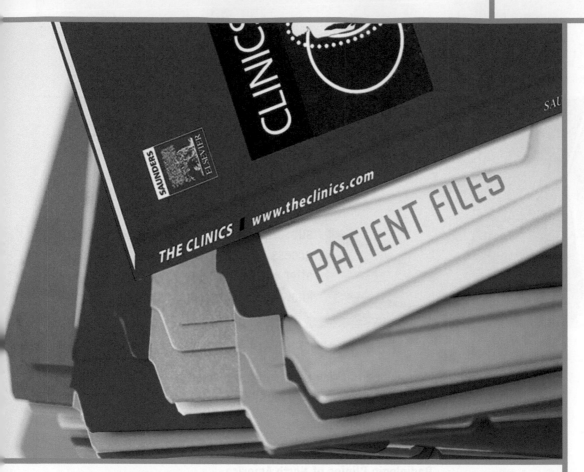

Every year brings you new clinical challenges.

Every **Clinics** issue brings you **today's best thinking** on the challenges you face.

Whether you purchase these issues individually, or order an annual subscription (which includes searchable access to past issues online), the **Clinics** offer you an efficient way to update your know how…one issue at a time.

Discover the Clinics in your specialty. Ask for them in your local medical book store • visit **www.theclinics.com** • or call 1.800.654.2452 inside the U.S. (1.314.453.7041 outside the U.S.) today!

Moving?

Make sure your subscription moves with you!

To notify us of your new address, find your **Clinics Account Number** (located on your mailing label above your name), and contact customer service at:

Email: journalscustomerservice-usa@elsevier.com

800-654-2452 (subscribers in the U.S. & Canada)
314-447-8871 (subscribers outside of the U.S. & Canada)

Fax number: 314-447-8029

Elsevier Health Sciences Division
Subscription Customer Service
3251 Riverport Lane
Maryland Heights, MO 63043

*To ensure uninterrupted delivery of your subscription, please notify us at least 4 weeks in advance of move.

Printed and bound by CPI Group (UK) Ltd, Croydon, CR0 4YY

03/10/2024

01040353-0005